TOPICS IN NEUROMODULATION TREATMENT

Edited by **José D. Carrillo-Ruiz**

Topics in Neuromodulation Treatment
Edited by José D. Carrillo-Ruiz

Published by InTech

Janeza Trdine 9, 51000 Rijeka, Croatia

Publishing Process Manager Vedran Greblo

Technical Editor Teodora Smiljanic

Cover Designer InTech Design Team

Additional hard copies can be obtained from orders@intechopen.com

Topics in Neuromodulation Treatment, Edited by José D. Carrillo-Ruiz
p. cm.
ISBN 978-953-51-0395-0

For EU product safety concerns:
IN TECH d.o.o., Prolaz Marije Krucifikse Kozulić 3, 51000 Rijeka, Croatia,
info@intechopen.com or visit our website at intechopen.com.

Meet the editor

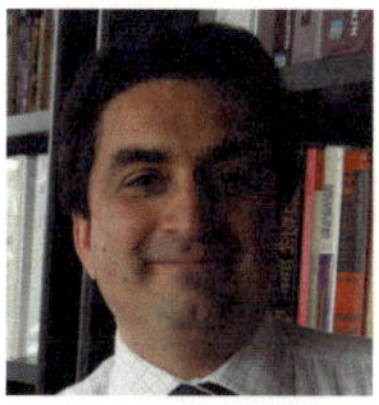

Dr José D. Carrillo-Ruiz has earned his M.D., M.Sc and PhD. from La Salle University and the National University of Mexico (UNAM). He also coursed his residency in Neurosurgery at Mexico General Hospital and UNAM, and made a fellowship in Stereotaxy and Functional Neurosurgery at Henri Mondor Hospital, Paris and Paris IV University, France. He belongs to the Stereotactic & Functional Neurosurgery and Radiosurgery Unit at Mexico General Hospital like staff physician and he is the Coordinator of Neuroscience Laboratory at Anahuac University in Mexico City. He is an expert in the area and has published several articles of basic and clinic research involving different neurological and psychiatric diseases including Parkinson´s disease, epilepsy, pain, depression and spasticity neuromodulation.

Contents

Preface

Neuromodulation is today an issue that has caused a great interest in recent years within the area of neuroscience and science in general. It has been defined as the application of electricity or chemicals in the central or peripheral nervous system for therapeutic purposes, i.e, is the procedure used in the nervous system to use the same way as neurons communicate among them to modify their anatomy and physiology, and therefore can change the pathophysiology of the disease. The reason for doing this is to modify the environment and improving neural function caused by cellular alterations in different diseases.

The ancient Chinese, Egyptians and Greeks used the electricity for therapeutic option, and it was followed in the Middle Age by some authors, but is taken up by Guillaume Duchenne in Paris, to treat some diseases such as facial paralysis and neurosis. During the eighteenth century to the sixties of the twentieth century there was great progress until a neurosurgery resident at the time, Dr. Norman Shealy, based on original work in dogs with the use of a pacemaker for conduction problems in the heart is proposed in the treatment of pain using neuromodulation in adapting this device for emitting a power source to the surface of the spinal cord to relieve pain. It was initially used to treat patients with malignancies (in other organs) and a short life expectancy, but it took nearly twenty years to gain experience and demonstrate that treatment was effective with the change of indications also. This experience showed incipient success so early attempts were made to treat others as epilepsy and Parkinson's disease to control seizures and tremor, respectively. The goodness of the use of neuromodulation clinched the next ten-years of experience in these three areas. It was significantly increasing the extension use for different symptoms of the disease and especially of different neurosurgical brain targets. The nineties and the dawn of the new millennium triggered an explosion of information in neurological and psychiatric illness which have been increasing over time. The application of electrodes in the brain, spinal cord or nerves has led to improve the signs or symptoms of pathological conditions such as dystonia, depression, obsessive-compulsive disorder, spasticity, including some of the most important. However this has been extended to other areas such as urinary and fecal incontinence, angina and vascular pain disease and every day there are other indications such as stroke that is very new.

In the case of substance use, within the nervous system have been confined mainly to pain with the application of intrathecal morphine and implementation of various analgesics for reducing the symptoms. The discovery of baclofen in the mid-eighties lessened spasticity in patients with spinal trauma or stroke. To date both drugs with their indications are valid. At present new substances have been used to improve pain and spasticity with limited results.

A new chapter has been opened to the treatment of these diseases by the magneto-therapy in which surgery is not necessary in the brain or spinal cord with results that still have to be proven whether they are comparable to those used in more invasive way .

The idea of this book is to give the reader a clear idea about these issues picking up the basics, indications for the use of neuromodulation in neurological, urological and vascular disease, expose complications and demonstrate the extensive experience of the clinical groups writing the book´s chapters.

This book "Topics in Neuromodulation therapy," aims to provide elements for the non-expert, but also to delve into some of these aspects of the diseases, mentioned above. The book has been divided into two sections: the first one, neuromodulation treatment that acts on the motor system which included epilepsy, urinary and fecal incontinence, and Parkinson's disease. In addition, a section that involves a sensitive part for the treatment of pain, and some in turn involving ischemia in the heart and brain.

The desire of the authors is that the readers will enjoy this text especially in helping to treat their patients.

Sincerely,

José D. Carrillo-Ruiz, M.D., M.Sc., Ph.D,
Associate Professor of Functional and Stereotactical Neurosurgery and Radiosurgery,
Faculty of Medicine, UNAM and Faculty of Health Science and Psychology,
Universidad Anahuac Mexico Norte,
México

Part 1

Neuromodulation Acting in Motor System

1

Neuromodulation Advances for Seizure Control

Ana Luisa Velasco[1], José María Núñez[1], Daruni Vázquez[1],
José Damián Carrillo-Ruiz[1], Manola Cuéllar-Herrera[1],
Rubén Conde[2] and Francisco Velasco[1]
[1]*Epilepsy Clinic, Neurology and Neurosurgery Service of the General Hospital of Mexico,*
[2]*Azteca Laboratories, Mexico City*
Mexico

1. Introduction

Epilepsy surgery has had an impressive development over the years, becoming a first option for many patients who have refractory seizures. The results of conventional surgery are

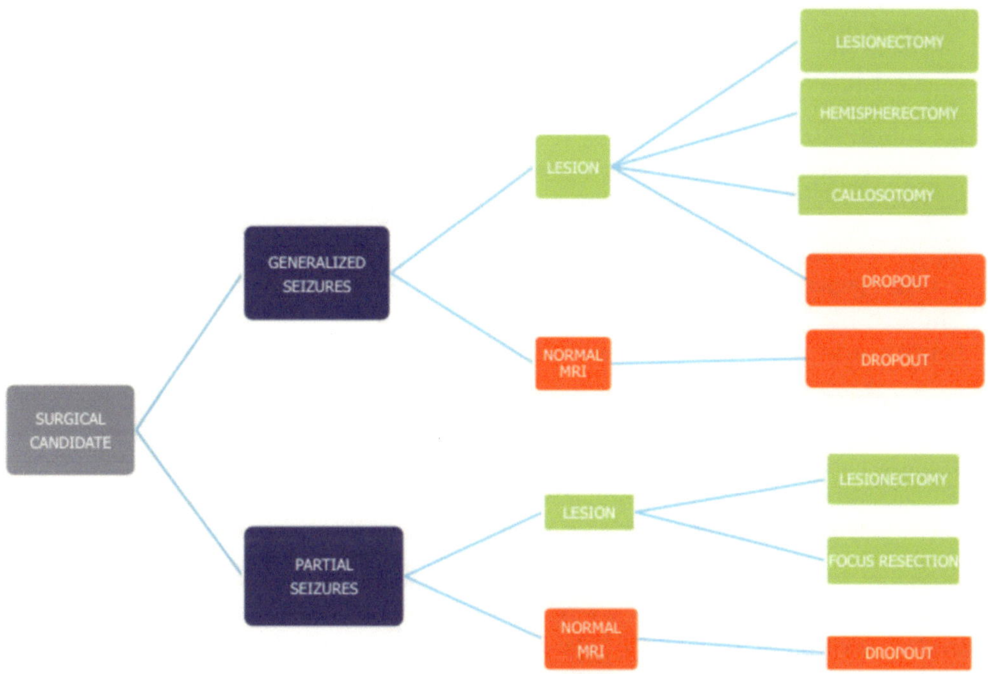

Fig. 1. Patients that are rejected from conventional epilepsy surgery
This flow diagram shows the usual route a patient follows to undergo a surgical procedure. In red are shown those patients who are rejected from surgery. Almost all patients who have none lesional MRI (magnetic resonance imaging) are almost always rejected (dropouts) since the diagnostic procedure is complicated and the outcome is not very reassuring. Patients who have lesions are sometimes rejected too. This is due to an involvement of primary functions with high risk of postsurgical neurologic deficit.

excellent thanks to experience, and better diagnostic and surgical techniques. Nevertheless, there are a number of patients who are rejected due to several reasons, for example bilateral or multiple epileptic foci, focus involving primary functional areas of the brain, generalized seizures or non lesional imaging studies. It has been calculated that there is a 30% of patients who need surgery that have to be rejected. These patients need a surgical alternative, and neuromodulation might be the answer to many of them. (Figure 1).

Even though neuromodulation has been proposed as an ideal surgical alternative for a number of neurological disorders, it's application for the control of epileptic seizures would seem to be the most appropriate therapeutic indication since epilepsy is considered in most cases a functional disorder. Several targets have been proposed to control seizures. Although there might be discrepancies about which target is the best, all authors agree that neuromodulation improves seizure control without deteriorating neurological functions. Many studies have been performed in different epilepsy surgery centers in the world proposing several seizure types that respond, different and stimulation modes. This chapter intends to discuss a number of questions that arise in the use of this method.

2. Who are the best candidates for neuromodulation?

As with all surgical procedures that are used to treat refractory seizures, patient selection is the first step to ensure a good outcome. If we err to recognize the appropriate candidate, even the best surgery is a failure. This principle applies to neuromodulation. Furthermore, neuromodulation is expensive and needs high to be performed.

In the future, neuromodulation might become the first option when considering a surgical method for refractory epilepsy. This is due to its low surgical risk and reversible qualities. But for now that ablative surgery is less expensive and shows good results. Criteria to select a patient are the following:

- Primary generalized seizures
- Multifocal or bilateral foci
- Seizures arising from eloquent areas (motor, memory and language for example)

In all the above clinical settings, conventional surgery has proven to be risky due to the fact that it can be a major surgery with high probability of infection, bleeding or loss of neural function. It is also less effective since surgeries tend to be restricted to avoid loss of function and hence residual seizures or relapses take place. If we add that there are a number of patients with non-lesional MRI, the risk and outcome is worse and patients are discarded from surgical options.

So the seizure type is decisive for the selection of the stimulation target. If we select a patient who has generalized seizures and we miss the fact that he has partial seizures with secondary generalized seizures, the patient will have a moderate improvement since generalized seizures will disappear but the partial and complex partial component will remain. So if we perform a seizure count, the number of seizures may turn out to be the same as before stimulation.

There are other considerations that we have to take into account. This procedure will need follow-up for several weeks to ensure good results. It is convenient that the patient and his caregiver understand the importance of follow-up appointments. It is desirable that the patient lives near the epilepsy center or at least has easy access to personnel that can check if the stimulator is working appropriately or to adjust the stimulation parameters. They must be willing to return with the caregivers if stimulation fails to ensure proper function of the whole system (see follow-up section at the end of the chapter).

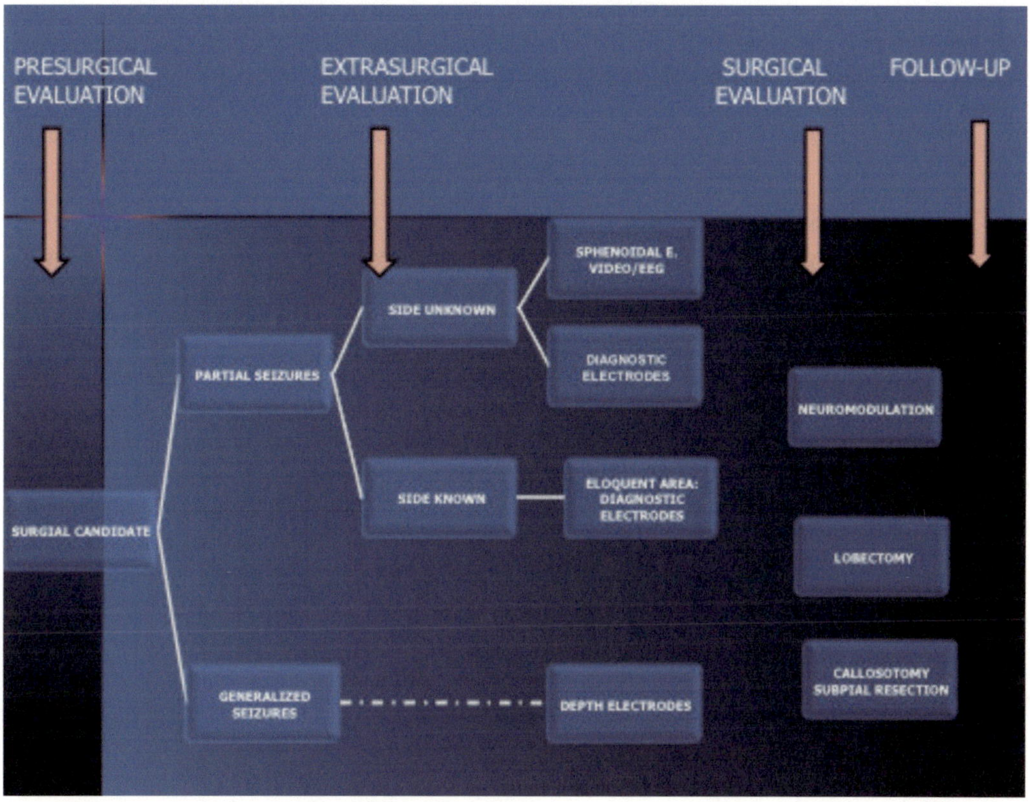

Fig. 2. Surgical evaluation of the epileptic patient
This figure depicts the clinical flow starting from the moment a patient is considered a surgical candidate. Presurgical evaluation in our Epilepsy Clinic includes a detailed medical history, EEG, in some cases video EEG with or without sphenoidal electrodes, MRI, PET/SPECT, functional MRI and neuropsyhcological testing. The extrasurgical evalation refers to phase II testing that includes continuous video EEG monitoring and brain mapping with electrical stimulation. Follow up includes the postsurgical testing: EEG, MRI, neuropsychological batteries.

Patient and caregivers must also have a clear idea of what to expect. Seizures do not disappear as soon as the stimulator is turned on. There is a variable period of time to obtain seizure reduction. This period of time varies according to the stimulated target and stimulation mode. If the cerebellum or *vagus* nerve are chosen, the best effect will take years to be reached, if the thalamus is stimulated, seizure reduction will take from 3 to 6 months to be achieved, if the target is hippocampal focus, the time span is reduced to 2 to 6 weeks if the hippocampus shows no signs of sclerosis in the MRI. If we stimulate the cortical epileptic focus in a programmed cyclic mode, seizures diminish in a matter of days (Velasco et al 2009) and if the mode is based on a closed loop fashion seizures take months to years to decrease (Fountas and Smith 2007).

3. What target should we stimulate?

Multiple targets that intend to achieve seizure reduction have been stimulated. At a first glance the amount of targets can be overwhelming and difficult to figure out. But basically, the different targets have been chosen based either on the idea of interfering with seizure propagation or generation (figure 3).

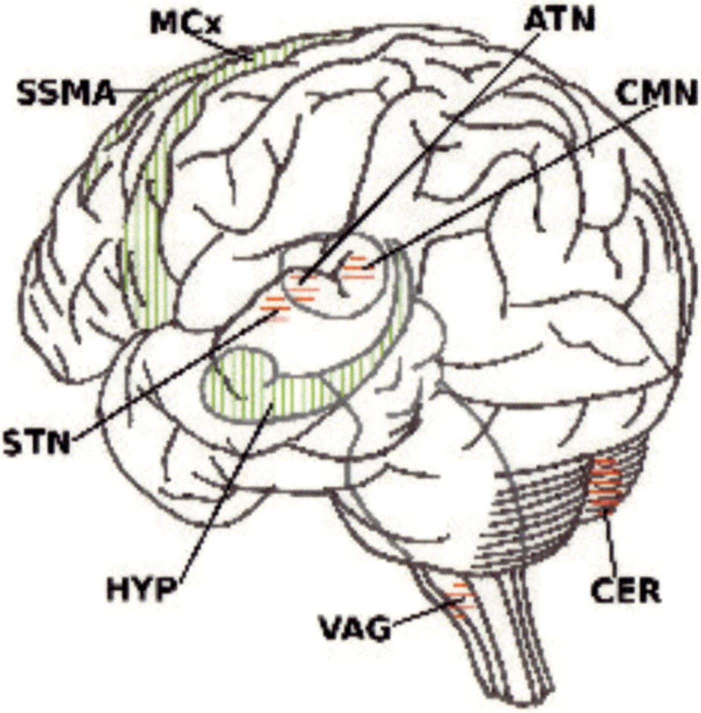

Fig. 3. Neuromodulation targets in epilepsy
Diagram shows some of the different targets for neuromodulation in epilepsy. In red are those targets whose stimulation interferes with seizure propagation: paravermian portion of the cerebellum (CER), vagus nerve (VAG), centromedian nuclei (CMN) and anterior nucleus (ATN) of the thalamus, subthalamic nucleus (STN). In green are the areas where epileptic foci can be located and stimulated to interfere with seizure generation: hippocampus (HIP), supplementary motor area (SMA), motor cortex (MCx)

3.1 Interfering with seizure propagation

This scope seems natural in generalized seizures but it has also been used in cases of partial seizures. In these scenarios, the rationale to select a target in which stimulation interferes with seizure propagation seems quite attractive. Several targets have been proposed: cerebellum, *vagus* nerve, thalamus (anterior, centromedian), and others such as subthalamic nuclei.

In 1973 the first report that suggested that low frequency stimulation of the cerebellar cortex (dorsal *paravermian* area) decreased seizures in humans was published (Cooper et al, 1973). The idea of stimulating the cerebellum was based in experimental findings in epileptic seizures induced in cats (Dow et al 1962). Even though results were controversial at first, a review of different studies with a total of 129 patients showed that 49% had significant seizure reduction, 27% being seizure free. This and other studies (Velasco et al 2005) have shown that the seizure type that best responds is primary generalized tonic clonic seizures and atypical absences and that even though there is an initial seizure reduction within the first two months of stimulation, the effect is not only maintained but there is a further decrease with time.

Vagus nerve stimulation is not very invasive since reaching the nerve at the neck level is a relatively simple procedure. It has been used in all types of refractory seizures. Its effects on seizure reduction are modest (~ 30 %). Even though the precise antiepileptic mechanism remains unclear, it appears that the thalamocortical relay neurons modulate cortical excitability, influencing seizure generation or propagation (Ben-Menachem 2002). It can produce dysphonia, headache and increases peptic ulcer and insulin dependant diabetes mellitus. It is not recommended for children under 12 years old.

According to the centro-encephalic theory by Penfield and Jasper (1954) high frequency stimulation of non-specific thalamic nuclei (such as centro-median or anterior thalamic nuclei) interferes with propagation of cortical or subcortically-initiated seizures. In 1984 Velasco et al performed the first bilateral centromedian electrode implantation in a 12-year-old boy with severe generalized seizures of the Lennox-Gastaut Syndrome. There was a considerable seizure reduction and impressive improvement in his intellectual status. Five years later they published a report of children and adults with generalized seizures of the Lennox-Gastaut Syndrome (Velasco 1989). The best results are obtained in the parvocellular portion. Neurophysiologic definition of the target is mandatory. This definition is based on electro cortical responses elicited by stimulation of the electrode contacts within different zones of the centromedian nucleus (Velasco F et al 2000, Velasco AL et al 2006). CM stimulation is more effective in generalized seizures and *epilepsia partialis continua*. When the patient selection as well as the anatomic and neurophysiologic criteria regarding the target localization are optimal, the results are >80% seizure reduction, some patients have become seizure free. An improvement in ability scales is also observed with no adverse effects.

As described above, the anterior nucleus is a non-specific thalamic nucleus and as such, interferes with propagation of cortical or subcortical initiated seizures but it also interferes with seizures initiated in mesial temporal structures and propagated through the *fornix*, mammillary body and anterior nucleus of the thalamus (Mirski and Fisher 1994). The SANTE study Group has reported the results of the bilateral stimulation of the anterior nucleus of the thalamus (Fisher et al 2010). Its best results have been obtained in complex partial and secondary generalized seizures, wich were reduced reduced by stimulation. By 2 years, there was a 56% median percent reduction in seizure frequency.

The subthalamic nucleus has been stimulated for seizure control based on the suppressive effects of pharmacological or electrical inhibition of the STN seen on different types of seizure in animal models of epilepsy (Chabardès 2002). It is considered that inhibition of the subthalamic nucleus causes activation of an endogenous epilepsy control system referred to as the nigral control of epilepsy system (Gale and Iadarola 1980). Patients with frontal lobe and myoclonic seizures are the best responders. Improvement varies from 30 to 80% (Vesper et al 2007). Mild facial twitching and paresthesias in legs and arms responded to adjustment of the stimulation parameters.

3.2 Interfering with seizure generation

Neuromodulation of the CM nuclei had already demonstrated anticonvulsive effects by stopping secondary tonic clonic generalized phase in patients with intractable mesial temporal lobe epilepsy but unfortunately it spared complex partial component that originated in the hippocampus (Velasco 1993a), thus patients continued to have disabling epilepsy. Based on the studies of Weiss et al (1998), Velasco et al (2000) started a project to demonstrate that the hippocampal stimulation would be a better alternative than trying to interfere with epileptic activity propagation.

Various authors (Boon et al 2007, Velasco et al 2007) have shown the beneficial effects in seizure reduction in patients with hippocampal foci stimulation; best responders are those patients whose epileptic focus can be pinpointed with hippocampal electrodes and thus stimulated directly and have non-lesional MRI. In these latter cases seizure reduction is >90% with several patients being seizure free.

Wyckhuys T et al (2007) found that high frequency stimulation of the hippocampus in kindled rats increases after-discharge thresholds with the consequent seizure reduction. There are some studies that have shown evidence that neuromodulation works by inhibiting the stimulated area. Clinical studies using neurophysiologic testing, single positron emission tomography and benzodiazepine receptor binding studies show that an inhibitory mechanism could explain seizure control (Velasco 2000, Cuéllar-Herrera 2004). Based in these observations, another challenge for epileptologists, the presence of intractable partial seizures arising from eloquent areas, was approached.

Cortical stimulation for motor seizures has been performed in two modes: an open (Velasco et al 2009) and closed loop (Sun et al 2008). The first step is to localize the epileptic focus implanting first a diagnostic grid and when done, implanting a permanent electrode directed to the focus. In case of the open loop mode, a significant (>90%) seizure decrease takes place over several days and effect persists thereafter, the stimulation mode is pre-established in a 24 hr cyclic 1 min ON, 4 min OFF. When the closed loop mode is used a seizure detection system is implanted too so that every time a seizure is detected, the stimulation therapy is delivered. In the latter mode, seizure reduction takes a longer period of time to produce a modest difference.

Interfering with:	Target	% seizure reduction
Propagation	Vagus nerve	30
	Centromedian nuclei	80-100
	Anterior nuclei	56 after 2 years
	Subthalamic nuclei	30-80
Generation	Hippocampal foci	80-100
	Motor foci	90-100

Table 1. Percentage seizure reduction
This table shows the percentage of seizure reduction according to the different targets. Note that the percentages are approximate and might vary according to the different techniques explained in the text.

4. How do we set the neural stimulation?

4.1 Verifying the chosen target

No matter what target we choose we must consider that there should be a neurophysiologic rationale in our reasoning. First we have to ask ourselves if we are able to detect the precise epileptic focus to be able to interfere with seizure generation, if not, we have to go for the disruption of the epileptic activity propagation. Either way we need to make sure we are in the correct location. From the anatomic point of view this should be easy, but several problems have to be faced. In case that we decide to go for seizure propagation we must target a precise anatomic region. The localization of the target is performed by the use of the current technology: stereotactic surgery, neuro-navigation, MRI, and neurophysiology. All expertise is needed to ensure the localization. Despite all these efforts, anatomy may be disrupted. This is particularly the case of reaching thalamic targets. We prefer patients whose thalamus and brainstem are intact and symmetric. MRI is used to verify position. Even so, the best-placed electrodes must have neurophysiologic confirmation.

In the case of centromedian stimulation, detailed analysis of incremental response morphology, polarity, peak latency, and cortical distribution may aid in defining the relation of the stimulated area with specific anatomophysiologic systems within the centromedian nucleus. Electrocortical responses produced by acute electrical stimulation along the centromedian nucleus or other structures are described in detail elsewhere (Velasco M, 1996).

To perform the physiologic confirmation of the electrode position in the parvocellular portion, the three pairs of combinations of the four contacts in each DBS electrode are stimulated (0–1, 1–2, and 2–3). Unilateral stimulation is performed at 6 Hz, 1.0 ms, 320–800 μA with 10-s duration to induce recruiting responses, and unilateral high frequency is conducted as well at 60 Hz, 1.0 ms, 320–800 μA to induce focalized desynchronization and negative DC shift of the EEG baseline. Scalp distribution analysis of electrocortical responses is performed. Within CM, suprathreshold stimulation in parvocellular subnucleus induces monophasic negative waxing and waning potentials, with peak latencies from 40 to 60 ms, recorded bilaterally in frontal and central regions, with emphasis on the stimulated side. Outside this subnucleus, incremental responses remain mainly biphasic positive-negative, with 16- to 20 ms latency, fixed amplitudes for the positive component, and distribution extending more toward the posterior leads. If the electrode is localized in the posterior and basal area of the centro median nucleus within boundaries with the parafascicular nucleus induces only short-latency positive potentials at low frequency and occasionally painful sensation at high frequencies (Velasco 1998).

In the case of epileptic focus stimulation, localizing the precise site where it is located is mandatory; it could make the difference in seizure outcome. In our Epilepsy Clinic, patients are implanted with externalized diagnostic multicontact intracranial electrodes, and recorded outside the operating room to be able to detect spontaneous seizures. This is to ensure we know where the focus is located (figure 4). In case of hippocampal stimulation we implant bilateral hippocampal electrodes, if the focus is unilateral, the diagnostic electrodes are explanted and only a single therapeutic permanent electrode is implanted; if the patient has bilateral foci, two electrodes, one in each hippocampus is implanted. The selected stimulation contacts are those that overlap with the epileptic focus (figure 5). All electrode implantations are verified with MRI.

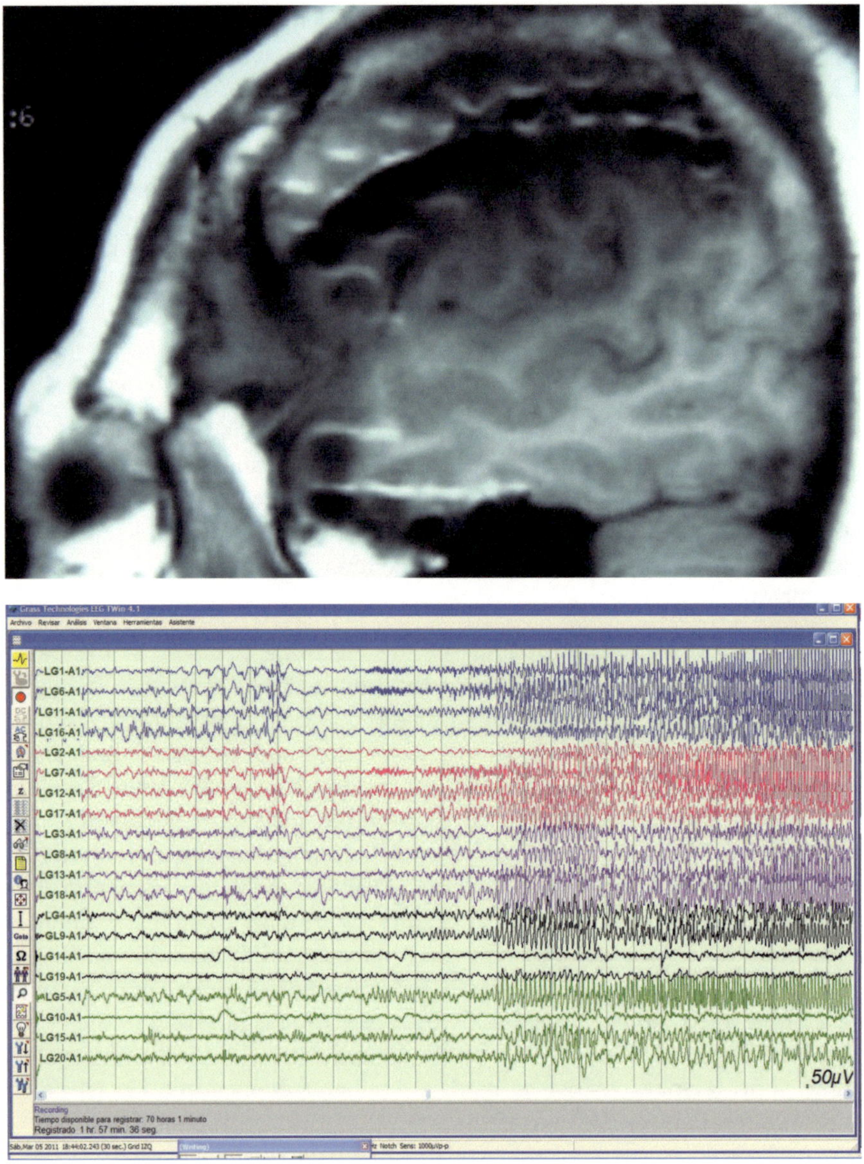

Fig. 4. Primary motor cortex epilepsy focus detection
This figure illustrates a patient with two grids localized in the right front central cortex to detect a seizure focus in the primary motor area of the right hand. 2A shows the patient's parasagittal MRI with the right hemispheric grids and 2B depicts the EEG recording of a spontaneous simple partial seizure of the left hand.

Maybe one of the topics that is most discussed and where no last word has been spoken refers to the stimulation parameters. We face many problems in this matter; probably the most important is the lack of sufficient financing resources that are required for the implementation of double-blinded protocols. To this problem we might add the necessity for more basic research data, multicentric studies, approval of FDA or similar agencies in different countries. Despite all this, there are some suggestions of the current parameters used for epilepsy:

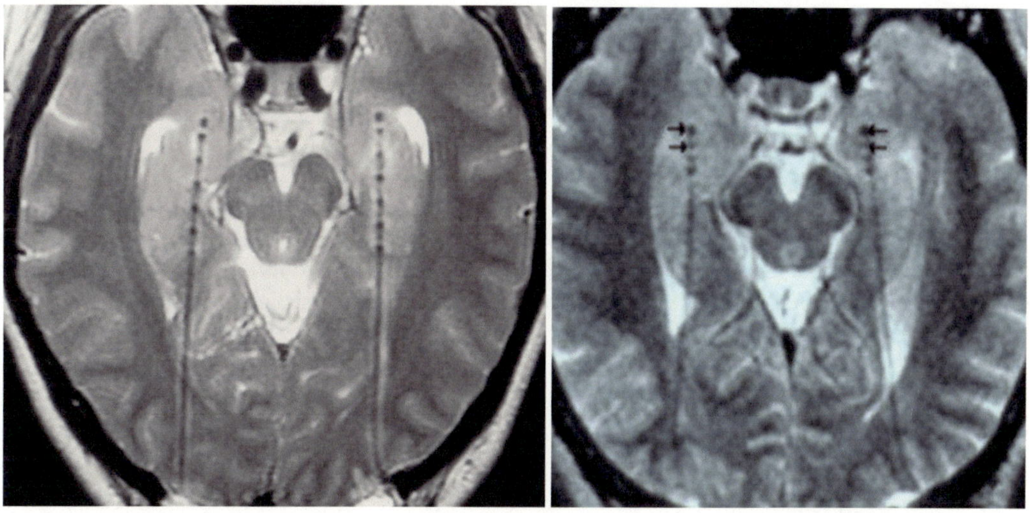

Fig. 5. Bilateral hippocampal electrodes for diagnosis and neuromodulation therapy
This figure depicts a patient with mesial temporal lobe epilepsy in whom bilateral hippocampal electrodes were implanted to determine focus. Recordings of spontaneous seizures demonstrated bilateral foci in most anterior contacts (left MRI); therefore bilateral 4 contact therapeutic electrodes were directed to the amygdalo-hippocampal areas to stimulate the patient in a bilateral fashion (right MRI)

4.2 Should we use cycling or continuous stimulation?

The electrical stimulation cycling mode of the nervous tissue was originally proposed to avoid electrical current overcharge in areas under or around electrodes, and therefore damaging neural tissue (Cooper, 1976). Discontinuous and cycling ES have been successfully used in treatment epilepsy (Ebner 1980, Davis 1992, George 2000). Although the main reason for using this mode of stimulation has been to save battery charge, its efficacy indicates that the beneficial effect outlasts each stimulation period.

4.3 What amplitude should we use?

Information derived from basic research has showed the importance of setting stimulation parameters that take into account principally the charge density-per-phase, which for safety's sake should not exceed 4 μC/cm2/phase (Babb 1977, Ebner 1980). In all of our CM stimulation cases, the stimulating pulse amplitude remained between 2.0 and 3.0 V while in hippocampus and motor cortex stimulation up to 3.5 V and only rarely were they changed during follow-up. This voltage represents between 50-80% of that which is necessary for inducing recruiting responses and DC shifts. It is important to mention that in cases with poor outcome, increasing the voltage 2 or 3 times the average did not improve efficacy.

4.4 Should we use high or low frequency stimulation?

Experience on neuromodulation studies in patients with movement disorders and those with pain, it is known that high frequency stimulation inhibits both. The same occurs in epilepsy; almost all studies use frequency in the range of 130 Hz. Velasco M et al (1997) demonstrated that low frequencies produced recruiting responses when stimulating the CM nuclei, and when bilateral stimulation at 3 Hz was performed in these *nuclei*, a typical absence seizure was reproduced. On the contrary, high frequency stimulation produced cortical inhibition of epileptic activity. In the case of neuromodulation of the subthalamic nucleus, low frequency has been used for good results (Chabardès 2002).

4.5 Open or closed loop mode?

Recent instances of clinical application of closed-loop seizure control, which are limited to stimulation with pulse trains in response to epileptiform activity, have been reviewed (Osorio et al 2001, Sun et al 2008). This method requires the implementation of a seizure detection algorithm to control the delivery of therapy using a suitable device. The theory is that stimulation therapy is provided as needed, potentially reducing the likelihood of functional disruption or habituation due to continuous treatment. It should also be better to save battery of the pulse generator reducing costs. Questions regarding the cost of a dual system (for detection and for stimulation) is one problem with this stimulation mode, we are currently dealing with the high cost of the stimulating system, most patients will not be able to pay for a detection system too. Secondly, there are currently no data that support that there is a potential likelihood of functional disruption with neuromodulation. Third, nowadays there are rechargeable batteries so the need to save energy should not be an issue. But more important is the fact that there are still many problems for precise seizure detection bringing as a result the application of unnecessary stimuli due to false positive detection or failure to stimulate if we modify seizure detection parameters to avoid the former. Probably this is the reason why studies have shown that stimulating with a closed loop mode takes much longer to reach best results. Further studies are mandatory to improve this methodology and solve issues regarding efficacy of the closed loop mode and cost of a implanting a dual system.

5. How can we make sure that neuromodulation is being adequately performed?

Neuromodulation in epilepsy has certain difficulties for its long-term assessment due to several reasons:

- The inherent characteristics of the symptoms (seizures)
- Patients do not experiment any sensations or secondary effects at all that indicate that stimulation is being delivered
- The time that neuromodulation takes to show a positive effect in seizure reduction
- "Carry on" effect
- Unlike movement disorders like tremor in Parkinson's disease, seizures appear once in a while and are not predictable, so it is not a matter of turning the pulse generator on or off and observing if seizures disappear to know if the stimulation system is working.

Except for the dysphonia that a few patients who undergo *vagus* nerve stimulation experiment when the stimulator is ON, other patients do not have sensations or secondary effects that could indicate if the stimulation is taking place. Two other important observations are that stimulation takes a variable time to show its effect, this period can take from several days to months; and that, when stimulation is stopped, there is a variable period of "carry-on" effect This term refers to the observed phenomenon in which the seizure reduction is maintained for days to months after the stimulator is turned OFF, the battery depletes or the stimulation is interrupted for any reason. Seizures reappear later in a progressive manner without reaching basal (before neuromodulation) level either in number or severity. Today, the neuromodulation community accepts the "carry-on effect".

These inherent characteristics carry the need to check the system every 6 to 12 months or when the patient returns to consult us because seizures are increasing in intensity or number. This check up consists in:

- Verifying pulse generator battery current: the pulse generator computer reader can tell us if the pulse generator has more than 50% or is running low.
- Checking electrode impedance (we have a comparative with our immediate post operatory measurements). If there is an increase, it could mean that that either the system extension or the electrode are broken or disconnected. In this case simple X rays are mandatory.
- Perform acute stimulation trial using the internalized stimulating system to generate recruiting responses. This will allow us to know that the system is working correctly and that the brain tissue is being stimulated, if not, either the system is broken or there is something in the tissue that is preventing a correct stimulation (blood, gliosis). Also the recruiting responses distribution in the scalp EEG can show us if the electrode moved from its intended placement. Within centromedian nucleus, suprathreshold stimulation in parvocellular subnucleus induces monophasic negative waxing and waning potentials, with peak latencies from 40 to 60 ms, recorded bilaterally in frontal and central regions, with emphasis on the stimulation side (Velasco 2006). Similar responses are found in hippocampal stimulation but are localized in ipsilateral temporal region and in motor cortex stimulation localized in ipsilateral frontal region.

6. What happens to the brain function if we stimulate it?

One of the main reasons to use neuromodulation is to preserve the functional areas of the brain. Neuromodulation in cases of abnormal movements or chronic pain has proven to be effective and to preserve function. Even when some undesirable effects are present, stimulation parameters and even the stimulated contacts can be changed and the adverse effects revert. When our group started stimulation of the centromedian thalamic nuclei for seizure control, we were dealing with patients with severe epilepsy, some of them Lennox-Gastaut patients with relentless psychomotor worsening due to the amount and severity of their seizures. The surgical options were not going to spare any function. So the functional implications of neuromodulation were not our main concern and we knew that the method was reversible. What we did not expect to find was an important improvement in the functions of these patients. We were surprised of how bed-ridden, totally dependent patients would start "learning" again. So we started evaluating their progress. Neuropsychological evaluation of this group was for the most part difficult in view of their deteriorated condition; several patients were in non-convulsive status, which made it impossible to apply a battery of standardized psychological tests in basal conditions. Nevertheless, the ability scales demonstrated that no patient had signs of neurologic or mental deterioration during electrical stimulation of the centromedian nuclei (Velasco et al 1993a, Velasco et al 2006), on the contrary, all patients improved their scales, some of them becoming independent and a couple of them seizure free and living a normal life. Patients with normal development before Lennox-Gastaut syndrome onset tend to regain their abilities regardless of convulsive syndrome severity (figure 6). Patients who had an early childhood onset had to learn everything from the start. The seizure and medication reduction added to the normalization of EEG background activity could explain this improvement (Velasco et al 1993b). Another explanation is that we are stimulating the reticular formation and thus improving the attention mechanisms of the brain, if a patient attends, he is able to learn new tasks.

In patients with neuromodulation of the hippocampal focus, using pulse amplitudes higher than needed, not only are the clinical benefits not increased but speech problems suchs as anomia can be produced. The problem disappears when the amplitude is decreased again (Nuche-Bricaire 2010).

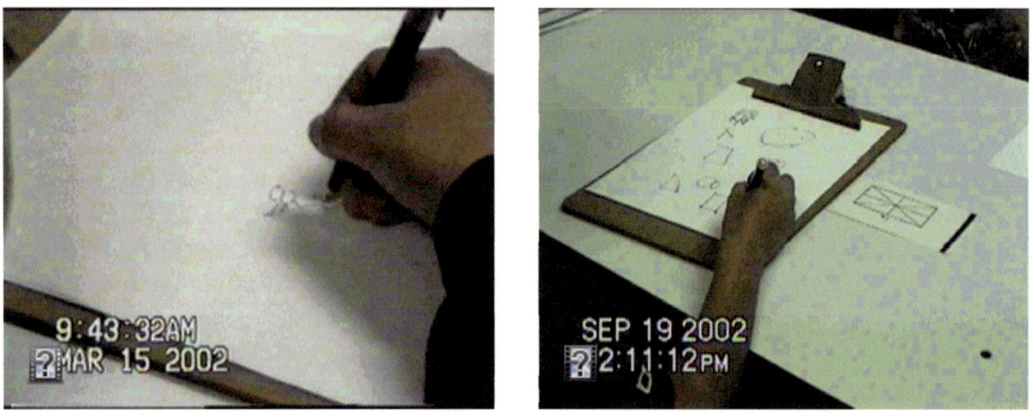

Fig. 6. Lennox-Gastaut syndrome response to neuromodulation
This figure illustrates the progress of a seven year-old patient with Lennox-Gastaut syndrome performing a neuropsychological battery. On the left image the patient has spent 5 minutes trying to copy a single figure with no success. The picture on the right shows same patient after 6 months with electrical stimulation of the thalamic centromedian nuclei. He is performing the same task but was able to copy several figures that were being presented to him in a couple of minutes paying attention to instructions and copying figures quite well despite they increased in difficulty and details.

In regard to stimulating the epileptic focus localized in the hippocampus, the groups mentioned above that have performed neuromodulation of the hippocampal foci have not reported a worsening of the memory function. Neuropsychological batteries for memory function (Table 2) have been applied and no deterioration has been found, and possibly a tendency to improve has occurred (Velasco 2007). The same thing happens with patients with stimulation of the primary or supplementary motor cortices, no decrease in motor function has been observed (Velasco 2009). Numbers or patients are small up to now and more studies need to be performed.

Function tested	Test
Attention and memory	*Neuropsi Attention and Memory Battery*
Verbal memory	*Rey verbal learning*
Verbal memory	*Digit Counting*
Verbal memory	*Logic memory*
Non verbal memory	*Visual reproduction*
Non verbal memory	*Wind Mill visual spatial Bezares Test*
Language dominance	*Dichotic listening test*

Table 2. Neuropsychological battery for memory function
This table illustrates the neuropsycological tests that are performed in a patient with intractable mesial temporal lobe epilepsy. In left column we point the function that testing is aimed for and on the right the specific test. This battery is accompanied with general testing as for example IQ and depression scales.

7. What have we learned about the possible mechanisms that explain why neuromodulation controls seizures?

In 2000 Velasco et al published the first results of subacute hippocampus foci stimulation in 10 patients. These patients had undergone intracranial electrode implantation as part of their surgical protocol to localize the epileptic focus; once localized, a two- to three-week trial of subacute stimulation was delivered before performing temporal lobectomy. This study design allowed the performance of a number of neurophysiologic (afterdischarges, paired pulse trials before and after stimulation), and single-photon- emission computed tomography (SPECT) studies comparing basal conditions with post-stimulation conditions. Since patients underwent lobectomy, stimulated tissue was recovered and analyzed using high- performance liquid chromatography (HPLC) techniques (Cuéllar-Herrera 2004). All studies suggested an inhibitory mechanism to explain seizure control (Figure 7). Wyckhuys T et al (2007) found that afterdischarges were inhibited and seizures disappeared in rats that had been kindled to induce epileptic seizures. None of the rats had an increase in seizure number.

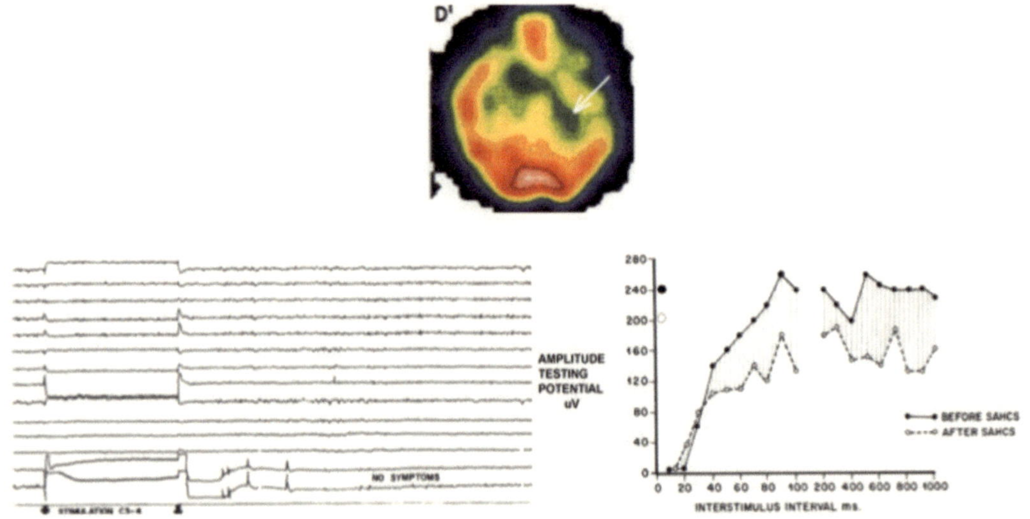

Fig. 7. Possible mechanisms that explain how neuromodulation works
This figure exemplifies the possible mechanisms through which neuromodulation works in hippocampal stimulation in man. Upper image is a single emission photon computerized study in a patient who underwent neuromodulation of the hippocampus for 3 weeks. At the lower left is the recording of afterdischarges in same patients in whom we apply maximum stimulation intensity in the epileptic focus and can no longer produce a clinical seizure and barely a few spikes instead of a prolonged afterdischarge accompanied by clinical symptoms of a complex partial seizure identical to the spontaneous ones presented by the patients. The lower right shows the difference between the recovery cycles before (continuous line) and after (broken line) neuromodulation. All three studies suggest an inhibitory effect of neuromodulation of the hippocampus.

8. Conclusion

This chapter shows a brief summary of the principal work that has been performed all over the world regarding neuromodulation for epilepsy. Results are encouraging; neuromodulation is a reversible surgical alternative that preserves neural function. It is capable of reducing seizure frequency and severity to a point that can be superior to what new generation antiepileptic medications have shown (Chadwik 2001, Van Rijckevorsel & Boon 2001) without their adverse effects. Patients tolerate it well, as a matter of fact, they are not even aware of being stimulated (except for vagus nerve stimulation). More concerns exist: are there other stimulation parameters worth trying (frequency, amplitude, pulse width), should they change according to the target; what is the best stimulation mode (open loop or close loop); are there other mechanisms that explain its antiepileptic effect? What will eventually happen in a longer follow up period?

Challenges are huge: exploring new targets, improving technology (better and cheaper stimulation and probably seizure detection systems, wider range of electrodes to choose from, smaller stimulating systems for younger children), improvement of surgical techniques so that we can find the focus and stimulate through the same electrode eluding unnecessary surgical procedures.

The main steps to be able to perform research in this matter have been taken; epilepsy expert groups tend to agree that neuromodulation is a field that can bring seizure relieve to patients. To be able to solve the questions and challenges, multidisciplinary, interinstitutional, worldwide projects with well thought designs are necessary.

9. References

Babb, T. L., Soper, H. V., Lieb, J. P., Brown, W. J., Ottino, C. A., & Crandall, P. H. (1977). Electrophysiological studies of long-term electrical stimulation of the cerebellum in monkeys. *J Neurosurg,* 47, 3, (Sept 1977), pp. 353–365, ISSN 0022-3085

Ben-Menachem, E. (2002). Vagus-nerve stimulation for the treatment of epilepsy. *Lancet Neurol,* 1, 8, (Dec 2002), pp. 477–482, ISSN 1474-4422

Boon, P., Vonck, K., De Herdt, V., Van Dycke, A., Goethals, M., Goossens, L., Van Zandijcke, M., De Smedt, T., Dewaele, I., Achten, R., Wadman, W., Dewaele, F., Caemaert, J., & Van Roost, D. (2007). Deep brain stimulation in patients with refractory temporal lobe epilepsy. *Epilepsia,* 48, 8, (Aug 2007), pp. 1551–1560, ISSN 0013-9580

Chabardes, S., Kahane, P., Minotti, L., Koudsie, A., Hirsch, E., & Benabid, A.-L. (2002). Deep brain stimulation in epilepsy with particular reference to the subthalamic nucleus. *Epileptic Disord, 4 Suppl 3,* (Dec 2002) pp. S83-93, ISSN 1294-9361

Cooper, I. S., Amin, I., & Gilman, S. (1973). The effect of chronic cerebellar stimulation upon epilepsy in man. *Trans Am Neurol Assoc, 98,* (1973) pp. 192–196, ISSN 0065-9479

Cooper, I. S., Amin, I., Riklan, M., Waltz, J. M., & Poon, T. P. (1976). Chronic cerebellar stimulation in epilepsy. Clinical and anatomical studies. *Arch Neurol, 33,* 8, (Aug 1976), pp. 559–570, ISSN 0003-9942

Cuellar-Herrera, M., Velasco, M., Velasco, F., Velasco, A. L., Jimenez, F., Orozco, S., Briones, M., & Rocha, L. (2004). Evaluation of GABA system and cell damage in parahippocampus of patients with temporal lobe epilepsy showing antiepileptic effects after subacute electrical stimulation. *Epilepsia,* 45,5, (May 2004), pp. 459–466, ISSN 0013-9580

Davis, R. & Emmonds, S. E. (1992). Cerebellar stimulation for seizure control: 17-year study. *Stereotact Funct Neurosurg,* 58, 1-4, (1992), pp. 200–208, ISSN 1011-6125

*Davis, R. (1998). Cerebellar stimulation for seizure control, In: Textbook of stereotactic and functional neurosurgery, Gildenberg, P., & Tasker, RR,. pp. 183-189, Publisher McGraw-Hill, ISBN 978-0070236042, Houston USA

Dow, R. S., Fernandez-Guardiola, A., & Manni, E. (1962). The influence of the cerebellum on experimental epilepsy. *Electroencephalogr Clin Neurophysiol,* 14, (Jun 1062), pp. 383–398, ISSN 0013-4694

Ebner, T. J., Bantli, H., & Bloedel, J. R. (1980). Effects of cerebellar stimulation on unitary activity within a chronic epileptic focus in a primate. *Electroencephalogr Clin Neurophysiol,* 49, 5-6 (Sept 1980), pp. 585–599, ISSN 0013-4694

Fisher, R., Salanova, V., Witt, T., Worth, R., Henry, T., Gross, R., Oommen, K., Osorio, I., Nazzaro, J., Labar, D., Kaplitt, M., Sperling, M., Sandok, E., Neal, J., Handforth, A., Stern, J., DeSalles, A., Chung, S., Shetter, A., Bergen, D., Bakay, R., Henderson, J., French, J., Baltuch, G., Rosenfeld, W., Youkilis, A., Marks, W., Garcia, P., Barbaro, N., Fountain, N., Bazil, C., Goodman, R., McKhann, G., Babu Krishnamurthy, K.,

Papavassiliou, S., Epstein, C., Pollard, J., Tonder, L., Grebin, J., Coffey, R., & Graves, N. (2010). Electrical stimulation of the anterior nucleus of thalamus for treatment of refractory epilepsy. *Epilepsia,* 51, 5,(May 2010), pp. 899–908, ISSN 0013-9580

Fountas, K. N. & Smith, J. R. (2007). A novel closed-loop stimulation system in the control of focal, medically refractory epilepsy. *Acta Neurochir Suppl,* 97, Pt 2, (2007), pp. 357–362, ISSN 0065-1419

Gale, K. & Iadarola, M. J. (1980). Seizure protection and increased nerve-terminal GABA: delayed effects of GABA transaminase inhibition. *Science,* 208, 4441, (Apr 1980), pp. 288–291, ISSN 0272-4634

George, M. S., Nahas, Z., Bohning, D. E., Lomarev, M., Denslow, S., Osenbach, R., & Ballenger, J. C. (2000). Vagus nerve stimulation: a new form of therapeutic brain stimulation. *CNS Spectr,* 5, 11, (Nov 2000), pp. 43–52, ISSN 1092-8529

Mirski, M. A. & Fisher, R. S. (1994). Electrical stimulation of the mammillary nuclei increases seizure threshold to pentylenetetrazol in rats. *Epilepsia,* 35, 6, (Nov-Dec 1994), pp. 1309–1316, ISSN 0013-9580

Nuche-Bricaire, A., Montes De Oca, M., Marcos-Ortega, M., Trejo, D., Núñez, JM., Vazquez, D. & Velasco, AL. (2010).Voltage-dependant Verbal Memory. Effects on the cognitive function through changing voltage parameters in deep brain stimulation. Proceedings of the 64th American Epilepsy Society Meeting. San Antonio, USA, Dec 2010.

Osorio, I., Frei, M. G., Manly, B. F., Sunderam, S., Bhavaraju, N. C., & Wilkinson, S. B. (2001). An introduction to contingent (closed-loop) brain electrical stimulation for seizure blockage, to ultra-short-term clinical trials, and to multidimensional statistical analysis of therapeutic efficacy. *J Clin Neurophysiol,* 18, 6(Nov 2001), pp. 533–544, ISSN 0736-0258

Penfield, W., & Jasper, H. (1954). Epilepsy and the functional anatomy of the human brain,: Publisher: Little Brown, ISBN 9780316698337, Boston USA

Sun, F. T., Morrell, M. J., & Wharen, R. E. J. (2008). Responsive cortical stimulation for the treatment of epilepsy. *Neurotherapeutics,* 5, 1, (Jan 2008), pp. 68–74, ISSN 1933-7213

Velasco, A. L., Velasco, M., Velasco, F., Menes, D., Gordon, F., Rocha, L., Briones, M., & Marquez, I. (2000). Subacute and chronic electrical stimulation of the hippocampus on intractable temporal lobe seizures: preliminary report. *Arch Med Res,* 31, 3(May-Jun 2000), pp. 316–328, ISSN 0188-4409

Velasco, A. L., Velasco, F., Jimenez, F., Velasco, M., Castro, G., Carrillo-Ruiz, J. D., Fanghanel, G., & Boleaga, B. (2006). Neuromodulation of the centromedian thalamic nuclei in the treatment of generalized seizures and the improvement of the quality of life in patients with Lennox-Gastaut syndrome. *Epilepsia,* 47, 7, (Jul 2006), pp. 1203–1212, ISSN 0013-9580

Velasco, A. L., Velasco, F., Velasco, M., Trejo, D., Castro, G., & Carrillo-Ruiz, J. D. (2007). Electrical stimulation of the hippocampal epileptic foci for seizure control: a double-blind, long-term follow-up study. *Epilepsia,* 48, 10, (Oct 2007), pp. 1895–1903, ISSN 0013-9580

Velasco, A. L., Velasco, F., Velasco, M., Maria Nunez, J., Trejo, D., & Garcia, I. (2009). Neuromodulation of epileptic foci in patients with non-lesional refractory motor epilepsy. *Int J Neural Syst,* 19, 3, (Jun 2009), pp. 139–147, ISSN 0129-0657

Velasco, AL. (2010) Developments in neurostimulation therapy for epilepsy. *US Neurology,* 5, 2 (Dec 2010), pp 78-81, ISSN

Velasco, F., Velasco, M., Ogarrio, C., & Fanghanel, G. (1987). Electrical stimulation of the centromedian thalamic nucleus in the treatment of convulsive seizures: a preliminary report. *Epilepsia,* 28, 4, (Jul-Aug 1987), pp. 421–430, ISSN 0013-9580

Velasco, F., Velasco, M., Velasco, A. L., & Jimenez, F. (1993). Effect of chronic electrical stimulation of the centromedian thalamic nuclei on various intractable seizure patterns: I. Clinical seizures and paroxysmal EEG activity. *Epilepsia,* 34, 6, (Nov-Dec 1993), pp. 1052–1064, ISSN 0013-9580

Velasco, F., Velasco, M., Jimenez, F., Velasco, A. L., Brito, F., Rise, M., & Carrillo-Ruiz, J. D. (2000). Predictors in the treatment of difficult-to-control seizures by electrical stimulation of the centromedian thalamic nucleus. *Neurosurgery,* 47, 2, (Aug 2000), pp. 295–304, ISSN 0148-396X

Velasco, F., Carrillo-Ruiz, J. D., Brito, F., Velasco, M., Velasco, A. L., Marquez, I., & Davis, R. (2005). Double-blind, randomized controlled pilot study of bilateral cerebellar stimulation for treatment of intractable motor seizures. *Epilepsia,* 46, 7, (Jul 2005), pp. 1071–1081, ISSN 0013-9580

Velasco, M., Velasco, F., Velasco, A. L., Lujan, M., & Vazquez del Mercado, J. (1989). Epileptiform EEG activities of the centromedian thalamic nuclei in patients with intractable partial motor, complex partial, and generalized seizures. *Epilepsia,* 30, 3, (May-Jun 1989), pp. 295–306, ISSN 0013-9580

Velasco, M., Velasco, F., Velasco, A. L., Velasco, G., & Jimenez, F. (1993). Effect of chronic electrical stimulation of the centromedian thalamic nuclei on various intractable seizure patterns: II. Psychological performance and background EEG activity. *Epilepsia,* 34, 6, (Nov-Dec 1993), pp. 1065–1074, ISSN 0013-9580

Velasco, M., Velasco, F., Velasco, A. L., Brito, F., Jimenez, F., Marquez, I., & Rojas, B. (1997). Electrocortical and behavioral responses produced by acute electrical stimulation of the human centromedian thalamic nucleus. *Electroencephalogr Clin Neurophysiol,* 102, 6, (Jun 1997), pp. 461–471, ISSN 0013-4694

Velasco, M., Brito, F., Jimenez, F., Gallegos, M., Velasco, A. L., & Velasco, F. (1998). Effect of fentanyl and naloxone on a thalamic induced painful response in intractable epileptic patients. *Stereotact Funct Neurosurg,* 71, 2, (1998), pp. 90–102, ISSN 1011-6125

Velasco, M., Velasco, F., & Velasco, A. L. (2001). Centromedian-thalamic and hippocampal electrical stimulation for the control of intractable epileptic seizures. *J Clin Neurophysiol,* 18, 6, (Nov 2001), pp. 495–513, ISSN 0736-0258

Vesper, J., Steinhoff, B., Rona, S., Wille, C., Bilic, S., Nikkhah, G., & Ostertag, C. (2007). Chronic high-frequency deep brain stimulation of the STN/SNr for progressive myoclonic epilepsy. *Epilepsia,* 48,10, (Oct 2007), pp. 1984–1989, ISSN 0013-9580

Weiss, S. R., Eidsath, A., Li, X. L., Heynen, T., & Post, R. M. (1998). Quenching revisited: low level direct current inhibits amygdala-kindled seizures. *Exp Neurol,* 154,1, (Nov 1998), pp. 185–192, ISSN

Wyckhuys, T., De Smedt, T., Claeys, P., Raedt, R., Waterschoot, L., Vonck, K., Van den Broecke, C., Mabilde, C., Leybaert, L., Wadman, W., & Boon, P. (2007). High frequency deep brain stimulation in the hippocampus modifies seizure characteristics in kindled rats. *Epilepsia,* 48,

2

Neuromodulation in Management of Overactive Bladder

Hitoshi Oh-Oka
Department of Urology, Kobe Medical Center, Kobe
Japan

1. Introduction

Symptoms of urgency and frequency, with or without incontinence, are collectively referred to as overactive bladder (OAB), that is particularly bothersome and worsens quality of life (QOL) (Cardozo et al., 2005). Patients' QOL is substantially impacted by OAB as social, psychological, occupational, domestic, physical, and sexual functioning are all affected (Abrams et al., 2000). Pharmacotherapy (anticholinergics) is the main treatment options in OAB. However, uncertainty still exists as to whether the effects of anticholinergics are worthwhile and which ones and which is the best route of administration. Neuromodulation is one of the non-drug alternatives of OAB managements like bladder training, pelvic floor muscle training (PFMT), and a combination of bladder training with biofeedback (Bergmans et al., 2005). Neuromodulation involves the use of either implanted or external electrodes to stimulate reflex inhibition of pelvic efferents or activation of hypogastric efferents to down regulate detrusor muscle activity (Alhasso et al., 2006). But, neuromodulation has not been widely accepted as first-line therapy because of few physiological and evidence based data. Patients with OAB are commonly treated using anticholinergics despite many adverse events (mainly dry mouth and constipation) (Abrams et al., 2006), possible poor medication adherence, and insufficient treatment satisfaction.

I review the current reports regarding neuromodulation and evaluate its efficacy and management mainly focused on interferential therapy (IF) in the treatment of OAB with and without urinary incontinence (wet & dry OAB).

2. Interferential therapy

2.1 History

IF utilizing effects of low frequency electrical stimulation was first conducted on the lower urinary tract in the treatment of urinary incontinence or urinary frequency, resulted in a clinical improvement (McQuire, 1975). The utility of this therapy for conditions such as urinary frequency, urge incontinence (UUI) and stress incontinence (SUI) was subsequently reported by several researchers (Dougall, 1985; Laycock and Green, 1988; Switzer and Hendriks, 1988). Yasuda reported the efficacy of IF over sham stimulation in double-blind cross over trial in Japanese patients regarding frequency, urgency and urinary incontinence

(UI) and revealed clinical efficacy of IF for neurogenic detrusor overactivity, idiopathic OAB and psychogenic pollakisuria (Yasuda et al., 1994). Suzuki reported the long term efficacy of IF with a mean follow-up of 6.7 months in 16 patients, with improvement rate 71.4% (Suzuki et al., 1994). Oh-oka reported clinical safety and efficacy of IF in the elderly wet OAB patients followed by treatment failure of anticholinergics (Oh-oka, 2008).

2.2 Basic principles/mechanisms

IF assumes the interference of two medium frequency currents producing a low frequency effect equal to the difference between the two currents around 4000Hz, that are applied to the body from different directions using four surface electrodes placed in the lower abdomen and lower buttocks, after that an interferential wave can be generated by the crossing of these two currents in the pelvic organs (bladder and pelvic floor). The mechanism for the treatment of OAB, including UUI, has been reported to include, 1) inhibition of efferent activities of the pelvic nerve through the somatosensory nerve stimulation in the pudendal region (action on the micturition center in the brainstem and the spinal cord) (Kimura et al.,1994; Sato et al., 1992), 2) increasing the pelvic blood flow (Nikolova, 1984), and 3) improving the urine storage function of the bladder and urinary tract through the sympathetic nerve (hypogastric nerve) (Kaeckenbeech, 1983). Of these, mechanism 1) appears to be most essential.

2.3 Clinical efficacy

A 20-minute treatment session was conducted twice a week for the first 3 weeks, and once every two weeks thereafter in Japan. Ease of usage and external application without giving harm to the superficial tissues are the main advantages of IF. The current and the intensity is well tolerated by the patients (Laycock and Green, 1988). Appropriate treatment frequencies of IF in patients with wet & dry OAB are generally 5 to 20Hz for reflex detrusor inhibition, but low frequencies such as 5 Hz may cause irritation (Yamanishi & Yasuda, 1988; Goode et.al., 2003), which can be resolved by reducing electric current. In patients with stress incontinence (SUI), frequencies ranging 20 to 50 Hz have been reported to be effective for urethra and pelvic floor (Yamanishi & Yasuda, 1988; Aukee et al., 2002). The frequency and period of stimulation vary according to investigators, from twice daily to once weekly, for 15 to 30 min. each, and from a month to 6 weeks, or 3-5 months (Yamanishi et al., 1997; Sand et al., 1995; Yamanishi et al., 2008). The optimal number of sessions required is still unknown, at least 10 treatments are recommended before the evaluation of clinical efficacy (Sand et al., 1995), and a session of 4-6 weeks is conventionally employed (Yamanishi et al., 1997; Li et al., 1992). For about the intensity of stimulation, the maximal tolerable intensity is usually employed (Yamanishi et al., 1997; Sand et al., 1995; Plevnik and Janez, 1979).

Yasuda et al. reported clinical efficacy of IF for patients with neurogenic detrusor overactivity (DO), idiopathic OAB and psychogenic pollakisuria. Subjective variables (patients' impression>good, improvement in urgency) and objective variables (improvement in pollakisuria, incontinence, 1-hr. pad test, overall improvement) had all improved significantly over sham stimulation. Furthermore, improvement was statistically significant in patients with neurogenic bladder ($n=32$, $p<0.01$) and urodynamic SUI ($n=17$, $p<0.01$) (Yasuda et al., 1994). Suzuki et al. reported clinical efficacy of IF with mean follow-up of 6.7±3.9 months in 16 patients with neurogenic DO, idiopathic OAB and psychogenic pollakisuria. Clinical efficacy of subjective variables (categorical scale of urinary frequency, urgency, patients' impression>good and overall improvement) were 46.7%, 53.3%, 81.3% and 71.4%, respectively. As for objective variables (urinary frequency, categorical scale of urinary incontinence (UI) frequency, incontinence volume) were 46.2%, 70.0% and 70.0%, respectively (Suzuki et al, 1994). Oh-oka reported the clinical efficacy of IF in 80 elderly non-neurogenic (idiopathic) OAB patients (69-78, median age 72.0) with UUI prospectively, for whom anticholinergics (propiverine hydrochloride) were not effective, who were provided with IF alone for three months (Table 1). In this paper he commented not only QOL score, but changes in lifestyle and plasma osmotic pressure (OP), brain natriuretic peptide (BNP). The average hours spent outdoors in one day, the one-day average radius of action increased, and the ADL scale score decreased; all these improvements were significant. Interviews from patients showed that all patients experienced increases in their amount of outdoor activities, time spent for shopping and hobbies, and time spent with their friends and close relatives. Also, OP increased significantly while BNP decreased significantly. These data indicate even in the absence of clinically evident cardiac disorders, OP and BNP levels can be high and that such levels are lowered in a relatively short period of time. IF can improve clinical symptoms of 'wet OAB' with relatively rapidly and thereby can improve ADL levels, implying a reduced load on left ventricular function. These features suggest that IF is a favorable treatment for the elderly, and for more than 1 year continuation of all 80 patients at their own request revealed satisfactorily compliance of IF (Oh-oka, 2008).

		baseline (pre IF)	post IF	p value
frequency of IF treatment required to show optimal effects	eight treatments (median)			
average weekly frequency of incontinence (times/week)		13.3 ± 5.2	3.6 ± 3.5	< 0.0001
60-min. pad test (gr.)		17.5 ± 2.1	3.1 ± 2.1	< 0.0001
daytime voiding episodes (times)		8.3 ± 2.4	7.0 ± 1.8	< 0.0001
nighttime voiding episodes (times)		1.8 ± 1.0	1.4 ± 1.0	0.0004
daytime voided volume (mL)		1199 ± 230	1220 ± 320	NS
nighttime voided volume (mL)		514 ± 185	464 ± 157	NS
IPSS		12.1 ± 5.3	6.3 ± 3.3	< 0.0001
QOL index		5.2 ± 0.8	2.4 ± 1.1	< 0.0001
Uroflowmetry variable				
voided vol. (mL)		170.2 ± 84.8	254.2 ± 60.6	< 0.0001
maximum flow rate (mL/sec.)		18.1 ± 6.8	25.7 ± 6.6	< 0.0001
average flow rate (mL/sec.)		8.9 ± 4.1	12.1±3.5	< 0.0001
postvoid residual urine volume (mL)		17.5 ± 24.0	14.5 ± 23.1	NS
specific gravity of urine		1.019 ± 0.007	1.016 ± 0.006	NS
The average hours spent outdoors in one day (hours)		1.5 ± 1.3	3.0 ± 1.4	< 0.0001
the one day average radius of action (meters)		400 ± 300	1200 ± 500	< 0.0001
ADL scale score		8.0 ± 1.2	3.4 ± 1.5	< 0.0001
Plasma osmotic pressure (mOsm/L)		295.1 ± 7.8	297.8 ± 3.6	< 0.0001
brain natriuretic peptide (pg/mL)		41.3 ± 38.7	19.2 ± 11.1	< 0.0001

IF; interferential therapy, IPSS; International Prostate Symptom Score, QOL; Quality of Life, ADL; Activities of Daily Living, NS; not significant

This data was modified from prior published work (Oh-oka, 2008, 2010)

Table 1. Amticholinergic resistant elderly wet OAB patients after 12 weeks of IF

Before and after IF, the follows were examined. 1) frequency of IF treatment required to show optimal effects, 2) average weekly episodes of incontinence, 3) 60-min. pad test, 4) episodes and voided volume in the daytime and nighttime, 5) fluid intake volume, 6) International Prostate Symptom Score (IPSS), QOL index, 7) Uroflowmetry, 8) postvoid residual urine volume (PVR), 9) specific gravity of urine, 10) average hours spent outdoors, 11) average radius of action and activities of daily life score, 12) standing blood pressure (BP) and heart rate, 13) clinical laboratory findings, 14) adverse events, 15) plasma osmotic pressure (OP), and 16) Brain natriuretic peptide. And the patients showed improvements for eight treatments (median). Improvement was observed in the followings; 2), 3), 4) voiding frequency, 6), 7) voided volume, maximal and average flow rate, 10), 11), 12) BP, 15) OP, and 16).

Demirtürk F et al. reported comparison to the effects of interferential current (0-100 Hz, 15 min., 3 times/week) and biofeedback applications (Kegel exercise, 15 min., 3 times/day) on incontinence severity in patients with 40 USI women and resulted both treatment modalities seemed to have similar effects on pad test (95% CI: -1.48 - 4.59), pelvic muscle strength (95% CI: -9.29 -1.78) and quality of life (95% CI: -11.91 - 5.31) outcomes (Demirtürk et al., 2008).

2.4 Challenges/future prospects

Currently, only interferential therapy using the Uromaster® is approved for use in the treatment of OAB and UI in Japan. IF reports regarding clinical efficacy or basic research in OAB are very few, and good, randomized, placebo controlled studies have rarely performed. Applying uniformly set treatment modalities (treatment parameters and schedules), long term data on the clinical outcome, also concerning the patients' characteristics (definition and duration of symptoms, previous treatment) is very important and urgently necessary (van Balken et al., 2004). Also combination effect with PFMT or anticholinergics should be further analyzed strictly to manage OAB for the future. On the other hand, advantages of IF include; the absence of complications such as increased episodes and (nighttime) voided volume resulting from more water intake to counter dry mouth, which is an bothersome adverse event observed with the use of anticholinergics including propiverine hydrochloride; and satisfactory compliance that can be achieved in patients who are not indicated for oral treatment or are incapable of oral ingestion. IF is suitable for short-term electrical stimulation for home use (portable IF devices are available, that are unauthorized for medical equipment in Japan).

3. Pelvic floor electrical stimulation

3.1 History

Caldwell reported the successful implantation of an anal sphincter stimulator for fecal incontinence, which proved to be effective for urinary incontinence (Caldwell, 1963). Anal plug electrodes were subsequently modified. Later Fall et al. provided reports regarding transvaginal electrical stimulation with urinary incontinence and interstitial cystitis (Fall et al., 1977, 1980, 1984).

3.2 Basic principles/mechanisms

Vaginal, anal, and surface electrodes are used for pelvic floor electrical stimulation. Vaginal electrode is popular for women, and anal electrode is usually used for men. The mechanism of these techniques was detrusor relaxation induced by afferent pathways including activation of hypogastric inhibitory neurons, inhibition of pelvic excitatory neurons with pudendal nerves (Lindström, 1983).

3.3 Clinical efficacy

Because of poor tolerability due to pain or discomfort of intravaginal and anal plug electrodes, surface electrical stimulation of dorsal nerve of penis or clitoris (transcutaneous electrical stimulation [TENS]) has been often adopted as low invasive modality for DO. The alternative TENS treatments was thought S2 or S3 dermatome, which might improve clinical outcome (Walsh et al, 1999). Comparison of neuromodulation to sham TENS, no TENS, other TENS including suprapubic or tibial nerve TENS, and medical treatment including anticholinergics is important. These studies resulted in a positive effect on detrusor instability (DI), an improvement in the first desire to void and increased bladder capacity on urodynamics. Some DI patients become stable, while in others the volume at first contraction improved significantly. For permanently decreasing incontinence TENS alone might be insufficient. Superiority of clinical efficacy between oxybutynin and electrical stimulation (intravaginal or TENS) in controversial (Soomro et al, 2001; Wang et al, 2006), but the prevalence of electrical stimulation devices might not enough (Walsh et al, 1999). Arruda RM et al. reported the effectiveness of oxybutynin, functional electrostimulation (transvaginal) and pelvic floor training for treatment of 64 women with DO after completion of 12 weeks of treatment and resulted all three treatments were equally effective for improvement rate of subjective symptoms, urgency and urodynamic cure (Arruda et al., 2008).

3.4 Challenges/future prospects

Intravaginal and anal plug are sometimes intolerable for many patients due to discomfort, mucosal injury (Yamanishi et al., 1997; Yamanishi & Yasuda, 1998) and high intensity stimulation for acceptable outcome, surface electrodes like TENS have been employed as less invasive treatment for OAB.

4. Electrical tibial nerve stimulation of the lower limb

4.1 History

During experimental studies in nonhuman primates with spinal cord injury to improve bipolar anal sphincter Stimulation, McGuire et al. found that detrusor activity inhibition was equally achieved by applying a positive current to the anal sphincter with a negative electrode placed over the posterior tibial nerve (McGuire et al., 1983). Similar results were obtained by applying current on the common peroneal or posterior tibial nerve and a ground electrode placed over the same nerves contralaterally. The idea of stimulating tibial nerve was based on the traditional Chinese practice of using acupuncture points to inhibit bladder activity (McGuire et al., 1983). Transcutaneous posterior tibial nerve stimulation was then evaluated in clinical trials with variable results.

4.2 Basic principles/mechanisms

Percutaneous tibial nerve stimulation (PTNS) delivers neuromodulation to the pelvic floor through the S2-4 junction of the sacral nerve plexus via the less invasive route of the posterior tibial nerve. Using the fine needle electrode insertion above the ankle, the tibial nerve is accessed. This area has projections to the sacral nerve plexus, creating a feedback-loop that modulates bladder innervation (Kohli & Rosenblatt, 2002).

4.3 Clinical efficacy

Govier et al. reported a safety and efficacy of PTNS for refractive OAB and/or pelvic floor dysfunction (Govier et al., 2001). Klingler et al. demonstrated reduction in pain and urodynamic improvement of DI, total bladder capacity, first bladder sensation, bladder volume at normal desire to void, and urinary frequency (Klingler et al., 2000). Peters et al. demonstrated the objective effectiveness of PTNS in OAB symptoms compared to extended-release tolterodine (Peters et al., 2009). PTNS is also effective for disease related DO (DO in multiple sclerosis, Parkinson's disease).

4.4 Challenges/future prospects

PTNS is less invasive, easily applicable, and well tolerated in all lower urinary tract conditions. Poor improvements in urodynamic studies, like other neuromodulation therapies, might be the main disadvantage, and it seems doubtful regarding the stable efficacy of chronic (over 10 to 12 weeks) treatment (van Balken et al., 2004). As in sacral root neuromodulation, PTNS seems less effective for improving chronic pelvic pain (van Balken et al., 2003).

5. Sacral nerve stimulation

5.1 History

In 1981 a group at the urological department at the University of California-San Francisco started a clinical program to evaluate the efficacy of sacral root electrode implantation in humans, leading to the humans (Tanagho & Schmidt, 1988; Schmidt, 1986). Since then, many reports regarding sacral nerve stimulation have been published as the technique has gained popularity.

5.2 Basic principles/mechanisms

SNS involves continuous electrical stimulation of the sacral nerves to inhibit or activate the neural reflexes that influence the bladder, urethral sphincter, and pelvic floor (Shaker & Hassouna, 1988; van Kerrebroek et al., 2007; Oerlemans & van Kerrebroek, 2008). Thus, SNS has been indicated for various types of lower urinary tract dysfunction refractory to conservative treatment, such as wet & dry OAB, pelvic pain syndrome and urinary retention (UR) (Oerlemans & van Kerrebroek, 2008; Shaker & Hassouna, 1998). In patients with OAB, SNS would restore the balance between inhibitory and excitatory control systems at various sites in the peripheral and central nervous system. This would involve activation of somatosensory bladder afferents projecting into the pontine micturition center, and/or activation of the hypogastoric sympathetic nerves (van der Pal et al., 2006). Also, Blok et al. reported changes in regional cerebral blood flow, using positron emission tomography, during chronic and acute sacral neuromodulation. They suggest chronic SNS influences, presumably via the spinal cord, brain areas previously implicated in detrusor hyperactivity, awareness of bladder filling, the urge to void and the timing of micturition (Blok et al., 2006). Furthermore, SNS affects areas involved in alertness and awareness.

5.3 Clinical efficacy

A percutaneous nerve stimulation (PNE) of the S3 roots for 1-4 weeks is used to select responders of neuromodulation, and patients who are eligible for permanent implantation shift to a chronic stimulation system (Chartier-Kastler, 2008). To prolong test period safely (reduce the risk of infection and surgical invasiveness) and to avoid false-negative results due to lead migration, PNE with the permanent tined lead under local anesthesia is also available (Spinelli et al., 2005). Schmidt et al. reported success rate of 63% (test stimulation) in 155 patients with refractory UUI. Sustained clinical benefit was reported at 18 months after implantation (Schmidt et al., 1999). Jonas et al. reported efficacy with refractory idiopathic UR who are refractory to other treatments. Success rate of SNS was 83%, including 69% who stopped using catheters at 6 months after implantation (Jonas et al., 2001). Shaker and Hassouna reported a marked reduction in leakage episodes from 6.49 to 1.98 times per 24 hours, and eight of 18 patients became completely dry after an average follow-up was 18.8 months (Shaker & Hassouna, 1988). Sutherland et al. reported their one institution's 11-year experience with SNS in 104 patients including dry, wet OAB and mixed incontinence. With a mean follow up of 22 months (range 3-162 months), sustained subjective improvement was >50%, >80%, and >90% in 69%, 50%, and 35% of patients, respectively. By QOL survey, 60.5% of patients were satisfied with current urinary symptoms (Sutherland et al., 2007).

To shorten operation time and decrease pain complaints at the stimulator site buttock placement was advocated. The unilateral SNS might result in malposition of the electrode or local fibrosis. Hohenfellner et al. recommended clinical efficacy of bilateral SNS than unilateral SNS (Hohenfellner et al., 1998). Aboseif et al. reported the efficacy and QOL improvement of SNS in patients with idiopathic, chronic, non-obstructive functional UR. Permanent implants were performed 20 patients who revealed more than 50% improvement in symptoms during the PNE test. Eighteen patients were subsequently able to void and no longer required intermittent catheterization. Average voided volumes increased from 48 to 198 ml and PVR reduced from 315 to 60 ml. Eighteen patients reported more than a 50% improvement in QOL (Aboseif et al., 2002). New approaches of bilateral caudal neuromodulation might yield excellent outcome in patients with urinary retention refractory to traditional, unilateral S3 stimulation (Maher et al., 2007).

5.4 Challenges/future prospects

Sacral nerve stimulation (SNS) is an established treatment for OAB. Adverse events related to SNS can be the physical presence of the device or adverse stimulation. Van Kerrebroek et al. reported adverse events seemed to occur in 102 patients (67%) at 5-year follow-up, and the most frequent events being new pain or undesirable change of stimulation (27%) (van Kerrebroek et al., 2007). Adverse stimulation does not necessarily require surgical intervention. It is often resolved by changing stimulation factors (pulse width, amplitude, mode of polarity etc.). Pain in implant site or scar pain could be adequately treated by antimicrobial agents, while device pain might require relocation of the device components. Hijaz et al. reported 10.5% of patients were explanted due to loss of efficacy or infection. In 16.1% of the patients, adverse events (implant site discomfort in 2.5%, lead migration in 0.6% and infection in 2.5%) or decreased efficacy (10.5%) could be managed successfully (Hijaz et al., 2006).

6. Magnetic stimulation

6.1 History

Magnetic stimulation has been used for experimental and clinical testing on the central and peripheral nervous systems (Barker et al., 1987). Compared to electrical stimulation, magnetic stimulation is useful to stimulate deep proximal nerves with little pain due to magnetic penetration of all body tissues without alteration. Also patients are not necessary to take off clothes during treatment because the magnetic field passes through clothes.

6.2 Basic principles/mechanisms

A varying magnetic field will induce an electrical field in any specified loop in its vicinity. The roots of sacral nerves S2-S4 provide the primary autonomic and somatic innervations of the urinary tract, including pelvic floor, urethra, bladder and other pelvic organs, and stimulation of these roots is an efficient way to modulate the pelvic floor and control functions of pelvic organs (Shafik, 2000). Magnetic stimulation can be applied both at the sacral root (Sheriff et al., 1996; Fujishiro et al., 2002) and the peri-anal region (Yamanishi et al., 2000; Galloway et al., 1999). However, the commercially available stimulator is usually a chair type and stimulates the peri-anal region including pelvic floor muscles because of difficulty to fix the coil to the sacral root for a long time.

6.3 Clinical efficacy

Reductions in the frequency of leakage and urodynamic improvement of maximum bladder capacity in UUI and increase in maximum urethral closing pressure in USI by continuous magnetic stimulation have been reported (Yamanishi et al, 2000a, 2000b). Unsal et al. reported the clinical efficacy of extracorporeal magnetic stimulation for the treatment of SUI and UUI in women (Unsal et al., 2003). Fujishiro et al. reported an investigational study and placebo controlled trial to evaluate the potential efficacy of magnetic stimulation of the sacral roots for the treatment of stress incontinence. They concluded significant efficacy for the treatment of UUI and SUI (Fujishiro et al., 2000 & 2002). Yamanishi et al reported a randomized comparative study investigating the urodynamic effects of functional magnetic stimulation (FMS) and functional electrical stimulation (FES) on the inhibition of detrusor overactivity, and concluded that both treatments were effective in the increase of first desire to void and maximum cystometric capacity. But the increase in the maximum cystometric capacity was significantly greater in FMS than FES group, also the inhibition of detrusor overactivity appeared greater in FMS than FES group (Yamanishi et al, 2000). Suzuki et al. reported the effect of functional continuous magnetic stimulation (FCMS) on urgency incontinence using a randomized, sham-controlled, crossover evaluation in 39 UUI patients.

They concluded magnetic stimulation was effective on UUI in comparison to sham stimulation (Suzuki et al, 2007). However, Culligan et al. reported no differences in pelvic muscle strength between patients receiving active or sham extracorporeal magnetic innervation treatments (ExMI) in the early postpartum period (Culligan et al., 2005). Voorham-van der Zalm et al. reported the clinical results of extracorporeal magnetic innervation therapy (ExMI) of the pelvic floor muscles with functional changes in the pelvic floor musculature, urodynamics and quality of life, and concluded ExMI did not change pelvic floor function (Voorham-van der Zalm et al., 2006). There are varying outcomes of several studies on ExMI stress the need for critical studies on the effect and the mode of action of electrostimulation and magnetic stimulation.

6.4 Challenges/future prospects

This type of stimulation cannot be applied for prolonged periods and unsuitable for long-term treatment, although it may be helpful for preliminary assessment of candidates for chronic sacral root neuromodulation. It is unclear if the exact mechanism of action is magnetic, nerve root, peripheral nerve, or intramural nerve stimulation. No prospective randomized studies to date have been performed to demonstrate this therapy's use in larger groups regarding UUI or USI.

7. Conclusions

Although the use of electrical stimulation and neuromodulation to treat patients with OAB has been widely investigated, in many reports important information is not enough and good randomized, placebo controlled studies are rare. The advent of various techniques of neuromodulation causes paradigm shift of treatment strategies of patients with OAB and other lower urinary tract dysfunction. We should compare various techniques and evaluate placebo effects overcoming unsolved aspects of the current treatment including neuromodulation. And our better approaches based on further understanding of voiding function and action mechanism of neuromodulatory techniques might lead more various types of patients with urinary tract dysfunction to more satisfactorily clinical outcomes. In consideration of these problems, I personally expect potential clinical efficacy of IF as short-term electrical stimulation, that has few adverse event, and improving not only QOL but ADL.

8. Acknowledgements

I thank Tomonori Yamanishi from the department of Urology of Dokkyo University School of Medicine for valuable advices on this paper.

9. References

Aboseif, S.; Tamaddon, K.; Chalfin, S. et al. (2002). Sacral neuromodulation in functional urinary retention: an effective way to restore voiding. *BJU Int*, 90, 662-665.

Abrams, P. ; Kelleher, C.J. ; Kerr, L.A. & Rogers, R.G. (2000). Overactive bladder significantly affects quality of life. *Am J Manag Care*, 6(11 Suppl), Jul, pp. S580-590.

Abrams, P.; Cardozo, L.; Chapple, C., et al.; 1032 Study Group (2006). Comparison of the efficacy, safety, and tolerability of propiverine and oxybutynin for the treatment of overactive bladder syndrome. *Int J Urol*, 13, 6, Jun, 692-698.

Alhasso, A.A.; McKinlay, J.; Patrick, K., et al. (2006). Anticholinergic drugs versus non-drug active therapies for overactive bladder syndrome in adults. *Cochrane Database Syst Rev*, 18, CD003193.

Arruda, R.M.; Castro, R.A.; Sousa, G.C., et al. (2008). Prospective randomized comparison of oxybutynin, functional electrostimulation, and pelvic floor training for treatment of detrusor overactivity in women. *Int Urogynecol J Pelvic Floor Dysfunct*, 19, 1055-1061.

Aukee, P.; Immonen, P.; Penttinen, J., et al. (2002). Increase in pelvic floor muscle activity after 12 weeks' training: a randomized prospective pilot study. *Urology*, 60, 1023-1024.

Barker, A.T.; Freeston, I.L.; Jalinous, R. et al. (1987). Magnetic stimulation of the human brain and peripheral nervous system: an introduction and the results of an initial clinical evaluation. *Neurosurgery* , 20, 100-109.

Bergmans, B.; Yamanishi, T., Wilson, P.D., et al. (2005). Adult conservative management. In: *Incontinence Edition 2005*. Edited by Abrams, P.; Cardozo, L., Khoury, S., et al. Paris: Health Publication Ltd, pp. 855-964.

Blok, B.F.; Groen, J.; Bosch, J.L. et al. (2006). Different brain effects during chronic and acute sacral neuromodulation in urge incontinent patients with implanted neurostimulators. *BJU Int*, 98, 1238-1243.

Caldwell, K.P. (1963). The electrical control of sphincter incompetence. *Lancet*, 2, 174-175.

Cardozo, L.; Coyne, K.S., & Versi, E. (2005). Validation of the urgency perception scale. *BJU Int* , 95, 4, pp.591-596.

Chartier-Kastler, E. (2008). Sacral neuromodulation for treating the symptoms of overactive bladder syndrome and non-obstructive urinary retention: >10 years of clinical experience. *BJU Int*, 101, 417-423.

Culligan, P.J.; Blackwell, L.; Murphy, M. et al. (2005). A randomized, double-blinded, sham-controlled trial of postpartum extracorporeal magnetic innervation to restore pelvic muscle strength in primiparous patients. *Am J Obstet Gynecol* , 192, 1578-1582.

Demirtürk, F.; Akbayrak, T.; Karakaya, I.C., et al. (2008). Interferential current versus biofeedback results in urinary stress incontinence. *Swiss Med Wkly*. 138, 317-321.

Dougall, D.S. (1985). The effects of interferential therapy on incontinence and frequency of micturition. *Physiotherapy*, 71, 3, March, 135-136.

Fall, M.; Erlandson, B.E.; Nilson AE et al. (1977). Long-term intravaginal electrical stimulation in urge and stress incontinence. *Scand J Urol Nephrol Suppl* , 44, 55-63.

Fall, M.; Carlsson, C.A. & Erlandson, B.E. (1980). Electrical stimulation in interstitial cystitis. *J Urol*, 123, 192-195.

Fall, M. (1984). Does electrostimulation cure urinary incontinence? *J Urol*, 131, 664-667.

Fujishiro, T.; Enomoto, H.; Ugawa, Y. et al. (2000). Magnetic stimulation of the sacral roots for the treatment of stress incontinence: an investigational study and placebo controlled trial. *J Urol* , 164, 1277-1279

Fujishiro, T.; Takahas.;, Enomoto, H. et al. (2002). Magnetic stimulation of the sacral roots for the treatment of urinary frequency and urge incontinence: an investigational study and placebo controlled trial. *J Urol*, 168, 1036-1039.

Galloway, N.T.; El-Galley, R.E.; Sand, P.K., et al. (1999). Extracorporeal magnetic innervation therapy for stress urinary incontinence. *Urology*, 53, 1108-1111.

Goode, P.S.; Burgio, K.L.; Locher, J.L., et al. (2003). Effect of behavioral training with or without pelvic floor electrical stimulation on stress incontinence in women: a randomized controlled trial. *JAMA*, 290, 345-352.

Govier, F.E.; Litwiller, S.; Nitti, V. et al. (2001). Percutaneous afferent neuromodulation for the refractory overactive bladder: results of a multicenter study. *J Urol* , 165, 1193-1198.

Hijaz, A.; Vasavada, S.P.; Daneshgari, F. et al. (2006). Complications and troubleshooting of two-stage sacral neuromodulation therapy: a single-institution experience. *Urology*, 68, 533-537.

Hohenfellner, M.; Schultz-Lampel, D.; Dahms, S. et al. (1998). Bilateral chronic sacral neuromodulation for treatment of lower urinary tract dysfunction. *J Urol*, 160, 821-824.

Jonas, U.; Fowler, C.J.; Chancellor, M.B. et al. (2001). Efficacy of sacral nerve stimulation for urinary retention: results 18 months after implantation. *J Urol*, 165, 15-19.

Kaeckenbeech, B. & Hublet, D. (1983) Urinary incontinence in women. *Acta Urologica Belgica*. 51, 104-223.

Kimura, A.; Suzuki, A.; Sato A., et al. (1994). Effects of Interferential Current Stimulation on Urinary Bladder Function in Anesthetized Rats. *Auton Nerv Syst* , 31, 316-321.

Klingler, H.C.; Pycha, A.; Schmidbauer, J. et al. (2000). Use of peripheral neuromodulation of the S3 region for treatment of detrusor overactivity: a urodynamic-based study. *Urology*, 56, 766-771.

Kohli, N. & Rosenblatt, P.L. (2002). Neuromodulation techniques for the treatment of the overactive bladder. *Clin Obstet Gynecol*, 45, 218-232.

Laycock, J. & Green, R.J. (1988). Interferential therapy in the treatment of incontinence. *Physiotherapy* 1988, 74, 4, April, 161-168.

Li, J.S.; Hassouna, M.; Sawan, M., et al. (1992). Electrical stimulation induced sphincter fatigue during voiding. *J Urol*, 148, 949-952.

Lindström, S.; Fall, M.; Carlsson, C.A. et al. (1983). The neurophysiological basis of bladder inhibition in response to intravaginal electrical stimulation. *J Urol*, 129, 405-410.

Maher, M.G.; Mourtzinos, A.; Zabihi, N. et al. (2007). Bilateral caudal epidural neuromodulation for refractory urinary retention: a salvage procedure. *J Urol*, 177, 2237-2241.

McGuire, E.J.; Zhang, S.C.; Horwinski, E.R., et al. (1983). Treatment of motor and sensory detrusor instability by electrical stimulation. *J Urol*, 129, 78-79.

McQuire, W.A. (1975). Electrotherapy and exercise for stress incontinence and urinary frequency. *Physiotherapy*, 61, 10, 305-307.

Nikolova, L. (1984) Effect of interference current and low-frequency magnetic field on tissue regeneration. *Vopr Kurortol Fizioter Lech Fiz Kult*. 3, 19-23.

Oerlemans, D.J. & van Kerrebroek, P.E. (2008). Sacral nerve stimulation for neuromodulation of the lower urinary tract. *Neurourol Urodyn*, 27, 28-33.

Oh-oka H (2008). Efficacy of interferential low frequency therapy for elderly wet overactive bladder patients. *Indian J Urol*, 24, 178-181.

Oh-oka H (2010). Neuromodulation in the Treatment of Overactive Bladder With a Focus on Interferential Therapy. *Curr Bladder Dysfunct Rep*, 5, 39-47.

Peters, K.M.; Macdiarmid, S.A.; Wooldridge, L.S. et al (2009). Randomized trial of percutaneous tibial nerve stimulation versus extended-release tolterodine: results from the overactive bladder innovative therapy trial. *J Urol*, 182, 1055-1061.

Plevnik, S. & Janez, J. (1979). Maximal electrical stimulation for urinary incontinence: report of 98 cases. *Urology*, 14, 638-645.

Sand, P.K.; Richardson, D.A.; Staskin, D.R., et al. (1995). Pelvic floor electrical stimulation in the treatment of genuine stress incontinence: a multicenter, placebo-controlled trial. *Am J Obstet Gynecol*, 173, 72-79.

Sato, A.; Sato, Y. & Suzuki, A.(1992). Mechanism of the reflex inhibition of micturition contractions of the urinary bladder elicited by acupuncture-like stimulation in anesthetized rats. *Neurosis. Res*, 15, 189-198.

Schmidt, R.A. (1986). Advantages in genitourinary neurostimulation. *Neurosurgery*, 19, 1041-1044.

Schmidt, R.A.; Jonas, U.; Oleson, K.A. et al. (1999). Sacral nerve stimulation for treatment of refractory urinary urge incontinence. Sacral Nerve Stimulation Study Group. *J Urol*, 162, 352-357.

Shafik, A. (2000). The role of the levator ani muscle in evacuation, sexual performance and pelvic floor disorders. *Int Urogynecol J Pelvic Floor Dysfunct* , 11, 361-376.

Shaker, H.S. & Hassouna, M. (1998). Sacral root neuromodulation in idiopathic nonobstructive chronic urinary retention. *J Urol*, 159, 1476-1478.

Shaker, H.S. & Hassouna, M. (1998). Sacral nerve root neuromodulation: an effective treatment for refractory urge incontinence. *J Urol*, 159, 1516-1519.

Sheriff, M.K.; Shah, P.J.; Fowler, C. et al. (1996). Neuromodulation of detrusor hyper-reflexia by functional magnetic stimulation of the sacral roots. *Br J Urol* , 78, 39-46.

Soomro, N.A.; Khadra, M.H.; Robson W., et al. (2001). A crossover randomized trial of transcutaneous electrical nerve stimulation and oxybutynin in patients with detrusor instability. *J Urol*, 166, 146-149.

Spinelli, M.; Weil, E.; Ostardo, E. et al. (2005). New tined lead electrode in sacral neuromodulation: experience from a multicentre European study. *World J Urol*, 23, 225-229.

Sutherland, S.E.; Lavers, A.; Carlson, A. et al. (2007). Sacral nerve stimulation for voiding dysfunction: One institution's 11-year experience. *Neurourol Urodyn*, 26, 19-28.

Suzuki, T.; Kawabe, K.; Kageyama, S., et al (1994). A long-term trial on instrument of interferential low-frequency wave "TEU-20" in pollakisuria, urinary urgency and urinary incontinence. *Jpn J Urol Surg*, 7, 529-540.

Suzuki, T.; Yasuda, K.; Yamanishi, T. et al. (2007). Randomized, double-blind, sham-controlled evaluation of the effect of functional continuous magnetic stimulation in patients with urgency incontinence. *Neurourol Urodyn*, 26, 767-772.

Switzer, D. & Hendriks, O. (1988). Interferential therapy for treatment of stress and urge incontinence. *Ir Med J*, 81, 1, Nov, 30-31.

Tanagho, E.A. & Schmidt, R.A. (1988). Electrical stimulation in the clinical management of the neurogenic bladder. *J Urol*, 140, 1331-1339.

Unsal, A.; Saglam, R.; Cimentepe, E. et al. (2003). Extracorporeal magnetic stimulation for the treatment of stress and urge incontinence in women-results of 1-year follow-up. *Scand J Urol Nephrol*, 37, 424-428.

van Balken, MR.; Vandoninck, V.; Messelink, BJ., et al (2003). Percutaneous tibial nerve stimulation as neuromodulation treatment of chronic pelvic pain. *Eur Urol*, 43, 158-163.

van Balken, MR.; Vergunst, H. & Bemelmans, B.L. (2004). The use of electrical devices for the treatment of bladder dysfunction: a review of methods. *J Urol*, 172, 846-851.

van der Pal, F.; Heesakkers, J.P. & Bemelmans, B.L. (2006). Current opinion on the working mechanisms of neuromodulation in the treatment of lower urinary tract dysfunction. *Curr Opin Urol*, 16, 261-267.

van Kerrebroek, P.E.; van Voskuilen, A.C.; Heesakkers, J.P. et al (2007). Results of sacral neuromodulation therapy for urinary voiding dysfunction: outcomes of a prospective, worldwide clinical study. *J Urol*, 178, 1844-1845.

Voorham-van der Zalm, P.J.; Pelger, R.C.; Stiggelbout, A.M. et al. (2006). Effects of magnetic stimulation in the treatment of pelvic floor dysfunction. *BJU Int*, 97, 1035-1038.

Walsh, I.K.; Johnston, R.S. & Keane, P.F. (1999). Transcutaneous sacral neurostimulation for irritative voiding dysfunction. *Eur Urol*, 35, 192-196.

Wang, A.C.; Chih, S.Y.; & Chen, M.C. (2006). Comparison of electric stimulation and oxybutynin chloride in management of overactive bladder with special reference to urinary urgency: a randomized placebo-controlled trial. *Urology*, 68, 999-1004.

Yamanishi, T.; Yasuda, K.; Sakakibara, R. et al. (1997). Pelvic floor electrical stimulation in the treatment of stress incontinence: an investigational study and a placebo controlled double-blind trial. *J Urol*, 158, 2127-2131.

Yamanishi, T. & Yasuda, K. (1998). Electrical stimulation for stress incontinence. *Int Urogynecol J Pelvic Floor Dysfunct*, 9, 281-290.

Yamanishi, T.; Kamai, T. & Yoshida, K. (2008). Neuromodulation for the treatment of urinary incontinence. *Int J Urol*, 15, 665-672.

Yamanishi, T.; Yasuda, K.; Suda, S. et al. (2000). Effect of functional continuous magnetic stimulation for urinary incontinence. *J Urol* , 163, 456-459.

Yamanishi, T.; Sakakibara, R.; Uchiyama, T. et al. (2000). Comparative study of the effects of magnetic versus electrical stimulation on inhibition of detrusor overactivity. *Urology* , 56, 777-781.

Yasuda, K.; Kawabe, K.; Sato, A.; et al. (1994). A double-blind cross-over trial on instrument of interferential low-frequency wave "TEU-20" in pollakisuria, urinary urgency and urinary incontinence. *Jpn J Urol Surg*, 7, 297-324.

3

Challenges in Sacral Neuromodulation

Mai Banakhar[1], Tariq Al-Shaiji[2] and Magdy Hassouna[3]
[1]*Clinical Fellow Toronto Western Hospital, King Abdul Aziz University*
[2]*Clinical Fellow Toronto Western Hospital*
[3]*Urology Toronto Western Hospital, Toronto University*
Canada

1. Introduction

Sacral neuromodulation (SNM) is an effective and increasingly used therapeutic option for refractory urge incontinence, chronic urinary retention and symptoms of urgency-frequency. The potential for neuromodulation has also been shown in patients with interstitial cystitis and neurogenic urge incontinence secondary to refractory detrusor hyperreflexia. With the increasing number of patients, obvious concerns and challenges raised. Young female patients who desire to conceive showed concerns pertaining to neuromodulation in pregnancy including possible teratogenic effect, symptom management during pregnancy & the effect of mode of delivery on the Sacral electrode. Another concern is the need for MRI follow up in neurogenic patients. Post operative troubleshooting raises another challenge in patient management. In our chapter, we will discuss these challenges in details.

2. Historical overview of neurostimulation

Knowledge of the neurological associations among spinal marrow, nerves, and the urinary bladder arose after the middle of the nineteenth century. In 1863 Giannuzzi stimulated the spinal cord in dogs and concluded that the hypogastric and pelvic nerves are involved in regulation of the bladder (Giannuzzi, 1863).The first attempt at bladder stimulation occurred in 1878, when Saxtorph treated patients with urinary retention by way of intravesical electrical stimulation (Madersbacher, 1999) After experimentations with various methods of stimulating the bladder such as the transurethral approach, direct detrusor stimulation (Boyce et al, 1964), pelvic nerve stimulation (Dees JE, 1965), pelvic floor stimulation (Caldwell KP, 1963), and spinal cord stimulation (Nashold et al, 1971) were carried out. Based on the work of Tanagho and Schmidt it was demonstrated that stimulation of sacral root S3 generally induces detrusor and sphincter action (Heine et al, 1977) (Schmidt et al, 1979) (Tanagho et al, 1982) (Tanagho, 1988).In 1988, Schmidt described the three stages of electrode placement (Schmidt, 1988). In 1988, a neuroprosthesis was first used for treatment of pelvic pain, and discomfort improved over 50% in 49% of patients (Schmidt, 1988). In 1990, Tanagho presented the results of Neurostimulation for incontinence, 70% of 31 patients with urge incontinence obtained subjective improvement of 50% or more, as did 40% of 25 patients with post prostatectomy incontinence (Tanagho, 1990). Two years latter, Tanagho published the results of neuromodulation in 27 children: five of seven children with meningomyelocele gained continence, as did four of six patients with voiding dysfunction and one of two patients with neonatal hypoxia (Tanagho, 1992). In 1998, Shaker and Hassouna evaluated the efficacy and safety of sacral root neuromodulation. They concluded that, for non obstructive urinary retention, sacral root neuromodulation is an appealing, efficacious treatment. Implantation is relatively simple and carries a low complication rate (Shaker & Hassouna, 1998).Finally, in October 1997, after two decades of experimentation with various approaches to sacral root stimulation, Sacral Neurostimulation (SNS) was approved by the Food and Drug Administration (FDA) for the treatment of Urge incontinence (UI) and Urgency –frequency syndrome (U/F). In 1999, it was approved for the treatment of non-obstructive urinary retention (NOUR). Since the approval, a number of technical advances has been made. The introduction of tined lead had made a dramatic change in surgical approach. Spinelli et al reported that the success rate of this technique in selective patients for the permanent implant is significantly higher (70%) than what is reported in the literature (50%). Outcomes of the implanted patients confirmed better patient selection with minimal complication. This technique allows the possibility of more accurate patient selection by using the definitive lead for longer test period before proceeding with the neurostimulator (IPG) implant (Spinelli et al ,2003) .

3. How does it work?

The Exact Mechanism of action in not well understood. A number of theories have been proposed to explain the effect of electrical neuromodulation which can be summarized as: somatic afferent inhibition of sensory processing in the spinal cord. Regardless of whether the lower urinary tract dysfunction involves storage versus emptying abnormalities, the pudendal afferent signaling serves as a common crossroads in the neurologic wiring of the system. Not only can pudendal afferent input turn on voiding reflexes by suppressing the guarding reflex pathways, pudendal afferent input to the sacral spinal cord also can turn off supraspinally mediated hyperactive voiding by blocking ascending sensory pathway inputs. (Kruse and Groat, 1993), (Thon et al, 1991), (Vadusek et al, 1986), (Groat et al, 1997), (Kruse et al, 1990), (Groat and Theobald, 1976)

Other possible mechanisms of sacral nerve stimulation include:

- Inhibits postganglionic neurons directly
- May inhibit primary afferents presynaptically
- Inhibits spinal tract neurons involved in the micturation reflex
- Inhibits interneurons involved in spinal segmental reflexes
- May suppress indirectly guarding reflexes by turning off bladder afferent input to internal sphincter sympathetic or external urethral sphincter interneurons
- Postganglionic stimulation can activate postganglionic neurons directly and induce bladder activity (induce voiding), but at the same time can turn off bladder-to- bladder reflex by inhibiting afferent- interneuronal transmission. (Wendy and Michael, 2005)

4. Indications for sacral nerve stimulation therapy

The US Food and Drug Administration (FDA) approved Sacral neuromodulation (SNM) for three main conditions: intractable urge incontinence 1n 1997, and for urgency- frequency and non obstructive urinary retention in 1999 (Shaker & Hassouna, 1998).Latter, the labeling was changed to include "overactive bladder" as an appropriate diagnostic category (Abrams et al, 2009). Patients in this group are considered candidates for SNS if they have chronic symptoms, refractory to medical therapy. (Apostolicism, 2011) (Knupfer, 2011)The Urodynamics study may or may not demonstrate uninhibited bladder contractions. Their symptoms include urinary urgency-frequency and urge incontinence (Al-Shaiji et al, 2011) (Abrams et al, 2003) (Siegel et al, 2000). Since its inception, widespread use for approved conditions has led to incidental improvements in other areas. Research is ongoing to channel the potential of neuromodulation into other applications.

4.1 Neurogenic disorders

Patients who have defined neurologic abnormalities such as multiple sclerosis (MS) or partial cord injury also may benefit from SNS, but studies in this population of patients have been few (Bosch and Groen, 1996)(Hassouna et al,2000). In spinal cord injured patients, detrusor hyperreflexia develops after spinal shock period resolves. Vastenholt reported (Vastenholt et al, 2003) a series of 37 patients with spinal cord injury who underwent implantation of sacral anterior root stimulation. He reported his 7 year follow-up of the group in which 87% continued using the implant for micturation control, 60% used it for benefits with respect to defecation. Of the 32 male patients, 65% were able to achieve a stimulator- induced erection. (Everaert etal, 1997) reported the urodynamic changes in 27 neuromodulation implanted patients with spastic pelvic floor syndrome, bladder neck dysfunction, sphincter hypertonia, sphincter dysfunction, detroser overdistenstion and hypercontractile detroser.

Other demyelinating disease as Guillain-Barre syndrome with voiding dysfunction has been reported to respond to sacral neuromodulation therapy (Wosnitzer et al, 2009). A study on incomplete spinal cord injured patients suffering from lower urinary tract symptoms showed that SNM is effective (Lombardi and Del, 2009). Chaabane et al reported a mean follow up of 4.3+/- 3.7 years, SNM is still effective in neurogenic bladder dysfunction group, and failures depend on the progression of the underlying neurological disease which usually are reported in the first year of follow up (Chaabane et al, 2001).

4.2 Interstitial cystitis (IC) and pelvic pain

IC per se is not an FDA approved indication for SNM; these patients have a set of symptoms of frequency, urgency and pelvic pain which in combination considered as characteristic of IC. A lot of studies showed patient symptoms relieve with SNM (Lukban et al, 2002) (Everaert et al, 2001) improved patient quality of life & narcotic requirements in refractory IC (Siegel et al, 2001) (Comiter, 2003).Peters reported total of 18 out of 21 interstitial cystitis patients who used chronic narcotics before Interstim, with the remaining three using non-narcotic analgesics. The mean narcotic use dropped from 81.6 mg/day Morphine Dose Equivalent (before implantation) that decreased afterward to 52.0mg/day (36%, P=0.015). Four of 18 patients ceased using all narcotics after permanent Interstim implantation (Peters, 2003). Ghazwani et al reported long term follow up of 21 female patients with painful bladder syndrome in which 52% showed response to PNE and proceeded for permanent IPG implantation. They had a significant improvement in bladder pain and voiding parameters at 1- year follow-up which was maintained at 5 years, with improvement in urgency & average voided volume. (Ghazwani et al, 2011). Gajewski and Al-Zahrani recommended SNM in these patients before any major invasive surgical interventions if the conservative measures have failed (Gajewski and Al-Zahrani, 2010).

4.3 Chronic genitourinary pain

SNM has been used to control a variety of forms of genitourinary pain. Chronic non bacterial prostatitis & chronic epididymo-orchalgia are a common challenge that had hope with SNM. Feler et al reported a 75% improvement in a 44y male diagnosed with chronic epididymitis and chronic non bacterial prostatitis (Feler et al, 2003).Vulvodynia consists of chronic vulvar discomfort including itching, burning and dyspareunia. Feler et al reported a 71y female who suffered of Vulvodynia for 9 years in which sacral neuromodulation provided excellent pain relief. (Feler et al, 2003).

4.4 Sexual function

There are few reported cases claiming improved sexual function in both male & females. Lombardi et al reported sacral neuromodulation for lower urinary tract function in male patients which showed impact on their erectile function. Total of 22 patients had their IEF-5 score shifted from 14.6 to 22.2 (Lombardi et al, 2008). In females, papers reported improvement in sexual function index of arousal and lubrication in voiding dysfunction female group (Lombardi et al, 2008). Pauls et al reported total female sexual function index improvement ($p=0.002$), and significant improvement domains of desire ($p=0.004$) and lubrication ($p=0.005$) in voiding dysfunction group (Pauls et al, 2006).However, all these reported papers were reported in voiding dysfunction group. No studies were constructed yet on any pure sexual dysfunction cases. Signorello et al claimed that the improvement in quality of sexual function in female patients with overactive bladder correlates with improvement in urinary symptoms (Signorello et al, 2011). In unpublished data from our center, female sexual function overall indices improved in voiding dysfunction female group P=0.028 (CI-23.14- -1.62), the parameters of satisfaction=0.037 (CI -4.9- -0.0177) & lubrication P=0.018 (CI -6.082 - -0.687) showed significant improvement in comparison to the other parameters (Banakhar et al, 2011)

4.5 Children

Similar to adults, children are faced with various degrees of lower urinary tract dysfunction that often deteriorate upper tract function. Usual treatment modality of intermittent catheterization & Anticholinergics are not uniformly successful and major reconstructive procedures are needed. Humphreys et al reported SNM in 16 children with refractory voiding dysfunction with mean age of 11 years. His study group showed 75% improved or resolved urinary incontinence, 83% improved their nocturnal enuresis, urinary retention improved in 73% of patients (Humphreys et al, 2004)

4.6 Non urologic indications

Angina pectoris (Van at al,2011), chronic migraine (Magis and Schoenen, 2011), fecal incontinence (Pascuall et al, 2011). The overall published results for SNM include all etiologies of fecal incontinence. Melenhorst et al reported 132 patients who had temporary stimulation. 100 were implanted (75%), the mean age was 75 years (26 -75 years) and the mean follow up was 25 months (2-63 months), the mean number of incontinence episodes decreased from 31 to 4.8 (P<0.0001) as documented in a bowel diary (Melenhorst et al,2007). SNM is also indicated for constipation (Van et al, 2011) .Masin et all reported results in 34 patients with chronic idiopathic constipation with a median follow-up of 12 months93-48). Cleveland Clinic Constipation score decreased significantly from (mean +/- SEM)14 +/- 8.3 to 7.5 +/- 4.9 (Masin et al, 2005) Other indications include deep brain stimulation for Parkinson's (Hilker, 2010) .

5. Contraindications

SNM is contraindicated in patients with anatomical bony abnormalities of the sacrum, in which transforaminal access may be difficult or impossible. Patients with mental incapacity or psychiatric illnesses rendering them incapable of operating the device Patients who have undergone an unsuccessful SNS Trial (test stimulation). Others include coagulation disorders and local acute sacrum infection. SNM appears to be safe in the presence of a cardiac pacemaker without cardioversion/ defibrillation technology (Wallace et al, 2007) (Roth, 2010). Some conditions are considered challenging as MRI & pregnancy; however, more details are discussed upcoming in the chapter.

6. Surgical technique

After complete clinical evaluation by history, examination & Urodynamics assessment, all patients need to fill up a voiding diary for minimum of 3 days (baseline), which will assess the number of voids, the voided volumes, the degree of urgency and in patients who experience inefficient voiding or retention, the amount voided versus catheterized volumes per 24 hours and the patient's sense of completeness of evacuation. Associated symptoms such as pelvic pain and bowel symptoms are also assessed. Latter, this diary will be used to assess the patient objective response to the test stimulation trial. Patients are counseled for the option of sacral neuromodulation and procedure risk and benefits are discussed with the patient. The first crucial step in determining if the patient is a good candidate for definite implant is a test stimulation trial. Test stimulation can be either percutaneous nerve evaluation (PNE) also called one- stage implant, or two staged implant in which the first step in two staged implant is the test trial.

6.1 One – Stage implant

Patients will undergo stimulation test trial named percutaneous nerve evaluation (PNE), which will determine if the patient is a candidate for permanent SNM. PNE is done as an outpatient procedure. It involves placement of a thin insulated wire into the third sacral foramen. Usually fluoroscopy is needed to localize the foramen during the PNE insertion. In our center, we perform it without any fluoroscopy, rather than that, we depend on the landmarks & patient sensory and motor response for localization table 1. After describing the procedure for the patient, marking of the boney landmarks are done while patient is in the prone position. The greater sciatic notch is palpated & marked bilaterally. The level of the notch marks the Y axis. The Medline is marked; one fingerbreadth laterally on each side marks the X axis .The meeting point of the Y & X axis resembles the third sacral foramen see figure 1. After cleaning & draping, local anesthesia is used for the skin & subcutaneous tissue. In our center, we use 1% plain Lidocaine, for both sides. Usually 10 cc will be enough but sometimes additional 10cc will be needed in some patients, however, the maximum total injected Lidocaine is 20 cc of 1% to avoid side effects.

> Tips
> *Be sure not to inject local anesthetic into the foramen, which will mask the desired response. To do so, we insert the needle until we hit bone before injecting which helps confirming that we are not passing through the halo of the foramen.
> *If the needle is inserted at the sciatic nerve, it would elect S3 stimulation response, to be sure that the needle is in the canal, use a second foramen needle and insert it just lateral to your target needle. If it hits bone, this confirms that your target needle is in the canal, but if not it means most probable you are not.

The procedure is done bilaterally, and the side giving better response will be chosen for wire insertion .Using the foramen needle, Long foramen needle is usually needed in obese patients, the third sacral canal is cannulated at the marked area. During insertion an angle of 60 degree should be maintained to access the canal. The sacral bone will be felt first; with minimal movement the canal can be cannulated. Then, the patient response is assessed by intermittent stimulation with external pulse generator (EPG). The target response of the thirds sacral foramen includes bellows contraction of the pelvic floor (e.g., rectum, vagina, scrotum and perineum) and planter flexion of the great toe, to some extent. S2 placement will result into planter flexion of the entire foot with lateral rotation, whereas S4 will reveal no lower extremity movement despite bellows response. Once the appropriate side and position is selected, the temporary unipolar lead is inserted through the needle and then connected to an external pulse generator and fixed with tape to the skin. At the end of the procedure the patient is given a voiding diary to fill up while the wire is in to assess her/his response for the stimulation. Patient is given instructions on how to manage the temporary lead during the test period to avoid any inadvertent migration or misuse. After a trial period of 3-5 days the patient will be assessed in the clinic for subjective and or, objective improvement by comparing the pre and post voiding diaries. If the patient developed 50% or more improvement (Subjectively or / and objectively), she/he will be considered as a candidate for permanent SNM implantation & removal of the temporary lead is done in the clinic. A baseline Sacrao-Coxygeal AP-Lateral X-rays are obtained to document lead position. If the patient claimed no benefit we question if they had intact sensation of the vibration at the target area, if not, a sacrao-coxygeal X-rays should be taken to rule out lead migration which is usually the cause of the false negative results. The maximum duration of this test is limited to 14 days to avoid bacterial contamination (Pannek et al, 2005). Antibiotic prophylaxis is not needed.

Limitations of this approach include lead migration, and potential discrepancy in clinical response with the permanent quadripolar lead implantation. Short term test stimulation period as well as lead migration probably explains the relatively low success rate of PNE, estimated at around 50% (Peter et.al, 2003)(Borawaski et.al , 2007).According to Everaert et.al false- positive PNE compose 33% of cases in home patients who have a beneficial test stimulation with a temporary lead do not continue to have a successful outcome after the permanent lead implantation (Everaert et al ,2004) . In our center, we adapted an algorithm to minimize the false negative cases that can gain benefit from SNM but their test trials were negative see figure 2.

Nerve root	Motor response	Sensory response
S2	Anal sphincter contraction (A-P pinching of perineum/ coccyx), leg/heel rotation, planter flexion of foot, calf contraction.	Sensory alteration of the base of penis or vagina.
S3	Bellows (inwards contractions), plantar flexion of great toe.	Rectal sensation, extending into scrotum or labia.
S4	Bellows	Rectal sensation only

Table 1. Sacral roots, motor and sensory response (Bullock and Siegel, 2010).

6.2 Two – Stage implant

If the patient is not a candidate for office-based test stimulation (e.g. obese, difficult anatomy, previous sacral surgery or unable to tolerate the procedure under local anesthesia) or did not respond to the in- office test, test stimulation may be performed in the operating room. Furthermore, the immediate implantation of a permanent lead aims to avoid lead migration and allows prolonged patient screening. (Kessler et.al. 2005)(Kessler et al, 2007). The procedure involves using the quadripolar leads which fix the lead into the foramen & avoid migration.

The test response can be performed using intravenous sedation, local anesthesia or general anesthesia. In case of general anesthesia, the anesthetist is reminded to avoid any long- acting muscle relaxants which may impair sacral nerve stimulation or visualize their motor response. Note that the upper body nerves recover earlier than the sacral nerve, the anesthetist may claim recovery of the muscle relaxant in the absence of sacral response may imply delayed recovery and the surgeon may need to wait more time (about 10 minutes) to have a response. Fluoroscopy C- arm is used to facilitate placement of the quadripolar permanent lead. Once it is inserted into the foramen, using the foramen needle, followed by guide wire & foramen dilator, it is tested by bipolar stimulation(by EPG, PW210, Rate 14, Amplitude 10 volts) in all 4 positions 0,1,2,3, for response. After which, the dilator sheath is withdrawn under fluoroscopic guidance figure 3. Fluoroscopy views are important and taken as baseline pictures to locate the S3 foramen in correlation with the greater sciatic notch and the skin marking which we made. Then during the lead insertion to confirm being in proper position & the last electrode is at the lower surface level of the sacral foramen. Finally, the dilator sheath is removed under continuous fluoroscopy to avoid electrode movement from its proper position ,and the last picture of the position will be considered as a baseline for future patient fellow-up if developed any complications figure 4.The lead is then tunneled deeply through the subcutaneous fat to the right or left buttock depending on the patient dominant hand side where the permanent implantable pulse generator (IPG) will be placed in the second stage if the patient is considered as a candidate. The lead is attached to the temporary connector and then tunneled through the subcutaneous fat to an alternative exit site. This is particularly an important step because if the patient developed superficial skin infection, then the alternative exit site would help prevent the infection from spreading to the lead and future permanent IPG location (Kohli and Patterson, 2009). Finally, the lead is connected to an external pulse generator and taped to the skin surface. A test period of 14 days is used to determine which patient meets the criteria to have the permanent IPG implanted. At the end of the test period the patient returns to the OR for either removal of the lead or implantation of the IPG, depending on the subjective and/ or objective responses, Figure 4D.

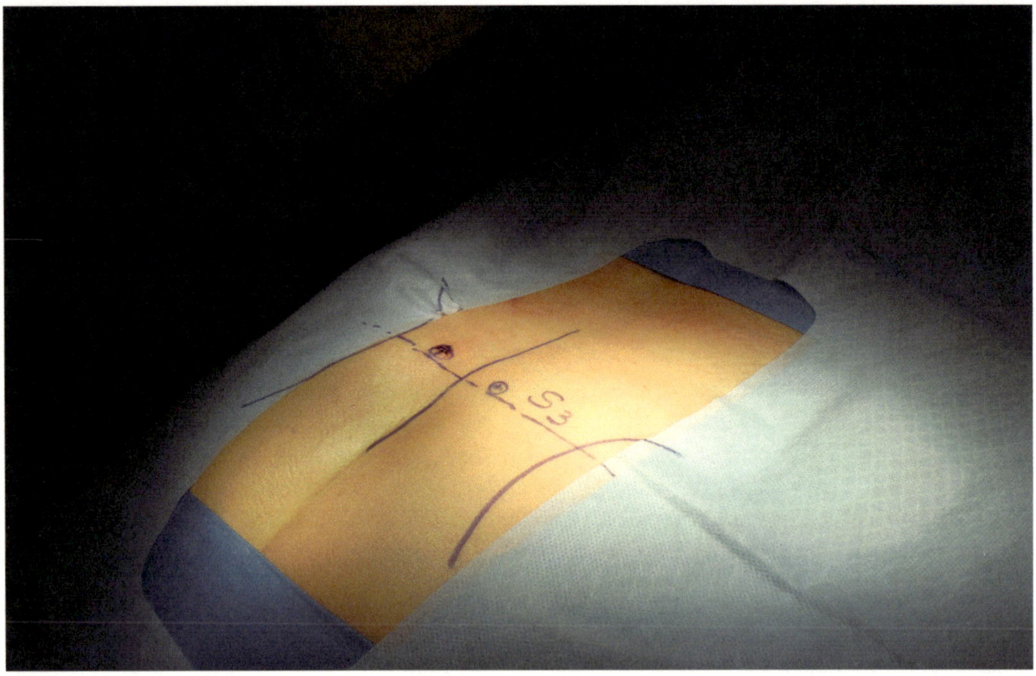

Fig. 1. Landmarks for S3. The curved line on each side resembles the greater sciatic notch which level corresponds for the Y axis, while one fingerbreadth from the marked midline is the X axis. S3 foramen is the joining point between the Y and X axis.

Tips

If no response can be demonstrated by the stimulation check the connection between the hook & the EPG, if it was well connected, check the battery of the EPG which can be expired. If all are working properly most probably the nerves are still under the effect of the muscle relaxant. Ask the anesthetist to reverse the effect of muscle relaxant if feasible & wait for the nerve to recover. Notice that the upper body nerves recover faster than the sacral nerves.

6.2.1 PNE versus staged testing

The PNE is a simple, safe, inexpensive, office- based procedure which is carried out under local anesthesia .A prospective randomized study showed that the two stage implant technique of SNM has a higher success rate compared to the one- stage method despite prior positive PNE in both short & long term (Everaet et al, 2004). Another important study by Borawaski et al reported significant positive results in the two stages procedures who proceeded with IPG implantation more that the PNE group in a randomized study (88% compared to 46%)(Borawaski et al, 2007).Other studies reported that the sensory response assessment at the time of implantation reduced the reoperation rate from 43% to 0% (Peters et al,2003) .The cost for the test protocol with the tined leads (two- stage procedure) are much higher compared to the PNE . Currently, the use of either one of the two screening options is arbitrary. In our center, one –stage procedure is the trend unless the two stage is indicated with difficult PNE (technical, anatomical, not cooperative patient).In our hands, most of the PNE has high success rate in comparison to two- stage procedure see table 2.

6.2.2 Unilateral versus bilateral test stimulation

Unilateral sacral nerve stimulation is the most widely used method of testing for suitability for permanent sacral Neurostimulation implantation. It has been proposed that based on the bilateral innervations of the bladder, bilateral sacral nerve stimulation may improve the efficacy of this therapy. In a prospective randomized crossover trial comparing unilateral with bilateral stimulation using PNE screening, bilateral stimulation appeared to offer no definite advantage over unilateral stimulation. However, 2 of 13 patients voided only with bilateral stimulation and remained in retention with unilateral stimulation (Scheepens et al, 2002).The authors concluded that bilateral test stimulation should be considered when unilateral stimulation fails. Further studies are needed to evaluate the role of bilateral stimulation during test stimulation trials, as well as during post implantation chronic phase.

6.3 Implantation

6.3.1 Position

Buttock placement (figure 4D) of the IPG has an attractive alternative to the subcutaneous implantation in the lower part of the anterior abdominal wall because of shorter operation time, avoidance of repositioning the patient during the operation and lower incidence of complications (Scheepens et al, 2001) .

6.3.2 Technique

After successful test phase, the patient is brought to the OR for implantation of the permanent implantable pulse generator (IPG).If the first test was one stage, fluoroscopy is needed for permanent lead insertion. Broad spectrum preoperative antibiotics as Ampicillin and Gentamicin are given intravenously. (We usually perform 5 minutes scrubbing of the operative field with dilute Povidone-iodine in addition to prepping with chlorhexidine). The quadripolar tined lead is inserted in a similar fashion on the side where the patient had the best PNE test response. The lead is then tunneled in the subcutaneous fat to a pocket formed in the left or right buttock region according to the patient hand dominant site. It is attached to the connector & IPG which will be buried deep in the subcutaneous pocket. On the other hand, if the first phase was two- staged procedure the implantation is done as the 2nd stage, it does not require fluoroscopy, and can be done under local or general anesthesia. The previous incision where the temporary connector was placed in the buttock is opened and the permanent IPG is connected to the lead after removal of the temporary connection system. A pocket is formed & irrigated with antibiotic mixed with sterile water to minimize infection risk. Then, the IPG is buried deep in the subcutaneous tissue in the buttock. Post operatively, the IPG is switched on and programming is done.

> Sterile water is used in irrigation and mixing with antibiotics, avoids electrical circuit formation & IPG erosion.

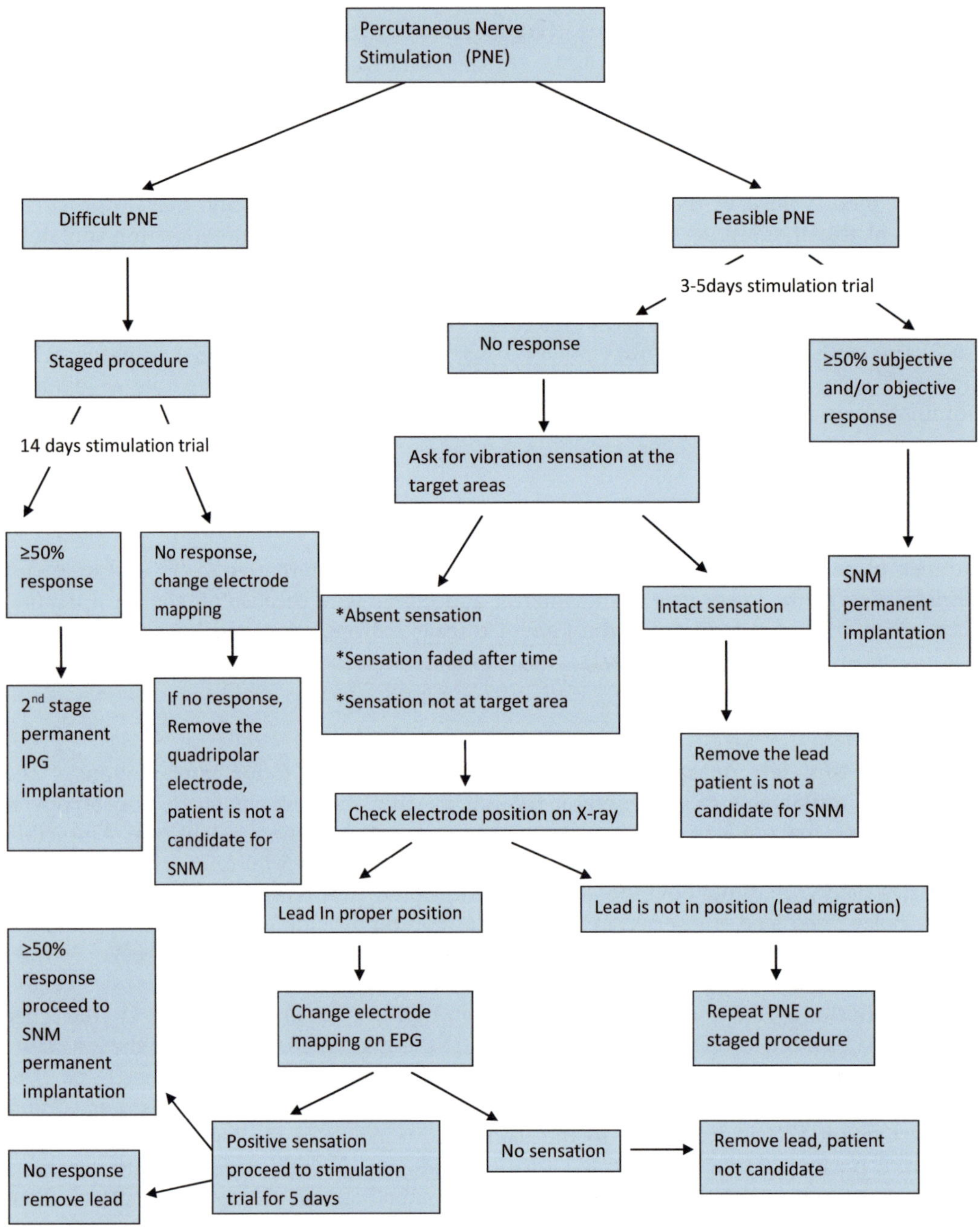

Fig. 2. Algorithm adapted by the Authors to minimize the false negative cases in Stimulation test trial

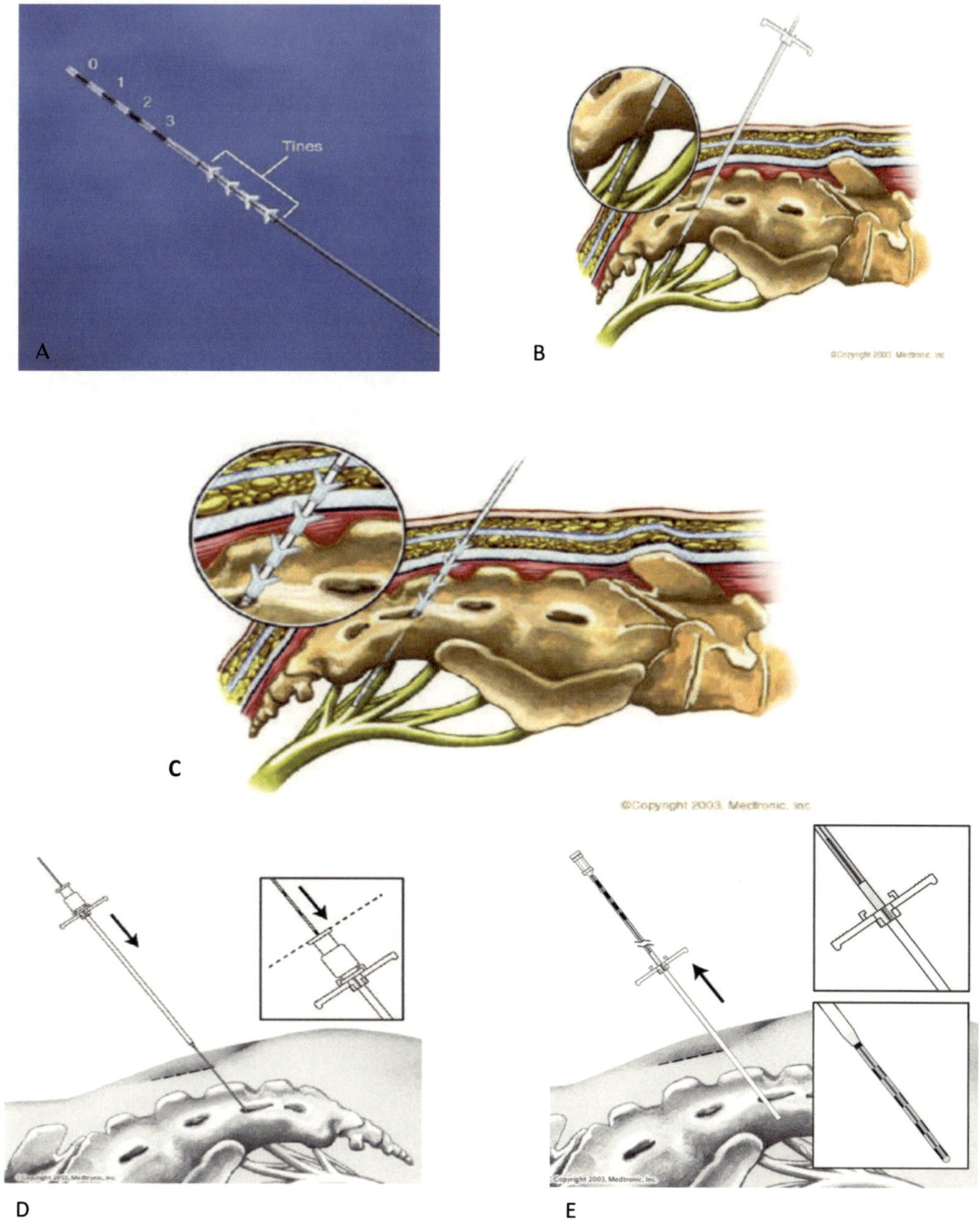

Fig. 3. A: Quadripolar tinned lead , the electrodes are shown, B: Sacral foramen needle is inserted and guided to the desired location, C: Location is verified by electrical stimulation to the needle, and fluoroscopy is used to confirm the position of the needle in the S3 foramen, D: The metal dilator is removed and plastic dilator is positioned, E: The quadripolar lead is introduced through the dilator plastic sheath into position which is confirmed by stimulation, the plastic dilator sheath in withdrawn carefully under fluoroscopic guidance Pictures adapted from Medtronic Inc, 2003.

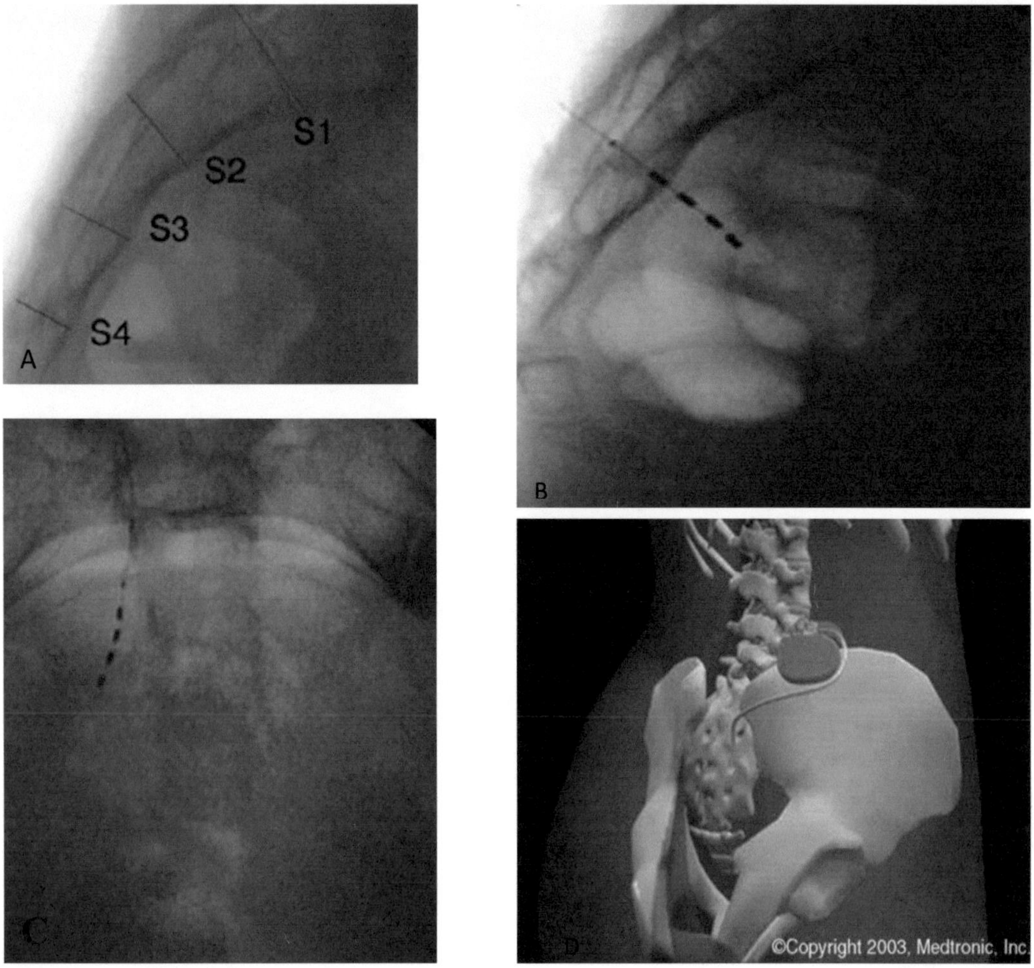

Fig. 4. A: Fluoroscopic view of the sacral foramens, B: Permanent electrode leads position; note that the last electrode is located at the lower surface of the sacral canal, C: A-P view of the electrode position ,D: IPG position. Pictures adapted from Medtronic Inc, 2003.

7. Complications

The Sacral Nerve Stimulation study group has published several reports on the efficacy and safety of the procedure for individual indications. Siegel summarized the reported efficacy and complications in the total patient group who were included in the trials conducted by the neuromodulation study group. The complications where pooled from the different studies because the protocols, devices, efficacy results and safety profiles were identical. Of the 581 patients, 219 underwent implantation of the Interstim system (Medtronic, Minneapolis, Minnesota).

The complications were divided into percutaneous test stimulation-related and post implantation related problems. Of 914 test stimulation procedures done on the 581 patients, 181 adverse events occurred in 166 of these procedures (18.2% of the 914 procedures).Most complications were related to lead migration (108 events, 11.8% of procedures). Technical problems and pain represented 2.6% and 2.1% of the adverse events. For the 219 patients who underwent implantation of the InterStim system (Lead and generator), pain at the neurostimulator site was the most commonly observed adverse effect at 12 months (15.3%) (Siegel et al, 2000) table 3.

Cleveland Clinic reported complication rate in 160 patients who proceeded to permanent IPG implantation from total of 214 lead implants. 17 patients (10.5%) had device completely removed for infection and failure of clinical response.26 patients (16.1%) underwent device revision for attenuated response, infection, IPG site pain and lead migration. The majority of patients with revisions due to poor response had an abnormal impedance measurement. As a result, the author strongly advocate impedance measurement in patient evaluation in patients with response related dysfunction (Hijaz et al, 2006)

PNE (one- stage)	Tined lead (Two -stage)
Advantages: • In-office, under local anesthesia. • Greater patient acceptance(Minimal invasive) • Removal of leads in office , no need for experience • Accurate patient feedback during insertion (no interference from IV sedation) • Less costly, more favorable reimbursement. • Less risk of infection since permanent lead and IPG will be placed in one sitting after successful PNE.	Advantages: • Less risk of lead migration during the test trial. • Greater comfort due to level of sedation for anxious or pain focused patients. • Quadripolar lead configuration allows for more precise placement and programming. • Symptom improvement remains unchanged when converted to chronic implant. • Longer trial period to assess for symptom improvement • Higher rate of true positives.
Disadvantages: • Higher rate of false negatives. Must do staged implant if equivocal. • Potential to place permanent lead in less favorable location, thus requiring re-operation.	Disadvantages: • Requires two surgeries even if trial is unsuccessful • Greater potential for infection due to increased length of trial and potential contamination of permanent lead. • More expensive if trial is unsuccessful

Table 2. Comparison of the advantages and disadvantages of one- stage (PNE) and two - stage implant (with tined lead) (Elizabeth et al 2010)

7.1 Lead migration

Lead migration can be simply resolved by reprogramming, reinforcing the lead or insertion of a new lead contra-laterally (Deng et al, 2006) some patients lose benefit due to accommodation to the stimulation, but contralateral placement can be attempted to overcome this phenomenon (Wagg et al., 2007)

7.2 Infection

When infection is diagnosed, the best management is explantation of the IPG, debridement of the infected tissue & antibiotics. The lead can be left behind but keeping in consideration that the infection may spread through it & if needed, may be removed. The wound is left to heal by secondary intention & the patient is covered with antibiotic for two weeks. Another IPG implantation can be considered after 6-8 weeks if inflammatory signs has resolved.

Complication	**Probability of occurrence (Siegel series)**
Pain at the Neurostimulation site	15.3%
New pain	9%
Suspected lead migration	8.4%
Infection	6.1%
Transient electric shock	5.5%
Pain at lead site	5.4%
Adverse change in bowel function	3.0%
Technical problems	1.7%
Suspected device problems	1.6%
Change in menestral cycle	1.0%
Adverse change in voiding function	0.6%
Persistent skin irritation	0.5%
Suspected nerve injury	0.5%
Device rejection	0.5%

Table 3. Reported complications with sacral neuromodulation therapy from the neuromodulation study group (Siegel et al, 2000)

7.3 Impedance related complications

Impedance describes the resistance to the flow of electrons through a circuit. Impedance or resistance is an integral part of any functioning circuit, but if there is too much resistance, no current will flow (Open). On the other hand, if there is too little resistance, an excessive current flow results in diminished battery longevity (Short). In the InterStim system, the circuit travels from the electrode through the patient tissue to another electrode (Bipolar) or through the patient tissue to the neurostimulator case (IPG) (Unipolar).

Impedance measurement is used as a troubleshooting tool to check the integrity of the system when the patient present with sudden or gradual disappearance of stimulation. Usually the normal measurement falls between 400 and 1500 Ω. High levels (>4000Ω) identify open circuit, usually is caused by fractured lead or extension wires, loose connections. In open circuits, the patient feels no stimulation. In these cases, the programmer which measures the impedance can be used to know which electrode is broken. Managing these cases can be done by reprogramming .The new mapping should avoid the broken electrode. If reprogramming is exhausted in these cases with no benefit, then revision is done. The aim of the revision is to identify the source of the open circuit (the electrode or connection).

On the other hand, low levels (<50Ω) identify short circuits which can be caused by body fluid intrusion into the connectors or crushed wires that are touching each other. Patients may not feel stimulation, or may feel it away from the correct area as the IPG pocket. Again, reprogramming followed by revision are the options in these cases.

7.4 Pocket (IPG site) pain, discomfort

IPG site pain is caused by either pocket -related, or output- related causes, see figure 5. To determine which is the case in the patient; turn the IPG off, if pain or discomfort persist, it means that the patient is having a pocket- related cause. Revision of the IPG and relocation can resolve the problem.

If the pain disappears, that implies an output- related cause. In these cases, check the patient mapping. If the patient is having a monopolar one change it into a bipolar (some patients are sensitive to the unipolar because the positive pole is the IPG). Another possibility is current leak, try reprogramming (Mapping, Pulse width, and rate). If it did not show any benefit, ask the patient if that discomfort is tolerable (burning sensation usually at the pocket and perineum), if not revision is advocated

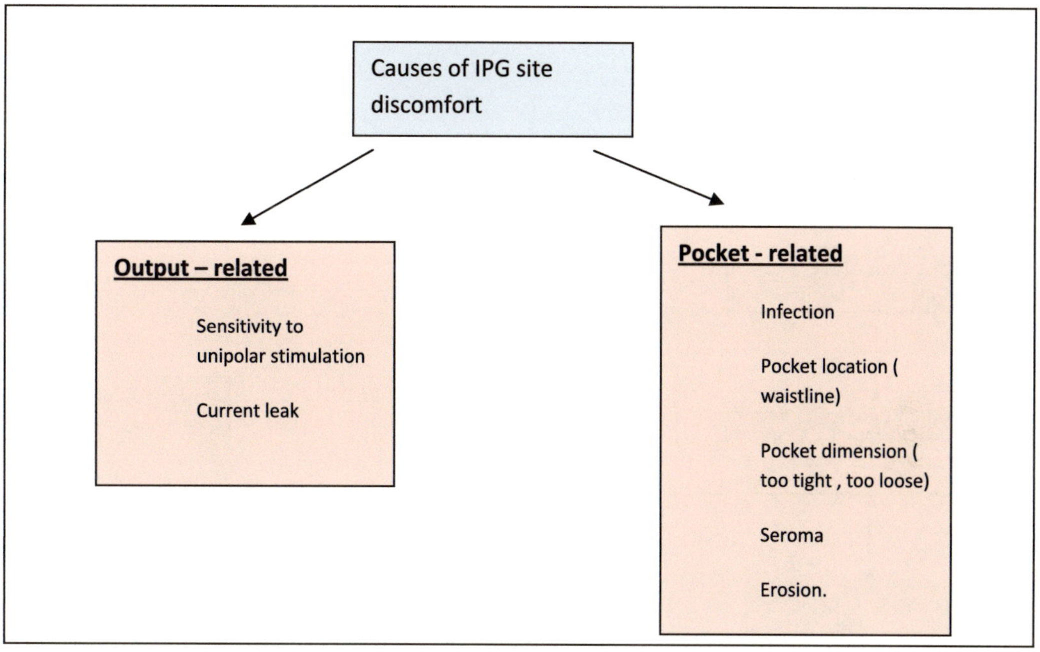

Fig. 5. Causes of IPG site discomfort (Hijaz et al, 2005)

7.5 Recurrent symptoms

When the patient presents with recurrent symptoms, we need to evaluate the impedance, battery, and stimulation perception. The impedance abnormalities were discussed previously. If the battery was low with decreased sensation, this warrants new IPG (battery) exchange (Anecdotally, the battery mean half life we have encountered ranged between 7 to 9 years, depending on the usage). The possibilities are that the patient perceives the stimulation in wrong area compared with the baseline, has no stimulation, or has intermittent stimulation, see management algorithm at figure 6

8. Contraindications for patients with implanted IPG

Contraindications for patients with implanted IPG include short wave diathermy, microwave diathermy or therapeutic ultrasound diathermy (Medtronic professional use manual, 2011). MRI & pregnancy are special conditions at which implanted Neurostimulation is contraindicated

8.1 Diathermy

The diathermy's energy anywhere in the body can be transferred through the implanted system and can cause tissue damage which could result in severe injury or death. Diathermy can also damage parts of the Interstim therapy system. This can result in loss of therapy from the Neurostimulation, and can require additional surgery to remove or place parts of the Interstim therapy system.

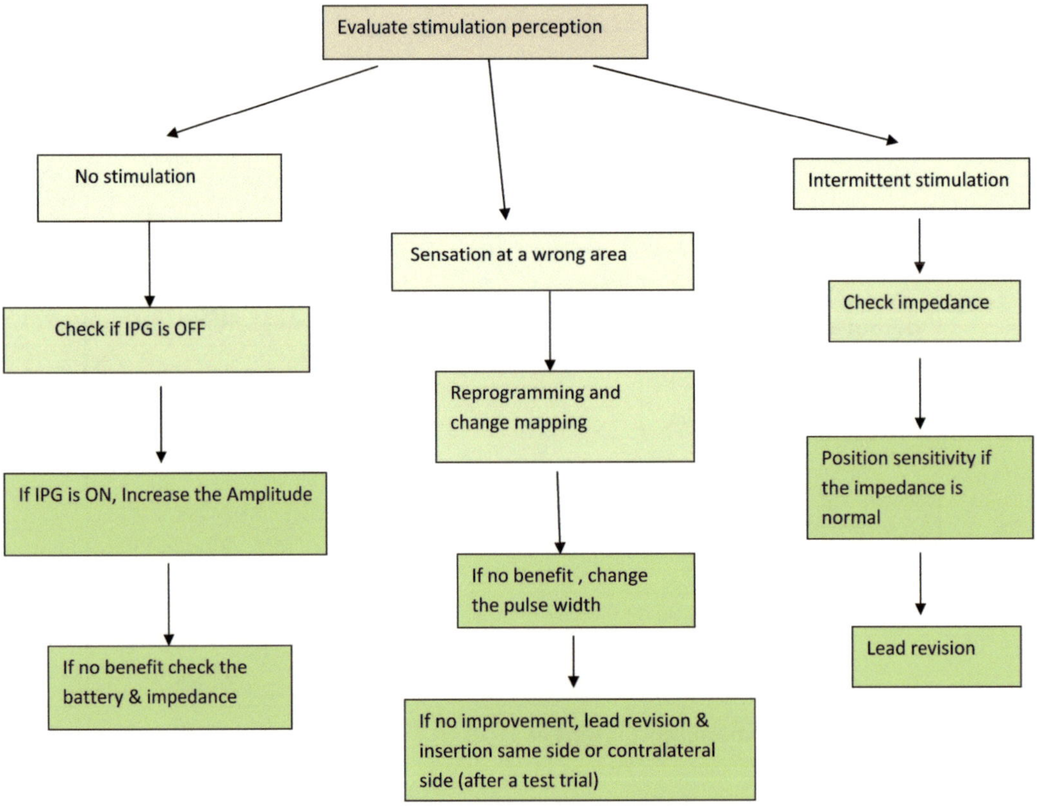

Fig. 6. Management algorithm for different stimulation perception (Hijaz et al, 2005).

8.2 Neuromodulation and MRI

MRI is a safe, non invasive and essential diagnostic tool. Currently the number of patients who have bladder Neurostimulation is growing rapidly. For many reasons, their conditions often need magnetic resonance (MRI) examination. However the current practice is to contraindicate patients with implantable devices (Shellock and Kanal, 1992) (Achenbach et al, 1997).Medtronic product technical manual indicates that exposure to MRI can potentially injure the patient or damage the Neurostimulator (Medtronic professional use manual, 2011). The induced electrical current from the MRI to the Interstim therapy system can cause heating, especially at the lead electrode site, resulting in tissue damage. The induced electrical current can also stimulate or shock the patient. The precaution is applied even if only a lead or an extension is implanted; it does not only apply to the IPG alone. Few factors increase the risk of heating and injury, but are not limited to, as high MRI Specific Absorption Rate (SAR) Radio Frequency (RF) power levels, MRI transmit coil that is near or extends over the implanted lead, implanted leads with small surface area electrodes, and short distance between lead electrodes and tissue that is sensitive to heat (Medtronic professional use manual). An MRI may permanently damage the neurostimulator, requiring to be removed or replaced .It also can reset the neurostimulator to power – on- reset values requiring reprogramming again. The Neurostimulation can move within the implanted pocket and align with the MRI field, resulting in discomfort or reopening of a recent implanted incision. In addition, the image details from MRI may be degraded, destroyed or blocked from view by the implanted Interstim system(Shellock, 2001)(Ordidge et al,2000)(Luechinger et al,2002)(shellock et al,1993). In contrast, many studies conducted on patients who underwent MRI examinations with implantable devices showed no clinical adverse effects (Luechinger et al, 2001) (Martin et al, 2004) (Gimbel et al 1996) (Buendia et al, 2011). Other concerns are associated with heating of the electrodes. Achenbach et al reported that temperature increase occurred at the tip of the pacing electrode (Achenbach et al,1997).However, Rezai et al reported that temperature elevations at the distal end of deep brain stimulation electrode of 25.3C occurred after 15 minute of MRI and noted that the use of clinically relevant positioning techniques for the Neurostimulation system and MRI parameters used for imaging the brain generated little heating (Rezai et al,2002).Furthermore, Martin et al reported in 2004 that they found no evidence that increase in SAR increase the likelihood that the pacemaker lead would heat and cause subsequent threshold changes (Martin et al, 2004). In the case of sacral nerve Neurostimulator, a variety of symptoms could develop if the lead is heated (e.g. urgency with pelvic pain, urinary frequency, incontinence for stool or urine and possible sexual dysfunction in both men and women). Furthermore, Sommer et al have showed a significant decrease in temperature in leads of the pacemaker when the center of the region to be imaged was located 30 cm or farther from the center of the lead loop (Sommer, 2000).

Nevertheless, Elkelini and Hassouna reported six patients with implanted sacral nerve stimulation who underwent eight MRI examinations at 1.0Tesla conducted in areas outside the pelvis (Elkelini and Hassouna, 2006). They examined the IPGs before and after the MRI procedure. All patients had their parameters recorded; then the IPGs were put to "nominal" status. Patients were monitored continuously during and after the procedure. During the MRI session, no patient showed symptoms that required stopping the examination. There was no change in the perception of the stimulation after reprogramming of the implanted sacral nerve stimulator, according to patients; feedback. Devices were functioning properly, and no change in bladder functions was reported after MRI examinations.

8.2.1 Concluding message

A lot of controversial issues arise in MRI safety in Neurostimulation implanted patients. There are no clear safety guidelines established yet. However, if a patient needs MRI it would be preferred to postpone the Neurostimulation implantation till patient is done with it. Patients should be instructed about the potential injury of MRI, and to stop the MRI if they fell any heat at the IPG site. Those who will undergo MRI should have their IPG explanted. If the patient is having the electrode left behind or part of the electrode (ghost effect) it can act as an antenna and result into the heat injury to the nerve, when so the MRI procedure should be stopped.

8.3 Neuromodulation and pregnancy

Sacral nerve stimulation has been increasingly used in females of child bearing age with various voiding dysfunctions. Nevertheless, electrical stimulation has been considered a contraindication in pregnant women. Medtronic product technical manual indicates that safety and effectiveness have not been established for pregnancy, unborn fetus, and delivery (Medtronic professional use manual,2011). Although no firm evidence exists, concerns pertaining to neuromodulation during pregnancy include negative effects on the fetus, conceiving mother, and the InterStim device itself as shown in table 4. Few animal studies have attempted to address this issue. In addition, data on human subjects is scarce and available in the form of case reports and small cases series.

8.3.1 Animal data

Wang and Hassouna were first to examine the effect of electrical stimulation on pregnant rats and fetuses (Wang and Hassouna, 1999). The authors divided 20 Sprague-Dawley pregnant rats into either electrical stimulation group (n = 10) or sham controls (n = 10). Rats in the stimulation group were stimulated 7 hours every day from Day 4 to Day 20 of gestation. Stimulation was done bilaterally at the level of S1, bipolar of 3 volts and frequency 20 Hz. The stimulation was adjusted to 80% of the value that induced a visible tail tremor. All pregnant rats were sacrificed and fetuses were examined at near term (Day 20 of gestation). The results showed that all pregnant rats were healthy during the gestation period and no abortions were observed. There was no significant difference between the stimulation group (2.27 +/- 0.51 gm.) and the sham group (2.13 +/- 0.51 gm.; p = 0.91) in terms of fetal body weight.

Fetus	Conceiving mother	InterStim device
• **Teratogenicity** • **Fetal malformation**	• Abortion • Premature labour • Irritation and ulceration of the stretched skin over the battery (depending on the site of the battery) • Obstetric and anaesthetic care difficulties / complications • Pain at the lead site	• Lead migration • Battery failure • Stretching the lead extender by the expanding abdomen

Table 4. Neuromodulation potential concerns during pregnancy (Wiseman et al, 2002) (Gaynor et al, 2006) (Nartowicz et al 1980),(Smimova et al, 1982) (Bernardini et al ,2010) (Saxena et al, 2009)

No significant difference was seen in the number of resorptions between both groups. All fetuses were alive at the time of caesarean section. No fetal malformation was observed in gross appearance, viscera and skeleton of all rats.

Karsdon at al. carried out an experiment to examine if uterine contractility during parturition can be inhibited with an electrical current (Karsdon et al, 2006). Electrical inhibition of in vitro spontaneously contracting preterm or term gestational rat myometrium tissue and in vivo spontaneously contracting uterus either directly in the rabbit and rat or transvaginally in the rat was studied. There was a decreased rat in vitro myometrial tension by 50%, decreased in vivo rabbit intrauterine pressure by 48%, decreased in vivo rat intrauterine pressure by 80%, and increased birth intervals (latency) by factors of 50 and 20. In addition, all electromyographic activity parameters were reduced significantly. The authors suggested that electrical inhibition may be a novel method to apply tocolysis in the human. These results, of course, argue against the concern premature labour induced by neuromodulation. In the same vein, Fujii et al. found that applying sacral surface electrical stimulation (ssES) treatment markedly decreased the peak power of uterine peristalses in comparison with that measured before ssES on the day of embryo transfer (ET)(Fujii et al,2008). Since the uterus at the time of ET is sensitive to ssES, the investigators speculated that electrical neuromodulation may be an effective method to induce uterine relaxation for ET.

8.3.2 Human data

Published data on human subjects is limited. It involves case reports and series of pregnant women undergoing a form of neuromodulation either for bladder or non-bladder related reasons. Saxena and Eljamel described 1 case report of young woman who had Spinal cord stimulation (SCS) implanted for chronic pain and then became pregnant (Saxena et al, 2009). In this case, the epidural SCS was high in the thoracic region with the epidural lead placed at T6 level. The IPG was implanted in the anterior abdominal wall being secured in a subcutaneous pocket. The patient had normal course of pregnancy and fetus development while the stimulation was on. However, she developed new severe pain at the side of the abdomen at the junction between the epidural lead and the lead extender, which became intolerable in the 25th week of gestation. Eventually, the lead extender wire was surgically cut in the 28th week of gestation under local anaesthesia. The rest of the pregnancy was uneventful. The authors suggested that if the IPG was implanted in a location that was unlikely to be affected by the enlarging gravid abdomen or if the lead extender was long enough, then she would have managed to continue her pregnancy without this mechanical related pain. Bernardini et al. also reported two female patients with complex regional pain syndrome I who were well managed with SCS and then became pregnant (Bernardini et al, 2010). In both cases, the leads were placed through the T12/L1 inter-space and the IPG was placed in the buttock region. In the first patient, the device was kept deactivated prior to pregnancy and maintained off for the entire duration of the pregnancy. The second patient became pregnant on two separate occasions, with active SCS for a portion of the first trimester (8 weeks) of her first pregnancy before turning it off. She went on to deliver a healthy full-term neonate via caesarean section under general anaesthesia. During her second pregnancy, she deactivated the device 5 weeks post conception, however the patient elected to use SCS at 30 weeks' gestation because the pain became intolerable. There were no obstetric or anaesthetic care complications related to the physical presence of the device. Rechargeable SCS systems were not affected when turned off during the duration of the pregnancy in both cases. In addition, intrauterine exposure to SCS was followed out for a minimum of two years and the developing fetuses were developmentally normal. Further reviewing of the literature also found two older case reports of SCS in the cervical spine to manage complex regional pain syndrome with concomitant usage during pregnancy to avoid the utilization of potentially teratogenic painkillers. In the first patient, there was a full term safe vaginal delivery despite the stimulator being switched on throughout pregnancy, labour, and delivery (Segal, 1999). In the second patient, she had SCS in the cervical spine 30 months before the pregnancy and had normal delivery under epidural anesthesia with no effects on the fetus or mother (Hanson and Goodman, 2006). One note regarding these patients is that the IPG was implanted in the subclavicular fossa. In 1988, Nanninga et al. reported the first case of the effect of sacral nerve stimulation for bladder control during pregnancy in a patient with myelodysplasia (Nanning et al, 1988). The patient activated the device to inhibit the bladder and deactivated it to allow voiding. Its use during pregnancy did not seem to have any adverse effect. In another report, a 30-year-old woman diagnosed with interstitial cystitis received a paddle lead (two lamitrode 44 paddles were placed in the sacrum such that they overlay at S2, S3, and S4 roots). The patient became pregnant but never used her stimulator during pregnancy (Feler et al, 2003). When Dasgupta et al. reviewed the long-term results of sacral nerve stimulation in the treatment of women with Fowler's syndrome over a 6-year period at one referral center, they found that there were 20 patients still voiding spontaneously at the time of review (with two having deactivated their stimulator because of pregnancy) (Dasgupta et al, 2004). There was no further elaboration regarding outcomes during or after pregnancy.

Sutherland et al. reviewed their 11 years experience with SNS for the management of refractory voiding dysfunction (Sutherland et al, 2007). Two patients in this cohort became pregnant after successful initiation of SNS therapy. One patient was treated for urgency and frequency 2 years prior to pregnancy. Pregnancy was carefully planned and neuromodulation was gradually decreased until it was deactivated. Nevertheless, her symptoms remained controlled during pregnancy. Following a successful vaginal delivery of a full-term baby, a temporary period of lead reactivation was needed due to postpartum idiopathic urinary retention and pain. Thereafter, the patient was free of symptoms, and remained so without neuromodulation. In the second patient, the same satisfactory efficacy was never obtained following postpartum device reactivation, and the device was eventually explanted. Lead migration during pregnancy and/or vaginal delivery was assumed to be the cause of decreased effectiveness, but this assumption was never confirmed radiographically.

Siegel presented an abstract regarding an internet-based survey of InterStim implanters pertaining to their views and approaches to neuromodulation in pregnant patients (Siegal, 2009). The survey showed that 66% of implanters have implanted a device in a woman younger than 30 years old. In patients that became pregnant, 2/3 decided to deactivate during the first trimester. Thirty-eight percent had patients with active devices during pregnancy, and 19% noted a change in efficacy after delivery. The survey concluded that there is likely little morbidity from having an active neuromodulation during pregnancy, however most implanters choose to deactivate on discovery of pregnancy. Perhaps the largest and most cited case series pertaining to SNS and pregnancy was published by

Wiseman et al. in 2002 (Wiseman et al, 2002). The authors obtained data on 6 women on SNS who then achieved pregnancy. The information was gathered using a standard questionnaire from 4 physicians known to treat patients on sacral neuromodulation. Data on indication for SNS, pregnancy course, the mode of delivery, neonatal health, the timing of implant deactivation and reactivation were all recorded. The results showed that in 1 patient, stimulation was switched off 2 weeks before conception and was never reactivated in the post partum period. In 5 patients the stimulator was deactivated between weeks 3 and 9 of gestation, after which 2 with a history of urinary retention had urinary tract infection, in which one of them also had IPG site pain and developed premature delivery at 34/40 weeks. Normal vaginal delivery was observed is 3 patients, including 1 in whom subsequent implant reactivation did not resolve voiding dysfunction. Elective caesarean section was carried out in the other 3 cases; in which 1 with urinary retention had to have the device switched back on at 19/40 weeks due to difficult catheterization without any complications during pregnancy. All neonates in the series were healthy. Based on their small cohort, the authors suggested few recommendations: 1) the device should be deactivated if a patient on neuromodulation becomes pregnant, 2) reactivation should be considered when deactivation leads to urinary related complications that threaten the pregnancy, 3) elective caesarean section should be discussed with the patient since it is possible for sacral lead damage or displacement to occur during vaginal delivery. Finally, Govaert et al. described a pilot study to assess the influence of SNS on endometrial waves of the non-pregnant uterus by using diagnostic ultrasound to study various aspects of uterine activity (Govaert et al, 2010). Six patients with an implanted SNS for faecal incontinence were included (3 premenopausal and 3 postmenopausal). Ultrasound recordings were performed with the stimulator turned off and in three stimulation frequencies. All premenopausal patients showed some form of endometrial activity when the stimulator was turned off. This activity was maintained when the stimulator was turned on in two patients, but disappeared in one patient. On the other hand, all postmenopausal patients had no endometrial activity with the stimulator turned off. Only one postmenopausal woman showed endometrial activity when the pacemaker was set at a frequency of 21Hz. The investigators concluded that in premenopausal women SNS seems to exhibit no effect or an inhibitory effect rather than an excitatory effect on uterine activity. Nevertheless, they were unable to recommend any guidelines for SNS usage during conception and pregnancy.

8.3.3 Concluding message

Not much is known about the effects of SNS on uterocervical function, pregnancy, and the developing fetus. Few studies on pregnant animals do not suggest any issues, but data on pregnant and non-pregnant women is scarce precluding the issuing of any firm recommendations or guidelines. Therefore, until such clear evidence exists, it is advised to turn off the stimulator during pregnancy or to wait with permanent implantation of the device until after family completion has been achieved.

9. Summary

Sacral neuromodulation offers minimally invasive treatment for voiding dysfunction. Despite many advances in the techniques of neuromodulation, the mechanism of neuromodulation remains undefined. Many technical challenges raised with the widespread use of this new therapy. Special attention is given for pregnant patients. Precautions should be followed to avoid complications in both pregnancy & MRI procedures in sacral neuromodulation patients.

10. References

Abrams P, Blaivas J, Fowler C, et al , The role of neuromodulation in the management of urinary incontinence ,BJU Int (2003) 91(4):355-9. erve

Achenbach S, Moshage W, Diem B, et al ,Effects of magnetic resonance imaging on cardiac pacemakers and electrodes, Am Heart: (1997), 134:467-73

Apostolidis A, Neuromodulation for intractable OAB, Neurourol Urodynami, (2011) Jun:30(5):766- 70.doi:10.1002/nau.21123

P. Abrams, K. E. Andersson, L. Birder et al., *4th International consultation on incontinence. Recomendations of the International Scientific committee: evaluation and treatment of Urinary Incontinence, Pelvic Organ Prolapse and fecal Incontinence, Health Publication Ltd, Paris, France, 4th edition, 2009*

Adonis Hijaz, Sandip Vasavada, *Complications and troubleshooting of sacral neuromodulation Therapy, Urol Clin N Am 32 (2005) 65-69*

Alshaiji Tariq , Banakhar Mai, Hassouna Magdy, Pelvic electrical neuromodulation for the treatment of overactive bladder symptoms, Adv Urol, 2011:2011:757454.Epub 2011 May 14

Al-Zahrani AA, ElZayat EA, Gajewski JB, Long -term outcome and surgical interventions after sacral neuromodulationimplant for lower urinary tract symptoms:14 years experience at 1 center, J Urol 2011 Mar:185 (3):981-6 Epib 2011 Jan 19

Boyce WH, Lathem JE, Hunt LD, research related to the development of an artificial electrical stimulator for the paralayzed human bladder: a review; J Urol 1964; 91:41-51

Banakhar Mai, Gazuani Yahya, Elkelini Mohamed, Al-Shaiji Tariq, Hassouna Magdy, Effect of sacral neuromodulation on female sexual function , abstract AUA 2011 May 14-19.

Bosch J, Groen J. Treatment of refractory urge urinary incontinence with sacral spinal nerve stimulation in multiple sclerosis patients. Lancet, 1996;348 (9029):7:717-9

Bernardini D.J, Pratt S.D, Takoudes T.C.and Simopoulos T.T ,Spinal cord stimulation and the pregnant patient specific considerations for management: Acase series and review of the literature. Neuromodulation,Technology at the neural Interface, 2010:13,270-274

Bullock TL, Siegel SW (2010) Sacral neuromodulation for voiding dysfunction in statskin D (ed) atlas of bladder disease.S pringer, Philadelphia, pp 1- 12

K. M. Borawski, R. T. Foster, G. D. Webster, and C. L. Amundsen,"Predicting implantation with a aneuromodulator using two different test implantation techniques: a prospective randomized study in urge incontinent women ,Neurourology and Urodynamics,2007,Vol 26,no 1, pp 14 -18

Bernardini, D. J., Pratt, S. D., Takoudes, T. C. and Simopoulos, T. T. Spinal Cord Stimulation and the Pregnant Patient-Specific Considerations for Management: A Case Series and Review of the Literature. Neuromodulation: Technology at the Neural Interface, (2010), 13: 270–274

Buendia F, Cano O, Sanchez-Gomez JM,IgualB, Osca J,Sancho-Tello MJ,Olague J,Salvador A, Cardiac magnetic resonance imaging at 1.5 T in patients with cardiac rhythm devices,Europace,2011,Apr 13(4):533-8.Epub2011 Jan11

Caldwell KP, The electrical control of sphincter incompetence ,Lancet1 963,:2:174-5

Chaabane W, Guillotreau J, Castel-Lacanal E, Abu-Anz S, De Boissezon X, Malavaud B, Margue P, Sarramon JP, Rischmann P, Game X: Sacral Neuromodulation for treating neurogenic bladder dysfunction:clinical and urodynamic study, Neuro Urol and Urodyna,2011,apr:30 (4):547-50.dio:10.1002/nau.21009

Comiter C.Sacral neuromodulation for the symptomatic treatment of refractory interstial cystitis: ap prospective study. J Urol 2003:169:1369-73

Dees JE. 1965. Contraction of the urinary bladder produced by electric stimulation : Preliminary report. Invest Urol 2:539-47

Dasgupta R, Wiseman OJ, Kitchen N, Fowler CJ. Long term results of sacral neuromodulation for women with urinary retention. BJU Int. 2004 Aug;94(3):335-7

De Groat WC, Kruse MN, Vizzard MA, et al, Modification of urinary bladder function after neural injury. Neurology, , 1997vol 72:347-64

De Groat WC, Theobald RJ, Reflex activation of sympathetic pathways to vesical smooth muscle and parasympathetic ganglia by electrical stimulation of vesical afferents, J Physiol, 1976:259:223

Elizabeth R., William and Steven W. Siegel" Procedural techniques in sacral nerve modulation , Int Urogynecol J ,2010, 21 suppl2,:s453-s460

Elkelini M S and Hassouna M.M, "Safety of MRI at 1.5 tesla in patients with implanted sacral nerve neurostimulator. European Urology,2006,vol 50,no 2,pp.311-316

Everaert K., Kerckhaert W., Caluwaerts H. et al., "A prospective randomized trial comparing the 1- stage implantation of a pulse generator in patients with pelvic floor dysfunction selected for sacral nerve stimulation, European Urology,2004,vol45,no5,pp.649-654

Everaert K, Devulder J, De Muynck M, et al. The pain cycle implications for the diagnosis and treatment of pelvic pain syndromes. Int Urogynecol J Pelvic Floor dysfunct,2001:12:9-14

Everaert K, Plancke H, Lefevere F, Oosterlinck W. The urodynamic evaluation of neuromodulation in patients with voiding dysfunction.Br J Urol. 1997; 79(5):702-7

Feler CA, Whitworth LA, Fernandez J. Sacral neuromodulation for chronic pain conditions. Anesthesiol Clin North America. 2003 Dec;21(4):785-95.

Fujii O, Murakami T, Murakawa H, Terada Y, Ogura T, Yaegashi N. Uterine relaxation by sacral surface electrical stimulation on the day of embryo transfer. Fertil Steril. 2008 Oct;90(4):1240-2

Gimbel JR, Johnson D, Levine PA, Wilkoff BL. Safe performance of magnetic resonance imaging of five patients with permanent cardiac pacemakers. Pacing Clin Electrophysiol,1996:19:913-9

Giannuzzi J, Recherches physiologiques sur les nerfs moteurs de la vessie. Journal de la physiologie de I'Homme et des animaux 1863, 6: 22-9

Gaynor-Krupnick DM, Dwyer NT, Rittenmeyer H, Kreder KJ. Evaluation and management of malfunctioning sacral neuromodulator. Urology. 2006 Feb;67(2):246-9

Govaert B, Melenhorst J, Link G, Hoogland H, van Gemert W, Baeten C. The effect of sacral nerve stimulation on uterine activity: a pilot study. Colorectal Dis. 2010 May;12(5):448-51.

Ghazwani YQ, Elkelini MS, Hassouna MM, Efficacy of sacral neuromodulation in treatment of bladder pain syndrome: long-term follow-up, Neurourol and Urodynam,2011 may 6.dio 10.1002/nau.21037

Heine JP, Schmidt RA, Tanagho EA,intraspinal sacral root stimulation for controlled micturition. Invest Urol, 1977:15:78-82

Hijaz A., VasavadaS.P, Daneshgari F., Frinjari F., Goldman H. and Rackley R., complications and troubleshooting of two stage sacral neuromodulation therapy: a single institution experience" Urology,2006, vol 68, no.3, pp 533-537

HumphreysM, Smith C, Smith J, et al. Sacral neuromodulation in children: preliminary results in 16 patients (Abstract) ,J Urol, 2004;171 (4)(suppl):56-57

Hassouna M, Siegel S, Nyeholt A, et al. Sacral neuromodulation in the treatment of urgency-frequency symptoms: a multicenter study on efficacy and safety.J Urol 2000:163;1849-54

Hilker R, Functional imaging of deep brain stimulation in idiopathic Parkinson's disease, Nervenarzt, 2010,Oct;81 (10):1204-7

Hanson JL, Goodman EJ. Labor epidural placement in a woman with a cervical spinal cord stimulator. Int J Obstet Anesth 2006;15:246–249.

Kohli N. and Patterson D., "InterStim therapy: a contemporary approach to overactive bladder' Reviews in Obstetrics and Gynecology, 2009,Vol 2, no 1 .pp.18-27

Kessler T.M., Madersbacher H., and Kiss G., "Prolonged sacral neuromodulation testing using permanent leads: a more reliable patient selection method? European Urology,2005 ,Vol.47, no.5,pp.660-665

Kessler T.M. , Buchser E., Meyer S. et al., "Sacral neuromodulation for refractory lower urinary tract dysfunction:results of a nationwide registry is switzerland, European Urology,2007,vol 51, no.5,pp.1357-1363

Knupfer S., Hamann M., Naumann CM, Melchior D, Junemann KP,Therapy- refractory overactive bladder: Alternative treatment approaches, Urologe A, 2011, Jul:50 (7):806-809

Kruse MN, Noto H, Roppolo JR, et al, ,Pontine control of the urinary bladder and external urethral sphincter in the rat,Brain in Res1990:532:182

Kruse MN, de Groat WC.,Spinal pathways mediate coordinated bladder/urethral sphincter activity during reflex micturation in normal and spinal cord injured neonatal rats, Neurosci let1993,152:141

Karsdon J, Garfield RE, Shi SQ, Maner W, Saade G. Electrical inhibition of preterm birth: inhibition of uterine contractility in the rabbit and pup births in the rat. Am J Obstet Gynecol. 2005 Dec;193(6):1986-93. Erratum in: Am J Obstet Gynecol. 2006 Feb;194(2):595.

Luechinger R, Duru F, Scheidegger MB, et al. Force and torque effects of a 1.5 telsa MRI scanner on cardiac pacemakers and ICDs. Pacing Clin Electrophysiol 2002:24:2

Luechinger R, Duru F, Zeijlemaker VA, et al. Pacemaker reed switched behavior in 0.5, 1.5 and 3 Tesla magnetic resonance imaging units: are reed switched always closed in strong magnetic fields? Pacing Clin Electrophysiol 2002:25:10

Lukban J, Whitmore K, Sant G. Current management o finterstitial cystitis: Urol Clin North Am, 2002: 29:649-60

Lombardi G, Mondaini N, Macchiarella A., Cilotti A, Del Popolo G: Clinical female sexual outcome after neuromodulation implanted for lower urinary tract symptom (LUTS), J Sex Med, 2008, Jun:5 (6):1411-7.Epub 2008 Mar 26

Lombardi G, Mondaini N, Giubilei G, Macchiarella A, Lecconi F, Del popolo G, Sacral neuromodulation for lower urinary tract dysfunction and impact on erectile function, J Sex Med, 2008 Sep;5(9):2135-40.Epub 2008 Jul 15

Lombardi G, Del Popolo G, Clinical outcome of sacral neuromodulation in incomplete spinal cord injured patients suffering from neurogenic lower urinary tract symptoms, Spinal cord,2009.Jun:47(6):486-91.Epub 2009 Feb 24

Madersbacher H .Konservative Therapie der neurogenen Blasendysfunktion, Urologe A 1999.:38:24-9

Magis D, Schoenen J., treatment of migraine: update on new therapies, Curr Opin Neurol, 2011 Jun:24 (3):203-10

Martin ET, Coman JA, Shellock FG, et al. Magnetic resonance imaging and cardiac pacemaker safety at 1.5 telsa, J Am Coll Cardiol 2004:43:7

Masin A, Ratto C, Ganio E, et al. Effect of sacral nerve modulation in chronic constipation. Ital J Public Health 2005;2:30

Melenhorst J, Koch SM, Uludag O, van Gemert WG, Baeten CG ,Sacral neuromodulation in patients with faecal incontinence: results of the first 100 permanent implantations. Colorectal (2007) Dis 9:725–730

Nashold BS JR, Friedman H, Boyarsky S.: electrical activation of micturition by spinal cord stimulation J Surg Res,1971; 11:144-7

Nartowicz, E., Burduk, P., Skowron, A., et al.: Pacemaker implantation in a pregnant woman. Pol. Tyg. Lek. 1980. 35: 541,

Nanninga JB, Einhorn C, Deppe F. The effect of sacral nerve stimulation for bladder control during pregnancy: a case report. J Urol. 1988 Jan;139(1):121-2.

Ordidge RJ, Shellock FG, Kanal E. A Y2000 update of current safety issues related to MRI. J Magn Reson Imaging 2000:12:1

Pauls RN, Marinkovic SP ,Silva WA, Rooney CM, Kleeman SD, Karram MM, Effects of sacral neuromodulation on female sexual function Int Urogynecol J Pelvic Floor Dysfunction 2007 Apr,18 (4):391-5.Epub 2006 Jul 26

Pascual l, Gonzalez, Gomez CC, Ortega R, Jimenez Toscano M, Marijuan JL, Lomas Espadas M, Fernandez Cebrian JM, Garcia Olmo, Pascual Montero JA, Sacral nerve stimulation for fecal incontevevce, Rev Esp Enferm Dig, 2011 Jul, 103(7):355-359

Product technical manual. http://professional.medtronic.com/therapies/sacral-nerve-stimulation-interstim therapy/indications safety-and-warnings/index.htm

Peters K.M , Carey J.M., and KonstandtD.B. , "Sacral neuromodulation for the treatment of refractory interstitial cystitis:outcomes based on technique"international Urogynecology Journal andpelvic Floor Dysfunction,2003, vol.14, no.4, pp.223-228

Peters K. Sacral neuromodulation decreases narcotic requirement in refractory interstitial cystitis, BJU Int, 2004:93 (6):777-9

J. Pannek, U. Grigoleit, and A. Hinkel, "Bacterial contamination of test stimulation leads during percutaneous nerve stimulation' Urology, 2005,Vol,65, no6,pp.1096-1098

Rezai AR, Finelli D, Nyenhuis JA, et al. Neurostimulation systems for deep brain stimulation: in vitro evaluation of magnetic resonance imaging-related heating at 1.5 Tesla, J Magn Reson Imaging 2002:15:241-5-

Roth TM, Sacral neuromodulation and cardiac pacemakers, Int Urogynecol J Pelvic Floor Dysfunct, 2010, Aug:21 (8):1035-7. Epub 2010 Jan 30

Schmidt RA, Bruschini H,Tanagho EA, Urinary bladder and sphincter responses to stimulation of dorsal and ventral sacral roots. Invest Urol,1979,,16:300-4

Saxena, A. and Eljamel, M. S. ,Spinal Cord Stimulation in the First Two Trimesters of Pregnancy: Case Report and Review of the Literature. Neuromodulation: Technology at the Neural Interface, (2009), 12: 281–283.

Scheepens W.A., Weil E.H.J., Van Koeveringe G.A. et al, Buttock placement of the implantable pulse generator: a new implantation technique for sacral neuromodulation a multicenter study, European Urology, 2001, vol.40,no.4, pp.434-438

Schmidt R , Application of Neurostimulation in Urology, Neurourol Urodyn1988 :7:585-92

Schmidit RA,Treatment of pelvic pain with neuroprosthesis, J Urol Abstract .1988,458:139:277A

Shaker HS, Hassouna M, sacral root neuromodulation in idiopathic nonobstructive chronic urinary retention J Urol 1998,:159:1476-8

Segal R. Spinal cord stimulation, conception, pregnancy, and labor: case study in a complex regional pain syndrome patient. Neuromodulation 1999; 1: 41–45.

Signorello D., Seitz CC, Berner L, Trenti E, Martini T, Galantini A, Lusuardi L,Lodde M., Pycha A,Impact of sacrl neuromodulation on female sexual function and his correlation with clinical outcome and quality of life indexes: a monocentric experience, J Sex Med, 2011, apr 8(4) :1147-55.dio:10.1111/j.1743-6109.2010.02189.x.Epub 2011 Jan 26

Shellock FG, Kanal E. SMRI Report: policies, guidelines and recomandations for MR imaging safety and patientsmanagement J Magn Reson Imaging 1992:2:247-8

Shellock FG, Morisoli S, Kanal E. MR procedures and Biomedical implants material and devices 1993: update. Radiology 1993: 189:587-99

Shellock FG. Pocket guide to metallic implants and MR procedures: update 2001. New York: Lippincott-Raven Healthcare.

Siegel SW, Catanzaro F, Dijkema H, et al. Longterm results of multicenter study on sacral nerve stimulation for treatment of urinary urge incontinence, urgency- frequency and retention. Urology, 2000:4(56 Suppl,1):87-91

Siegel S, Paszkiewicz E, Kirkpatrick C, et al. Sacral nerve stimulation in patients with chronic intractable pelvic pain.J Urol 2001:166(5):1742-5

Steven Siegal, SUFU 2009 - Use and Management of InterStim&#174 Sacral Neuromodulation in Pregnant Patients: A Survey of Active Implanters - Session Highlights. *Urodynamics & Female Urology (SUFU) 2009 Winter Meeting, February 25 - 28, 2009 - Las Vegas, NV, USA*. SUFU 2009 - Use and Management of InterStim®

Sacral Neuromodulation in Pregnant Patients: A Survey of Active Implanters - Session Highlights.

Sutherland SE, Lavers A, Carlson A, Holtz C, Kesha J, Siegel SW. Sacral nerve stimulation for voiding dysfunction: One institution's 11-year experience. Neurourol Urodyn. 2007;26(1):19-28; discussion 36.

Scheepens WA, de Bie RA, Weil E, et al.: Unilateral versus bilateral sacral neuromodulationin patients with chronic voiding dysfunction ,J Urol 2002,168:2046-2050

Smimova, L. M., Glukhova, P. A., Pavlova, S. S., et al.: Pregnancy and labour in patients with electric cardiac pacemaker. Akush. Ginekol. (Mosk) 1982. 5: 31,

Saxena, A. and Eljamel, M. S. , Spinal Cord Stimulation in the First Two Trimesters of Pregnancy: Case Report and Review of the Literature. Neuromodulation: Technology at the Neural Interface, 2009, 12: 281–283.

Thon WF, Baskin LS, Jonas U, et al, Surgical principles of sacral foramen electrode implantation, World J Urol,1991:9:133

Tanagho EA, Schmidit RA, Bladder pacemaker:scientific basis and clinical future. Urology1982:20:614-9

Tanagho EA, Neural stimulation for bladder control, semin Neurol1988 :8:170-3

Tanagho EA, Electrical stimulation.J Am Geriatr Soc, 1990, 38:352-5

Tanagho EA,Neuromodulation in the management of voiding dysfunction in children,J Urol1992 :14802 pt2):655-7

Torsten Sommer, Vahlhaus C, Lauck G, et al. MR imaging and cardiac pacemaker: in vitro evaluation and in vivo studies in 51 patients at 0.5 T1 Radiology, 2000:215;869-79

Vadusek DB, Light JK, Liddy JM, Detrusor inhibition induced by stimulation of pudendal nerve afferents, Neurourol urodyn1986,:5:381

Vastenholt JM, Snoek GJ, Buschman HP, et al.A 7 year follow- up of sacral anterior root stimulation for bladder control in patients with spinal cord injury: Quality of life and users experiences, Spinal cord @003:41;397-402

Van Kleef M, Staats P, Mekhail N, Huygen F, Chronic refractory Angina Pectoris, Pain Pract, 2011, Mar 16 . doi: 10.1111/j.1533-2500.2010.00444.x.

Van Wunnik BP, Baeten CG, Southwell BR, Neuromodulation for constipation: sacral and transcutaneous stimulation, Best pract res Clin Gastroenterol, 2011 Feb;25(1):181-91.

Wang Y, Hassouna MM. Electrical stimulation has no adverse effect on pregnant rats and fetuses. J Urol. 1999 Nov;162(5):1785-7

Wiseman OJ, v d Hombergh U, Koldewijn EL, Spinelli M, Siegel SW, Fowler CJ. Sacral neuromodulation and pregnancy. J Urol. 2002 Jan;167(1):165-8.).

Wagg A., Majumdar A., Toozs-Hobson P., Patel A. K. , Chapple C. R., and Hill S., Current and future trends in the management of overactive bladder, International urogynecology Journal and pelvic Floor Dysfunction 2007, vol.18,.no.1,pp.81-94

Wallace PA, Lane FL, Noblett KL, Sacral Nerve veuromodulation in patients with cardiac pacemakers, Am J Obstet Gynecol, 2007, Jul,197 (1):94.e 1-3

Wendy W.Leg, Michael B. Chancellor, How Sacral Nerve stimulation Works,Urol Clin N Am, 2005, 32:11-18

Wosnitzer MS, Walsh R, Rutman MP, The use of sacral neuromodulation for the treatment of non-obstructive urinary retention secondary to Guillain- Barre syndrome, Int Urogynecol J Pelvic floor Dysfunction, 2009, Sep:20(9);1145-7.Epub2009 Mar 11.

4

Prelemniscal Radiations Neuromodulation in Parkinson Disease´s Treatment

José D. Carrillo-Ruiz[1,2], Francisco Velasco[1], Fiacro Jiménez[1], Ana Luisa Velasco[1], Guillermo Castro[1], Julián Soto[1] and Victor Salcido[1]
[1]Unidad de Neurocirugía Funcional, Estereotaxia y Radiocirugía, Hospital General de México
[2]Departamento de Neurociencias de la Universidad Anáhuac México Norte México

1. Introduction

The early experience, in 80´s, of the use of electrical stimulation in thalamus (Vim and Voa/Vop nucleus) and Globus pallidus internus (GPi) to treat Parkinson´s disease (PD) promoted the well known performance in subthalamic nucleus (STN) neuromodulation. More recently, in 2000´s, the reutilization of old targets (utilized in lesions procedures) like Prelemniscal radiations (Raprl) and motor cortex, and new targets like Pedunculopontine nucleus (PPN) and Zona Incerta (Zi) complemented the tools to treat PD. The use of neuromodulation in thalamus, Gpi and STN in the treatment of Parkinson disease are spread around the world and strongly reinforced the electricity´s utilization in different brain nuclei, not only for clinical aspects but also in physiopathological basic research. By otherwise, the emergent targets need to demonstrate they use and effectiveness like a tool in the treatment of the illness.

This chapter is focused in the study of Raprl neuromodulation to ameliorate the symptoms and signs of PD, analyzing the anatomical and physiological background in this area (Carrillo-Ruiz et al, 2007; Ito, 1975; Velasco F et al, 1972, 2009). Trough this article is demonstrated that exists clear evidence that Raprl is a good surgical point to treat PD patients.

2. Anatomy

Subthalamic area is part of diencephalum. It is constructed like a pyramid with base in the bottom and has an upper trunked-vertex. This space is formed by nucleus and fibers in a small compact volume of few cubic milimeters. Nuclei are divided in two: 1) Subthalamic area nuclei that included STN, Zi and sustantia Q of Sano. 2) Extended nuclei from mesencephalum, that corresponded to Sustantia Nigra (SN) and Red Nucleus (RN or Ru). In the other side, fibers could be considered more complex and numerous. If it named from anterior to posterior, it could be described as follows: ansa lenticularis, Forel´s Fields (H, H1 and H2), Raprl, perirubral fibers, rubrothalamic fibers, among others (Velasco F, 2009).

2.1 Nuclei

The nuclei extend from the midbrain area to midbrain diencephalon and involved SN and RN.

2.1.1 Substantia nigra

The substantia nigra is a great motor nucleus located between the tegmentum and the bases of the stem along the midbrain, extending into the subthalamic region of the diencephalon. The core is formed for medium-sized multipolar neurons. It is divided into two parts: one part compacta (SNc) and reticular portion (SNr). The portion is containing cytoplasmic inclusions in compact form of granules of melanin pigment, which is an area rich in dopamine, being more abundant in primates and especially in man. The granules are sparse at birth but rapidly increase in childhood and more slowly in the rest of life. In the reticular portion, the cells are not pigments but contain large amounts of iron demonstrable by histochemistry. Neurons in the pars reticulata are crossed by axons of neurons in the pars compacta. Afferents originate from the axons of caudate and lenticular found in the telencephalon and fewer of the subthalamic nucleus and midbrain raphe nuclei and the pontine reticular formation. The efferent fibers that originate in cells of the compact area go mainly to the caudate nucleus and putamen and some end up in the amygdala temporal lobe. The cells of the reticular portion are projecting into neostriatum, the ventral anterior nucleus and ventral lateral thalamus and superior colliculus.

2.1.2 Red nucleus

Ru is an important component of tegmental motor area. This nucleus has an ovoid shape (round is cross-shaped), extending from the caudal boundary of the superior colliculus to the subthalamic region of the diencephalon. The nucleus has a pinkish color in fresh specimens having a greater blood supply than the surrounding tissue. The core looks red dotted cuts with Weigert and Weil method, due to the myelinated fibers of the same. The red nucleus is divided into two regions: the caudal region that is phylogenetically the oldest, and consists of large cells and is known as magnocellular portion. The rostral is more recent and is especially developed in humans, is formed of small cells, so called parvicelular portion. As afferents can say that those in the cerebellum and cerebral cortex have been the best studied. The fibers that originate in the cerebellar nuclei (mainly the dentate nucleus) form the superior cerebellar peduncles and enter the midbrain. Some fibers end in the Ru and others around him on his way to thalamic nuclei (ventral lateral nucleus) and from this point toward the motor areas of the frontal lobe. These same areas give rise to numerous afferent fibers and there cortico-rubral pathways through the superior colliculus to the red nucleus. Efferent connections of the red nucleus are rubrospinal tract fibers that cross the median plane in the ventral tegmental decussation (Forel) and continue in the brainstem and the lateral funiculus of the spinal cord. Some fibers terminate in the facial motor nucleus and lateral reticular nucleus projecting to the cerebellum, some fibers end in the inferior olivary nuclei. There are also some other fibers involved like emboliform and globose nuclei of the cerebellum.

The other two nuclei are described in the next lines:

2.1.3 The subthalamic nucleus or body of Luys

STN or Sth is pink, is located at the junction of the cap of the midbrain and hypothalamus, below the thalamus. The upper and lower faces are convex. The outer edge is in contact with the internal capsule, and its rear end is above the locus niger, the upper surface is separated from the underside of the thalamus in the Zi and lenticular fasciculus. There are two types of neurons: a smaller than 10 µ and larger ones occupying the outside.

The Sth or STN is one of the motor nuclei and is best developed in advanced mammals. The connections of the subthalamic nucleus are reciprocal to the Gpi, these fibers are the subthalamic fasciculus that cuts through the internal capsule. The subthalamic nucleus also receives some pedunculopontine nucleus afferents and sends some to the SNr efferent pathways (Figure 1).

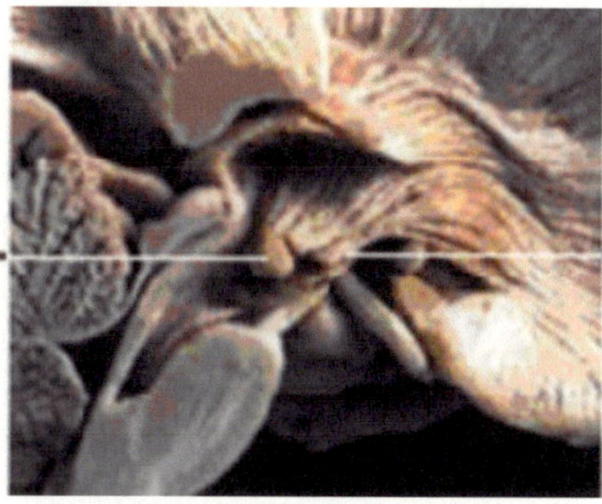

Fig. 1. Red nucleus and subthalamic nucleus. The position of the red nucleus is posterior to the back of subthalamus, however, the subthalamic nucleus is anterior. (Modified from England & Wakely, 1992).

2.1.4 Zona incerta

Zona incerta (Zi) was first described by Forel. It is a core derived from ventral thalamus, is a different heterogeneous nucleus that remains in the base of the thalamus. It is a very thin core of serpentine shape, starting from the base of the SN to the dorsal region of the diencephalon and ends in the posterior nuclei of the hypothalamus. It is located immediately above the STN, between the fiber bundles in the Forel´s fields and Raprl. The Zi is divided into four sectors: rostral, dorsal, ventral and caudal. The rostral component extends over the dorsal and medial STN, while it caudal or motor remains posterior to the STN. The Zi receives afferent exit points of the basal ganglia, which is the globus pallidus and substantia nigra pars reticulata, the ascending reticular activating system and motor areas, associative and limbic cortex. In contrast, the Zi sends efferent ways to the parafascicular and centromedian nucleus of the thalamus, ventral anterior nucleus, ventral lateral nuclei of the thalamus, midbrain extrapyramidal area, output nuclei of the basal ganglia and the cerebral cortex. Different sections have different functions Zi: rostral sector has been attributed to visceral control, dorsal sector in the wake, ventral area is under the guidance of the eye and head movements, and the posterior sector in the generation of axial flow and proximal members, including locomotion (Plaha, 2006).

2.1.5 Substance Q of Sano

Substance Q of Sano was described by the Japanese neurosurgeon Pr. Keiji Sano. It is located below the Zi and also immediately adjacent to the SN. Its function is not well elucidated; it may be part of the reticular formation.

2.2 Fibers

The efferent fibers of the globus pallidus are contained in two tiny beams, different between them, the lenticular fasciculus and the lenticular loop. The lenticular fasciculus consists of fibers that cross the internal capsule to reach the subthalamus, where they form a band of white substance known as H2 Forel´s field. Most of the constituent fibers change direction in the area prerrubral or H (Haube= cap in german) Forel´s field, and penetrate the thalamic fasciculus or H1 Forel´s field, ending in the ventral lateral nucleus and ventral anterior thalamus. At a higher level, the handle forms a lenticular sharp curve around the medial border of the internal capsule and ends in the nuclei ventral lateral and ventral anterior thalamus. Only some fibers of the globus pallidus veer caudally and terminate in the pedunculopontine nucleus, which is one of the lateral group nuclei of the reticular formation located between the union between midbrain and pons. Mesencephalic reticular formation continues in the subthalamus where Zi appears between the lenticular and thalamic fascicles.

The subthalamus contains sensory tracts, extensions rostral midbrain nuclei (Ru and SN), and fibers´ bundles of the dentate nucleus of the cerebellum and globus pallidus, and STN. The sensory tracts are half lemniscus tract, and spinothalamic tracts that are extended immediately below the ventral intermediate nucleus, where the fibers ending.

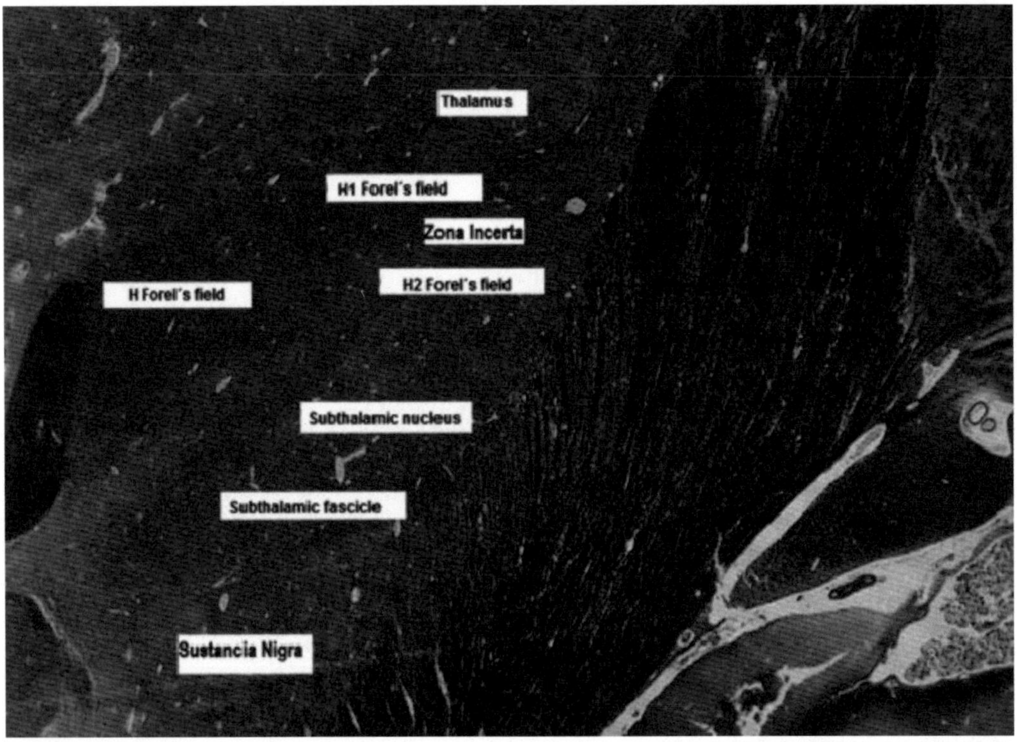

Fig. 2. Subthalamic area includes nuclei and fibers. It shows the nuclei of the basal ganglia: substantia nigra, subthalamic nucleus, the motor thalamus and Zona Incerta. Among them, the respective fibers: subthalamic fascicles; H, H1 and H2 of Forel´s fields. The cut is rostral, therefore the Ru or the Raprl are not seen (modified from England & Wakely, 1992).

Dentothalamic fibers that cross the median plane through the decussation of superior cerebellar peduncles surround and traverse the Ru and continue forward in the H Forel´s field or prerrubral area. The fibers help to form dentothalamic tracts and terminate in the thalamic nucleus ventral oral posterior (Vop) of the ventral lateral nucleus of the thalamus.

2.2.1 Prelemniscal radiations

Among the midbrain and diencephalon are found towards the back of subthalamus in the mesencephalic tegmentum (Figure 3), an area of white matter containing a bundle of fibers located and arranged so oblique and ventrolateral well the half lemniscus (Lm), this set of fibers are the most posterior and superior to the Zi and for being right in front of Lm are called prelemniscal Radiations or in latin Radiatio Praelemniscalis (Raprl).

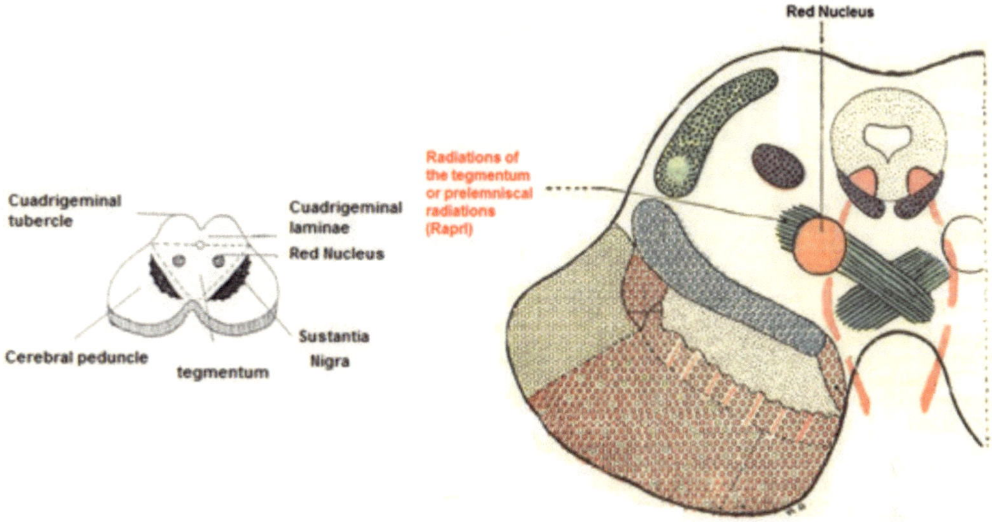

Fig. 3. Mesencephalic tegmentum. On the left, the tegmentum is located between the cerebral peduncles in front, and an imaginary horizontal line that crosses the aqueduct, forming a triangle. On the right side, we see the red nucleus and radiation from the tegmentum, which are Raprl (Modified from Testut, 1948).

Forel described in 1877, the position of Raprl. Originally he called them like BA Th, and clearly distinguishing them from his H fields (more medial and anterior), and they shown in the diagram below in Figure 4. The original name was aported by Cécile Vogt-Mugnier, in 1909, to refer to Raprl as radiation from the cerebellum in front of the lemniscus (prelemniscal) and Hassler, as her pupil in 1959, included it in the description of his stereotactic atlas. Also, in 1960, Talaraich included Raprl in his atlas.

2.2.1.1 Raprl definition

When it considered exclusively Raprl like a target structure, this could be understand like a compact group of fibers located in the white posterior subthalamic area, in front of the sensory lemniscus, that brings its own name. But in this moment, the real origin remains uncertain. Nevertheless, anatomic studies demonstrated that probably they come from three different sites: 1) Axons growth from the cerebellar nuclei to the thalamus 2) Fibers crossing from pallidum to motor thalamus, and 3) Neurons projecting from reticular formation nuclei in ascendant pathway The whole fibers run obliquely from the posteroinferior to anterosuperior way forming a funnel, beginning in mesencephalic reticular nuclei passing through Substantia nigra to the thalamus (Vim and Voa/Vop) and ascending between Ru and STN and Zi. (Modified from Testut, 1947). See figure 1.

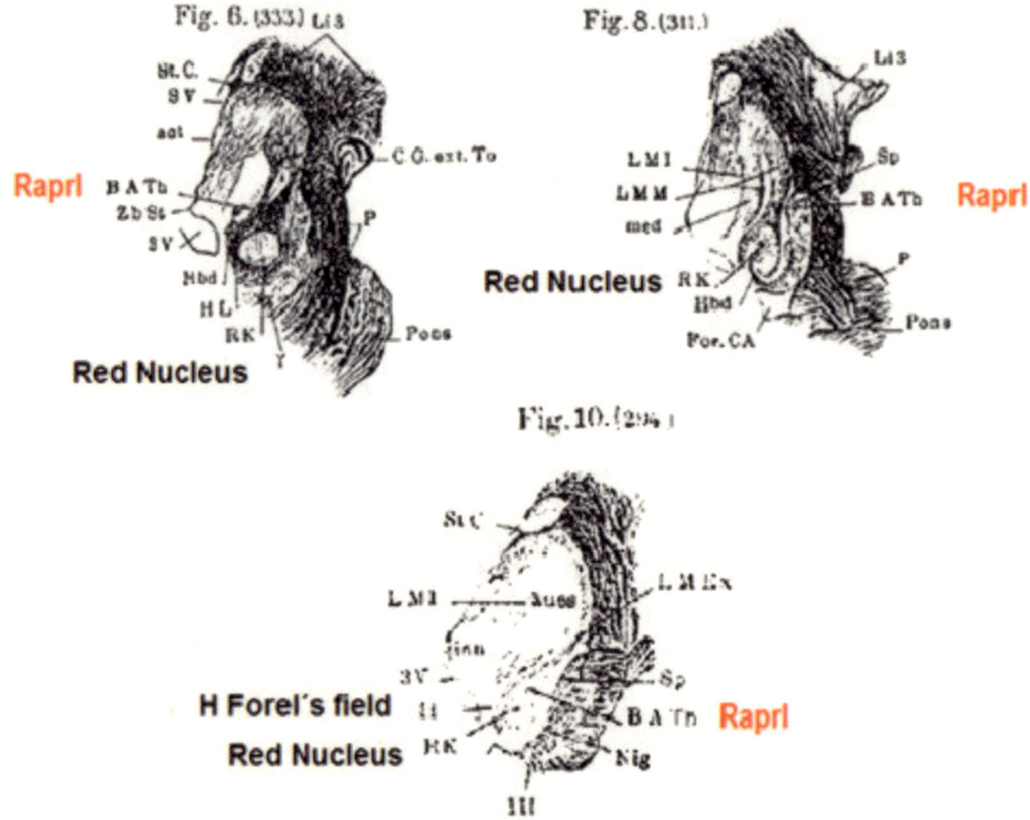

Fig. 4. Forel's original description of the subthalamic region. Coronal cut with some obliquity. In Fig. 6 (333), fig 8 (311) and fig. 10 (294), are located at Raprl as Bath, RK: Red Nucleus. In the last figure, perfectly distinguishes H Forel´s field of Raprl (Forel, 1877).

1. Projections of the basal ganglia. Globus pallidus are connected to the motor thalamus, by the lenticular bundle and Forel´s fields (H, H1 and H2), also interfacing with other structures such as the STN and Zi. Importantly, the fields are above and rostral to Raprl, and there is no absolute division between them: mainly with the fields H1 and H in medial face, making their way to the thalamus are intertwined. In addition there are fibers connecting the STN and SN by subthalamic fasciculus, which also passes through this area. Ru nuclei have reciprocal connections with STN, which also are compacted here. See figure 7.

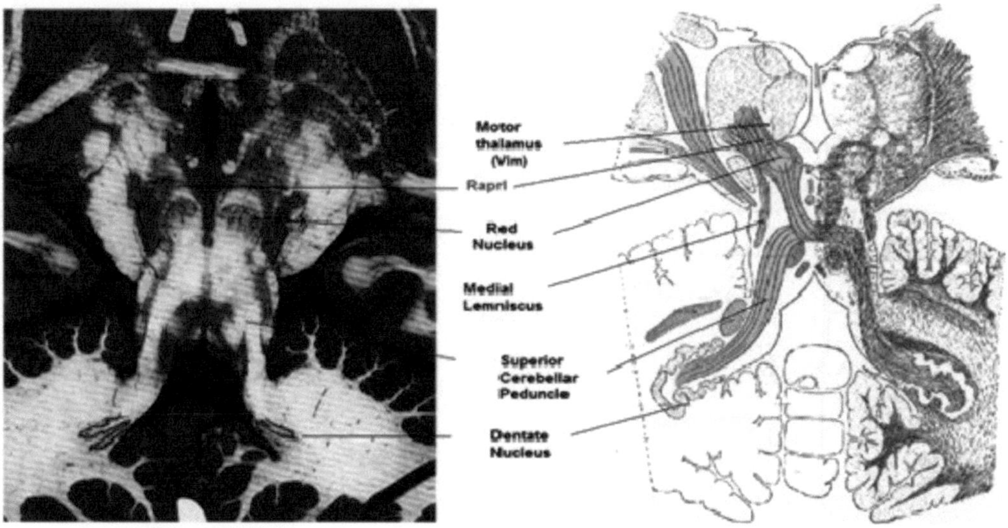

Fig. 5. Dentorubric and rubrothalamic-dentothalamic fibers of Raprl. This Flesching or horizontal cut, in a brain (left) and its schematization (right) form a funnel of Raprl fibers from different parts of the cerebellum and red nucleus. Note the anterior location of Raprl over the medial lemniscus (Modified from Testut, 1947 and England and Wakely, 1992).

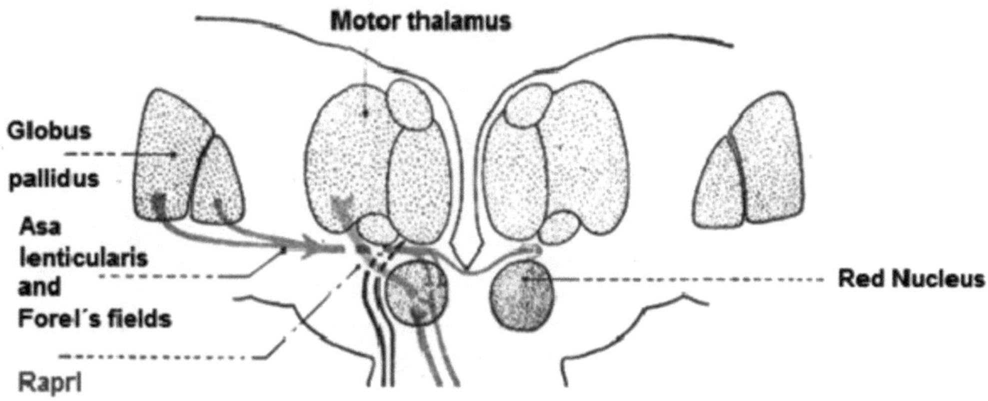

Fig. 6. Component fibers of the basal ganglia on Raprl. Note to Raprl on arrival to the thalamus via rubrotahalamic and dentorubric pathways and, along with tracks from the lenticular loop and fibers of the Forel´s fields H, H1 and H2 that cross in the posterior subthalamic region (Adapted from Barr, 2005).

2. Projections of the reticular formation. The nuclei of the reticular formation (medulla, pons and midbrain) come down to two important centers in their connections with the thalamus. The first is Zi, in which reticular formation ends and the other is the thalamic reticular nucleus. Zi is adhered to the Raprl virtually its entire course, so leave this core fibers are directed towards the thalamus. There is also an important Zi connection with a motor nucleus of the reticular formation which is the pedunculopontine nucleus. Anatomical studies in cats have shown that, although they have the same name as in humans, this area belongs to the reticular formation of fibers emanating from the

mesencephalic tegmentum and the ventral oral nucleus of the pons and terminate in the thalamus (Nauta and Kuypers, 1958). In the monkey, the same area corresponds to midbrain reticular nuclei (Ward et al, 1948). See Figure 8B.

3. Various projections. There are also other nuclei and fibers that are smaller and are located in the tegmentum of midbrain, which also could be part of Raprl. Some of these are: intercommissural fibers between STN, Gudden´s tegmentum bundle, which connects the hypothalamus with the thalamus; internal capsule fibers of accessory nucleus, among others. See figure 7.

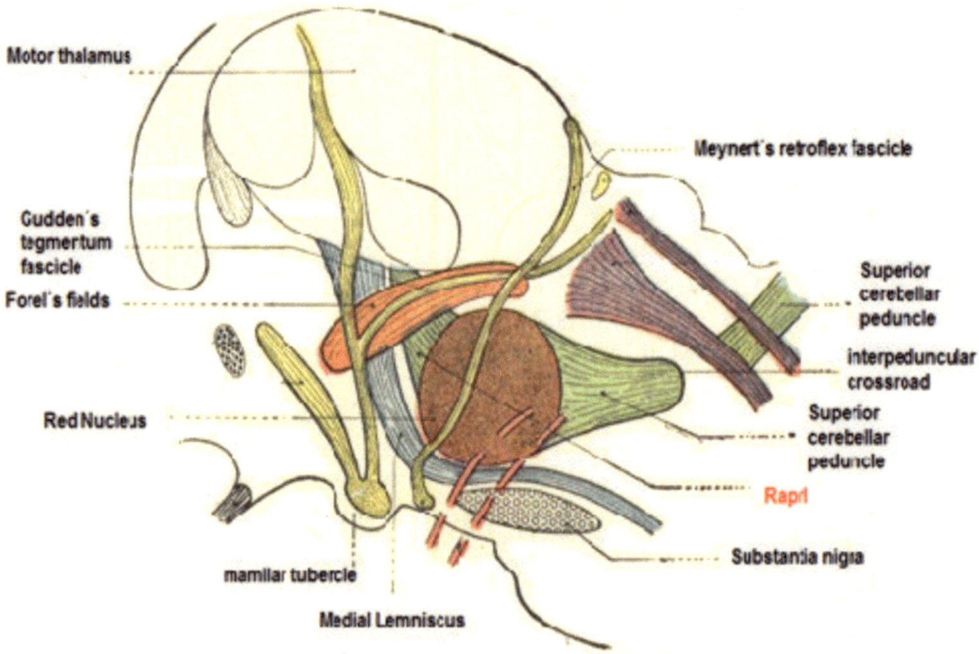

Fig. 7. Various connections are the Raprl. It is noted that the area of the Raprl exists confluence of several other structures such as the Gudden´s tegmentum bundle, among others. Note again, as are adjacent to the lemniscus Raprl and their relationship to Forel´s fields (Adapted from Testut, 1947).

2.2.1.2 Raprl´s stereotactical ubication

Then, in the three spatial planes would be the following relations (Schaltenbrand and Bailey, 1959):

a. In the coronal plane, the Raprl are located below the Voa and Vop thalamic nuclei; Vimi and Vimeo, inferior is placed the substance Q of Sano; externally is the thalamic reticular nucleus, the STN and cPCI; medially Ru is ahead with the Forel´s fields: H1, H2 and H immediately, and in dorsal area is placed the Lm. (Figure 8A).
b. In the sagittal plane are located: rostrally thalamic nuclei already discussed, in caudal part of the STN, SN and substance Q; forward shows the Zi and Forel´s fields medially; and the lemniscus is back. Laterally is located the STN and the internal capsule, medially the brachium conjuntivum (BCJ) and Ru (Figure 8B).

c. Finally, in the axial plane, shows from top-down as follows: outside the Raprl the lenticular nucleus and thalamus divided both by the internal capsule. Thalamic nuclei are Voa, Vop and Vim, and behind the Vce. Laterally, it is located the STN and Zi, and medially the BCJ and Ru, and more anterior Ha, H, and H1 Forel´s field.(Figure 8C)

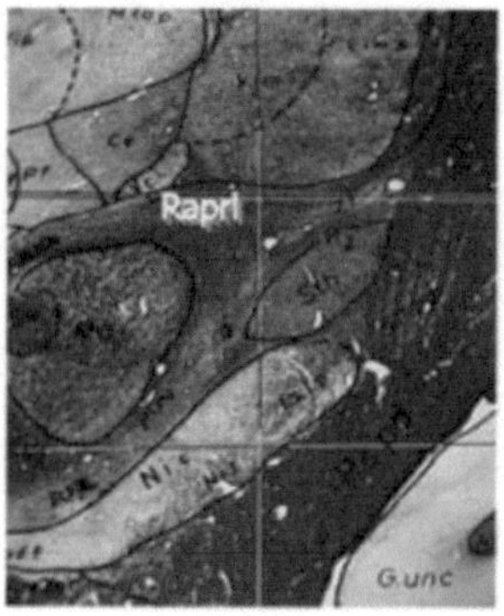

A

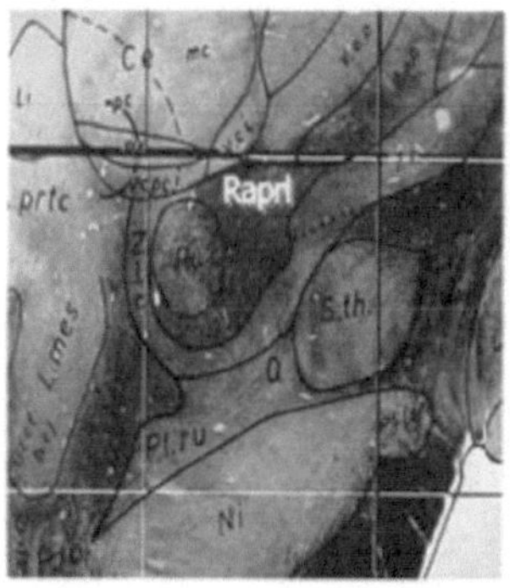

B

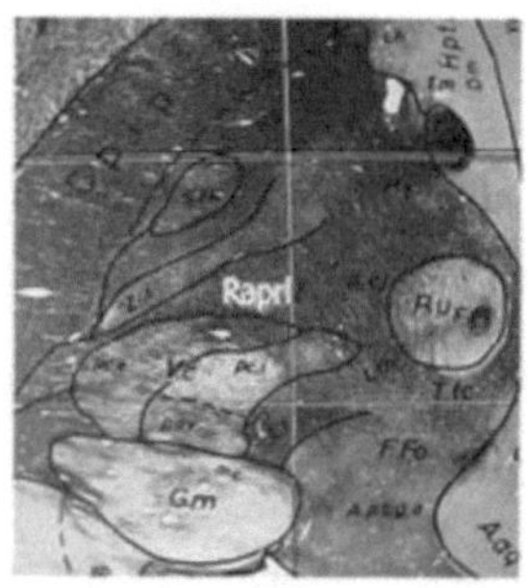

C

Fig. 8. Brain stereotactical sections to locate Raprl in humans. A) Coronal, where Zi, internal capsule and the STN stands externally, Ru stays medially; in cephalic area the thalamic nuclei are seen (Vimi and Vimeo, Ce); caudally substance Q, Ru and SN. B) Sagittal section shows where is the oblique arrangement of the fibers with the direction of thalamic nuclei (Vim, Voa and Vop). Ru and SN are observed caudally. Rostrally is finding the STN.
C) Axial section puts the Ru and Raprl between the medial and posterior part of the Zi and the STN. (From Atlas for Stereotaxy of the Human Brain, Schaltenbrand y Bailey,1959).

3. Physiology

If it is considered the anatomical aspects described below, Raprl´s functional aspects belong to diverse systems. The anterior component, which is part of basal ganglia, regulates the postural control. The inferior component has relation with reticular activation and in this sense with selective attention and motor orienting response; and the cerebellar component is involved into the dento-thalamo-cortical system to modulate muscular tone and coordinated voluntary movements. Dysfunction of these systems originated postural abnormalities, tremor, rigidity and probably bradykinesia (Bertrand, 1969; Velasco M, 1986).

Electrophysiological studies in Raprl that have previously been shown that intraoperative microelectrode records under local anesthesia without sedation have reported that the area 2 to 3 mm below the output of motor thalamus has a unitary activity in the not show any neuronal firing, just listening to background activity that is organized from time to time with bursts of 4 to 6 cps, similar to the frequency of tremor parkinsonism (Velasco et al 1973, 1975), also reported by others (Birk and Struppler, 1989; Luecking et al, 1971). These bursts of rhythmic activity resemble those reported in Vim (Jasper, 1966) and Voa (Tasker, 1967) of the thalamus, but are less frequent and prominent. Besides neurons were triggered with morphology completely different to STN. See Figure 9.

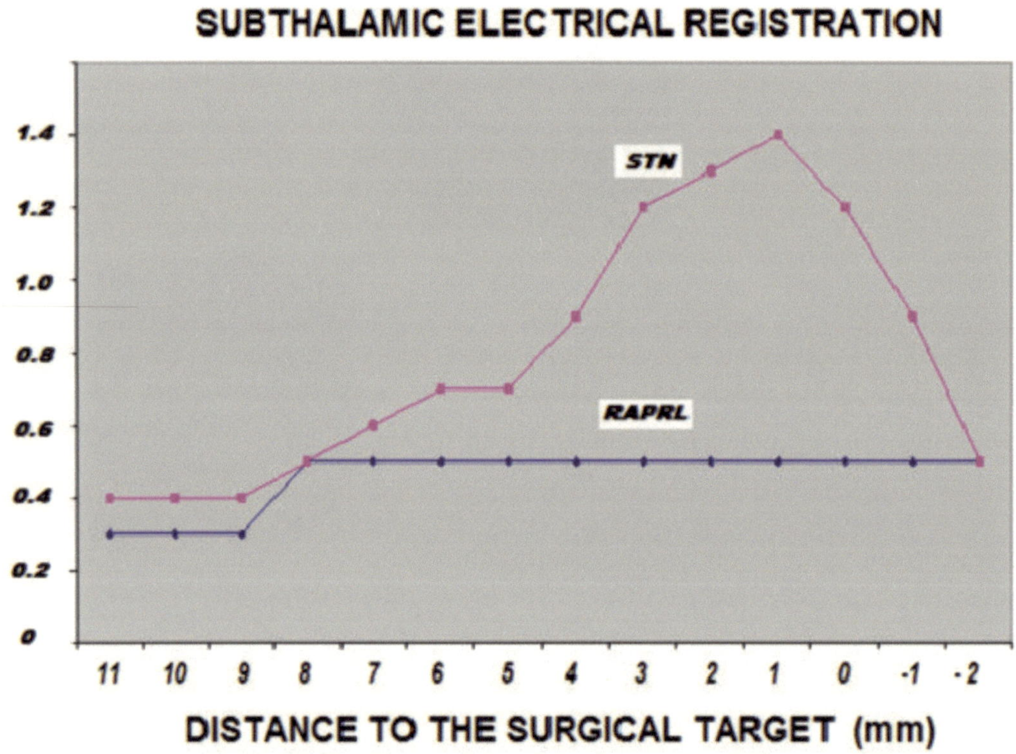

Fig. 9. STN and Raprl register comparison. Voltage difference seen at the site where the neurons firing in the STN when is compared to the Raprl. There is practically a physiological noise corresponding to fibers and a few neurons firing.

In addition, getting late evoked potentials already described previously (Velasco et al, 1988) confirms the involvement of the reticular formation in PD. Events related to somatic evoked potential (SEP) induced by median nerve stimulation during selective attention paradigm when an electrode located in the Raprl. In this area, only the late components (P200, P300), but not early (N20) were recorded. The late components vary significantly in amplitude for the effect of attention, so there is maximum amplitude during selective attention and new and there is minimal amplitude during habituation and distraction (Velasco et al, 1975, 1979, 1986; Jiménez et al, 2000). In contrast, the SEP recorded immediately posterior and medial lemniscus show a prominent N20, but not later P200 and P300 components. These findings place the Raprl as an extralemniscal system and are in contradiction with other reports (Birk and Struppler, 1989; Luecking et al, 1971, Momma et al, 1980). Similar components without component P200 were recorded early in the mesencephalic reticular formation (Velasco et al, 1979). Moreover, in monkeys with radiofrequency lesions made in an area equivalent to Raprl that corresponds to subthalamic and mesencephalic reticular formation, diminishing the contralateral limb tremor produced by lesions previously located in the SNc (Velasco et al, 1979). Also in humans (Andy et al, 1963, Velasco et al, 1980) and in experimental animals (Adey et al, 1962, Watson et al, 1974) lesions of this area can produce a "lack of spontaneous use" of contralateral extremities called **neglect.**

In humans, this appears to only occur when there is an additional subcortical atrophy in the thalamus (Velasco et al, 1986). In view of these observations, the existence of a reticulo-thalamic that mediates attention and tremor was proposed (Velasco et al, 1979).

4. Targeting and surgical technical aspects

Nowadays stereotactic surgery is refined in the precise identification of Raprl, since it is a very small target. In ancient times the ventriculography was commonly performed, and was changed by tomography scanner/magnetic resonance fusion with specific computational software. Patients are operated under local anesthesia, since patient collaboration and the commonly seen decrease or arrest of tremor in the moment of electrode´s insertion is an important clinical guide of the correct placement, and this is corroborated with macroestimulation when the electrode is connected to screening test machine. Coordinates for Raprl target are: lateral 11-13 mm, inferior to AC-PC line 4-5 mm and posterior to midline point in AC-PC line of 6-9 mm. Should electrodes' contacts are anterior or superior to Raprl target, the results in controlling tremor and rigidity are incomplete or null; if the contacts are posterior, contralateral paresthesias are elicited, and if the contacts are displaced medially macrostimulation induces gaze deviation (Bertrand 1969, 2004; Velasco 1982).

Before discussing what the effect of stimulation on the sign in concrete, it is worth explaining that it reproduces what happens in the Raprl when the single insertion of the electrode produces a decrease or disappearance of the sign on the side contralateral to the site of electrode´s introduction. This happens dramatically with tremor and rigidity, and for bradykinesia also presented a decrease, and it is difficult to assess the other two signs (gait and posture) with the patient is supine. The explanation of this phenomenon has been described from thalamotomy or subthalamotomy, where the insertion of the radiofrequency electrode to the distance and the tip of the instrument on the nerve tissue, causes that the motor circuit the is blocked by the physical presence of the object. Once in the post-operative, clinical signs reappear in the patient. The same happens with the introduction of a single electrode first, by modifying the above signs, and introducing the second electrode there is also the same effect on the opposite side of implantation.

In some cases of a second (bilateral) electrode implantation, it is also worth discussing the transient impairment of consciousness after the introduction of it. It happens when it introduces in the left side, but when he gets on the contralateral side, the patient must be alert, is immobilized and has transient aphasia comprehension and expression. The patient presents an excessive sleepiness that lasts even after the surgery a few hours to 48 hours. The way that can explain this is to prevent access of information by ascending activating system, leading to a consequent loss of consciousness and awake. This effect is transitory and after this time the patient is recovered the alert state.

5. Surgery indications and contraindications (Bertrand 1969, Carrillo-Ruiz 2003, Velasco, 1972, 2001; Espinosa 2010)

The next are the indications to choose patients to Raprl neuromodulation:

1. Patients diagnosed with idiopathic PD.
2. Good response to Levodopa test.
3. Age between 35 to 80 years.
4. Intact cognition or discrete alterations of mood.
5. Tremor is the predominant symptom.
6. Rigidity accompanies tremor.
7. Acral bradykinesia.

On the other side, the issues below are contraindications:

1. Rigidity/bradykinetic signs exclusively.
2. Severe unbalance or gait disturbances.
3. Traditional surgical contraindications (coagulopathies, high anesthesic risk ASA > 3, etc…).
4. Patients with previous brain lesions, mainly in subthalamus.

6. Results

6.1 Neuroimaging

The next images demonstrated the site of the electrodes between the Ru and Zi. Figure 10 shows an axial image where the electrodes are observed in Raprl. The electrodes are located between STN and Ru nuclei, being one tenth below the line intercommissural. On the right side is illustrated a diagram of the structures, with the names of the most important structures.

Figure 11 shows coronal and axial sections of MRI in T2 sequence, where the electrodes are observed bilaterally that are lateral to the midline, some of them displayed three to four other contacts as rounded hypointense images with a white halo, which is located between the Ru and STN.

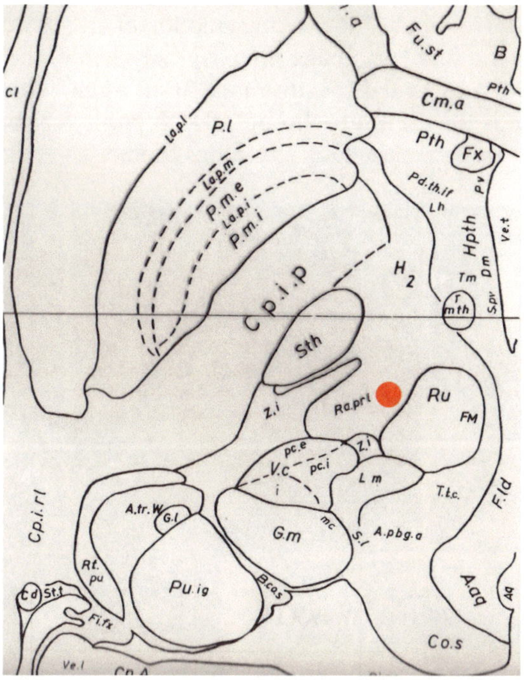

Fig. 10. Position of the electrodes. The image seen in an axial section of the atlas of Schaltenbrand and Bailey, the position where the electrode is located (red circle) between the STN and Ru which it corresponds to Raprl. It transposes the same level on MRI.

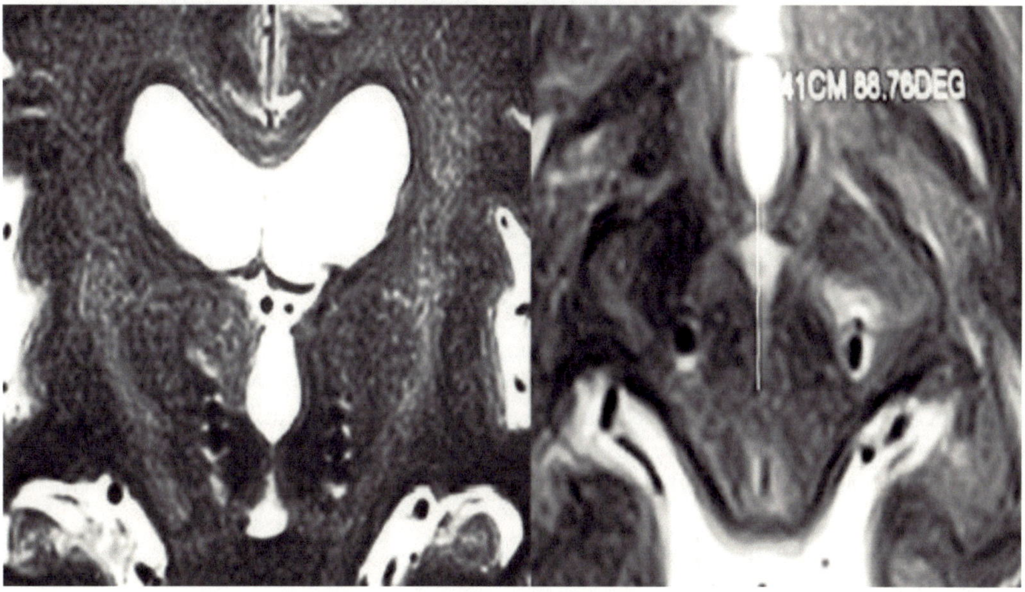

Fig. 11. Position of the electrodes in the MRI. Here is a coronal (left) and axial (right) sections. In the first corresponded to 2.5 to 5 mm anterior to the PC on both sides, the different electrode contacts. In the second, two ovoid hypotenses images 2 to 3 mm below the AC-PC line level. Note the electrodes are immediately lateral red nucleus.

In figure 12, it shows a three dimensional representation of an electrode in Raprl target with different projections. In the first MR image, in a sagittal section; the second, third and fifth with an oblique/anterior and in the fourth image at an angle with a posterior projection, that shows very clearly as the electrode through the trephine reaches the stem brain to the midbrain, showing the location of the four electrodes contacts.

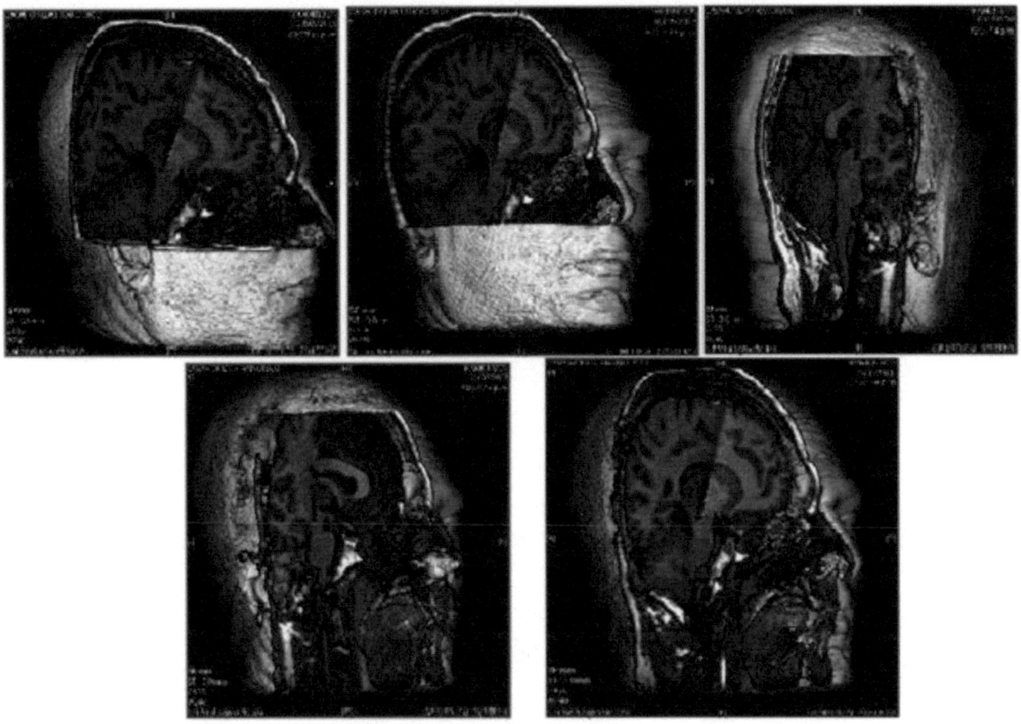

Fig. 12. Three dimensional reconstruction of an MRI demonstrated in a case position of the electrodes in Raprl. It is noted as the electrode enters oblique anteroposterior manner, following a midbrain-thalamic region. The tip is located in the midbrain tegmentum of the patient. The rest of the contacts found in midbrain-subthalamic union in the posterior third of subthalamus.

It has been described in several articles the position of the electrode when it was located in Raprl target. It is interest to note that groups with implantation in STN had reported the best points of stimulation with effectiveness in amelioration of the signs as outside of STN that corresponded to the white posterior subthalamic zone (Yokohama et al, 2001; Yelnik et al, 2003; Hamel et al, 2003). Undoubtedly this is corresponded to Raprl and Raprl/Zi area.

6.2 Clinimetric results in lesional era

During stereotactic lesional era (60´s to 80´s), Raprl leucotomy showed an important effect to arrest tremor with the simple insertion of the leucotome in the fibers that was optimized in the moment of fibers´ coagulation itself. There is little information on the effect in other signs (Bertrand, 1969, 2004; Ito, 1975; Velasco F, 1972).

6.2.1 Tremor

The unilateral lesion in Raprl from yesteryear, has demonstrated a significant effect on this sign. Andy et al demonstrated a decrease of 50% (1963), Bertrand et al (1969) 60% to 90% (1974), Mundinger et al (1965) of 75%, Hassler et al with a decrease of 61.5% (1965) to 90-100% (1970); Houdart et al (1966) with a decrease of 75% Hullay et al (1971) with 95% decrease of the tremor, Velasco et al 44% (1972) to 100% (1975), Struppler et al (1972) with an unspecified data, Driollet et al (1974) with an unspecified data, Ito (1975) with 93% decrease and Bubnov (1975) with an unspecified percentage.

6.2.2 Rigidity

In attention, there are few lesional studies that mention the improvement in rigidity in addition to the tremor. One of them is the work of Mundinger et al (1965), also referred to greater improvement in this sign of 85% vs. 75% of the tremor when the Raprl-Zi damaged. Ito (1975) also mentions an improvement close 100%. Other lesional studies mentioned improvement in rigidity: those of Andy et al (1962), Houdart et al (1965) and Driollet et al (1974) though not in the numbered percentage of improvement.

6.2.3 Bradykinesia and other PD signs

Only one study indicating the presence lesional assessment of akinesia after radiation injury of the skull unilaterally, that is to Houdart et al (1965), where no change of akinesia in patients, it is clear that at that time there were scales clinimetric as we now know it is difficult to reach other conclusions. There were no other studies for evaluating gait, posture or other non-motor and vegetative symptoms in the literature.

It is relevant express there is no statistical analysis established in lesional results to confirm differences between controls and patients with lesion in Raprl.

6.3 Clinimetric results in neuromodulation era

In the first report of Raprl stimulation, the lesional effect was reproduced with the arrest or amelioration in tremor (94%) and was consistent over 1 year; but the rigidity (90%) was also stochastically improved. Bradykinesia was unchanged because was not relevant in those patients (Velasco et al, 2001). The next studies indicated effectiveness in unilateral or bilateral tremor, rigidity and bradykinesia, with less improvement in gait and posture disturbances. In this moment the percentage of symptom alleviation is indicated for tremor 91% ($p<0.001$), rigidity 94% ($p<0.001$), bradykinesia 64% ($p<0.05$), gait 40% and posture 35% (Carrillo-Ruiz 2007, 2008).

6.3.1 Tremor

Unilateral tremor was disappeared with the simple insertion of the electrode in the Raprl target. The results in the acute state were also satisfactory that was permanent when the patients were studied along one year. The effect of stimulation on tremor is indisputable and overwhelming. Unilateral and bilateral Raprl electrical stimulation shows that between 85% and 90% of the PD patients have diminished the tremor. Looking at the figure specified for tremor, there is a significant decrease of the tremor of all four limbs and head. This applies equally to a large percentage of decrease from 85 to 94% in one year. See figure 13.

6.3.2 Rigidity

If there is a unilateral effect of acute and long term improvement in the tremor, the effect of Raprl stimulation on rigidity perfectly clear and even much higher percentage of improvement, with a very important statistical significance. This is demonstrated in our previous study (Velasco et al, 2001) with a decrease of 93%, also reproduced by the Japanese group (Murata et al, 2003) from 95 to 100%. Like unilateral stimulation in the case of bilateral stimulation, the improvement is very similar being 95 to 100% at the prevailing effect. See figure 14.

6.3.3 Bradykinesia

Bradykinesia and akinesia is not the principal factor to study in the first articles of neuromodulation, because the patients, who was implanted unilaterally, had low or null braykinesia, so the analysis was no relevant. One of the main contributions of next study is to elucidate the effect of bilateral stimulation of the Raprl on bradykinesia, akinesia, gait and posture, because none of the previous studies mentioned any effect on these items, since patients had no alterations in this part. See figure 15.

6.3.4 Gait and posture

So it is fruitful results of the bilateral implantation in patients with advanced PD, noting that the patients had a major alteration to walk with confinement to bed or wheelchair (Hoehn-Yahr of 5) and to improve their scores decreasing by half can walk with difficulty. This is significant from a statistical point of view only up to six months. Then there is the decline and likely to change. If it consider gait, the improvement is a moderate decrease in the rate of 35%, with statistical significance in the ninth month, but with a decrease in the time scale.

In this moment our group is analyzing the data at long follow-up. The scales of subitems in UPDRSIII for each sign are verifying to determinate the exact differences at 4 years. It is important extern that a persistent effect has seen in the next years to implantation and stimulation, but the efficacy was diminished through the time.

7. Other groups experiences

Raprl Neuromodulation is extended to other neurosurgical teams over the world. Murata and coworkers, in Japan, reported that tremor was suppressed by monopolar stimulation not only to PD, but also for different tremor cases including essential tremor. The effect in rigidity and bradykinesia was decreased and it were reported qualitatively and diminished for tremor from 78.3% to 90%, and rigidity 92.7% (Murata et al, 2003, 2007; Kitagawa et al, 2005). Espinosa and cols, in Colombia showed the same effect over UPDRSIII and diminished in tremor and rigidity (from 70% to 100% for both signs), and reported that improvement was sustained over the time (Espinosa & Arango, 2005, Espinosa et al, 2010).

Fytagoridis & Bloomstedt, in Sweden, demonstrated the amelioration in tremor, in an important manner (91%) and also in rigidity and bradykinesia when stimulation in Raprl was used (Fytagoridis & Bloomstedt, 2010).

By other side Plaha reviewed the exactly position of the electrodes in his PD patients with STN electrical stimulation. He described that the best contacts corresponded to electrodes behind the STN. This area corresponded to Zi caudalis (Plaha et al, 2007), that is near to Raprl, how it was strongly discussed. See table.

Author	Year	Site	Number of patients	Disease	Uni/Bil	UPDRS III relief	Trem	Rigid	Brady Kinesia	Gait	Posture
Velasco et al	2001	Raprl	10	PD	Uni	60%	94%	90%	30%	Na	Na
Murata et al	2003	Raprl /Zi	8	ET	Uni	Na	90%	Na	Na	Na	Na
Kitagawa et al	2005	Raprl /Zi	8	PD	Uni	44.3%	78.3%	92.7%	65.7%	NP	NP
Espinosa et al	2005	Raprl	3	PD	Bil	40%	NP	NP	NP	NP	NP
Murata Et al	2007	Zi/ Raprl	18	PD	Uni	NP	NP	NP	NP	NP	NP
Carrillo-Ruiz et al	2007	Raprl	20	PD	Uni/Bil	75%	81-90%	88-100%	50-60%	Na	Na
Herzog et al	2007	Raprl	21	ET	Uni	Na	99%	Na	Na	Na	Na
Hamel et al	2007	Raprl	11	ET	Bil	Na	68 to 73%	Na	Na	Na	Na
Carrillo-Ruiz et al	2008	Raprl	5	PD	Bil	65%	90%	94%	75%	40	35
Blomsted et al	2009	Raprl /Zi	5	ET	Uni	89%	Na	Na	Na	Na	Na
Espinosa et al	2010	Raprl	26	EP	Uni/Bil	NP	70-100%	70-100%	NP	NP	NP
Fytagoridis et al	2010	Raprl /Zi	35: 27/8	ET/PD	Bil	NP	91%	NP	NP	NP	NP

PD: Parkinson´s disease; ET: Essential tremor; NP: Not presented; Na: Not applied; Uni: unilateral; Bil: bilateral; Trem: tremor, rigid:rigidity; Zi: Zona incerta caudalis; Raprl: Prelemniscal Radiations.

Table 1.

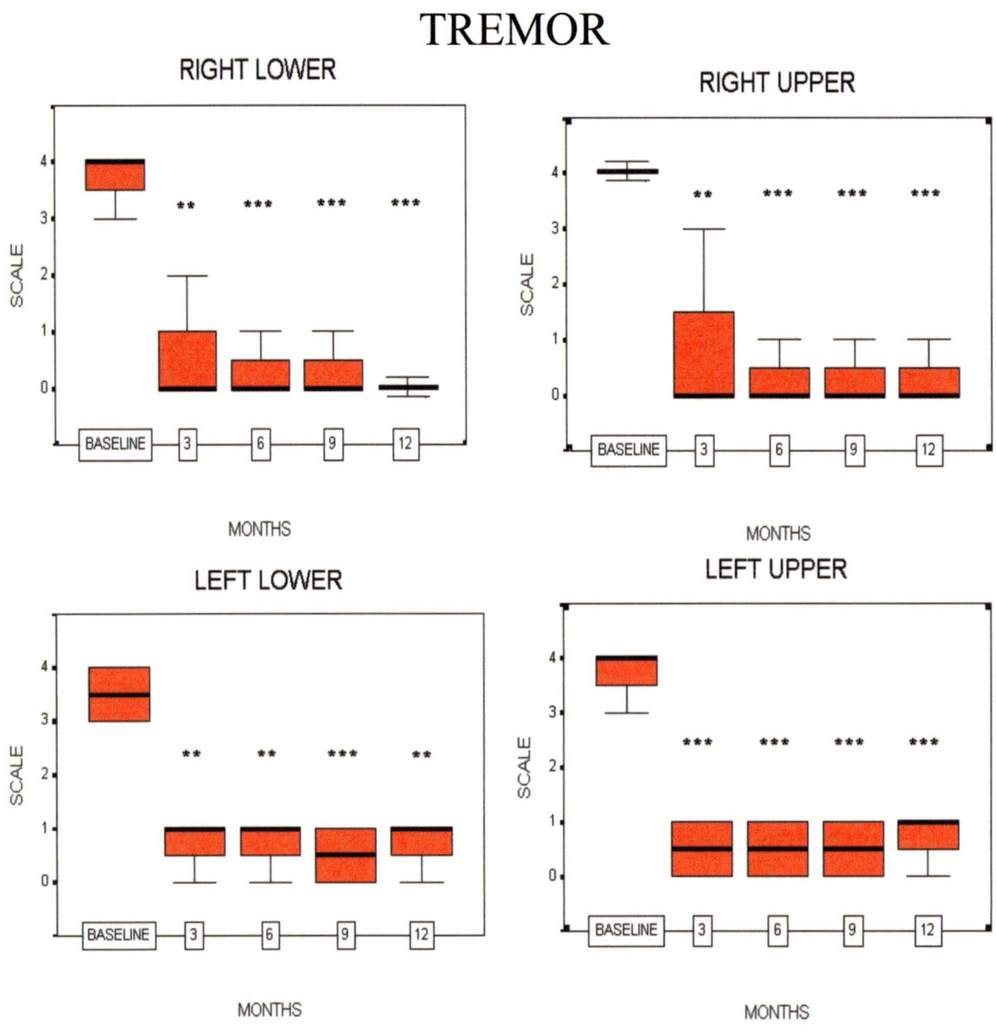

Fig. 13. Clinimetric changes for Tremor. Longitudinal assessment of the tremor is seen by using the subitem 20 of the UPDRS part III. A and B corresponded to superior limbs. C and D for inferior limbs. The evaluation is presented in baseline, 3, 6, 9 and 12 months. Box plot represents the 75% of all patients; the bar illustrates the median and the outliers, maximum and minum values. Asterisks show statistical significance (*p<0.05, ** p<0.01,***p<0.001), (Carrillo-Ruiz, 2003).

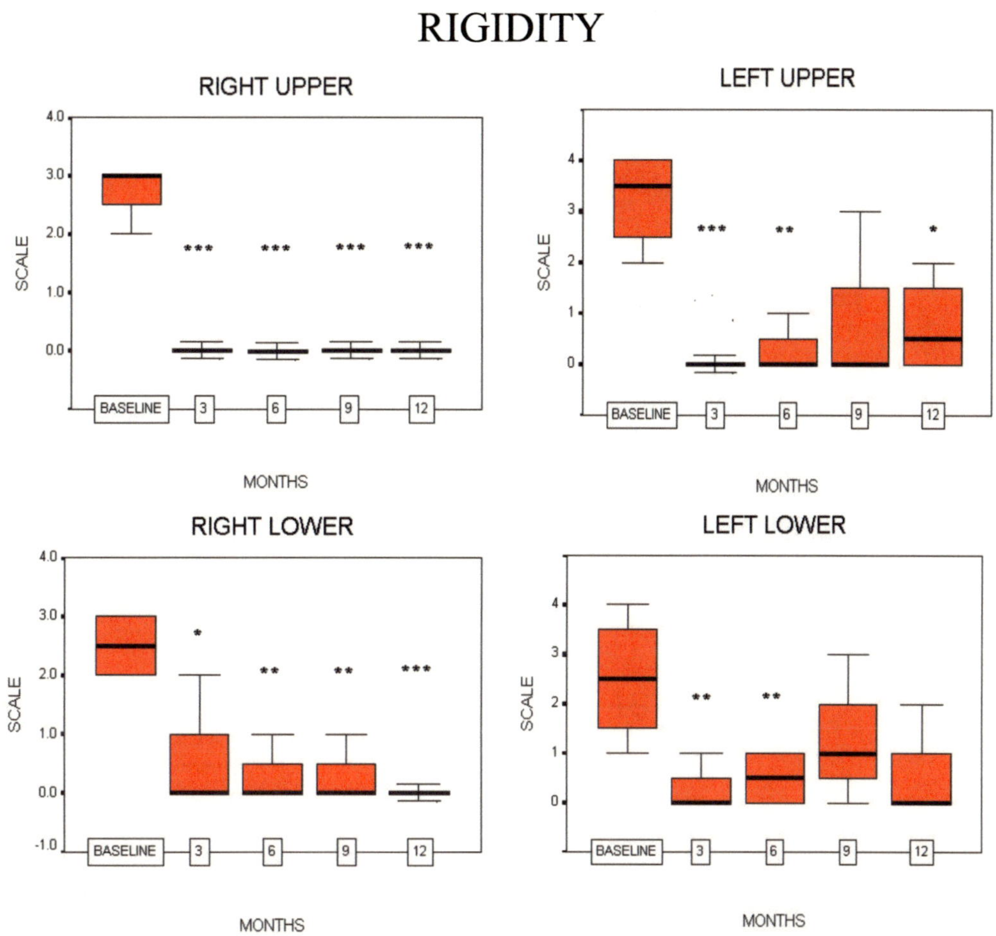

Fig. 14. Clinimetric changes for rigidity. Longitudinal evaluation of the stiffness is seen by using the number 23 of the UPDRS part III. The same elements presented of figure 13. Remarkable as tremor, the amelioration of rigidity in the evolution of the Raprl stimulation that is highly significative (Carrillo-Ruiz, 2003).

8. Comparision of Raprl vs STN, Gpi and thalamus as surgical targets

Fibers once they reach the thalamus are distributed in a fan in the Vim, Vop and Voa. This is why despite being effective suppression of tremor by thalamotomy or electrical stimulation of the Vim, the best place to suppression of tremor is the thalamo-subthalamic rim, corresponding to each Raprl core and along or separately (Tasker et al, 1967, Nguyen et al, 1993; Benabid et al, 1996). STN tremor improved, from 60 to 80% in the studies but is not the ideal target to treat tremor (Krack et al, 2003) and even international level is preferred to use Vim stimulation on the STN when the patient presents only tremor and other symptoms of the disease.

The GPi is a target that does not diminish surgical beyond 50% of the tremor, which is not a good anatomical site to remove the ipsilateral or contralateral tremor.

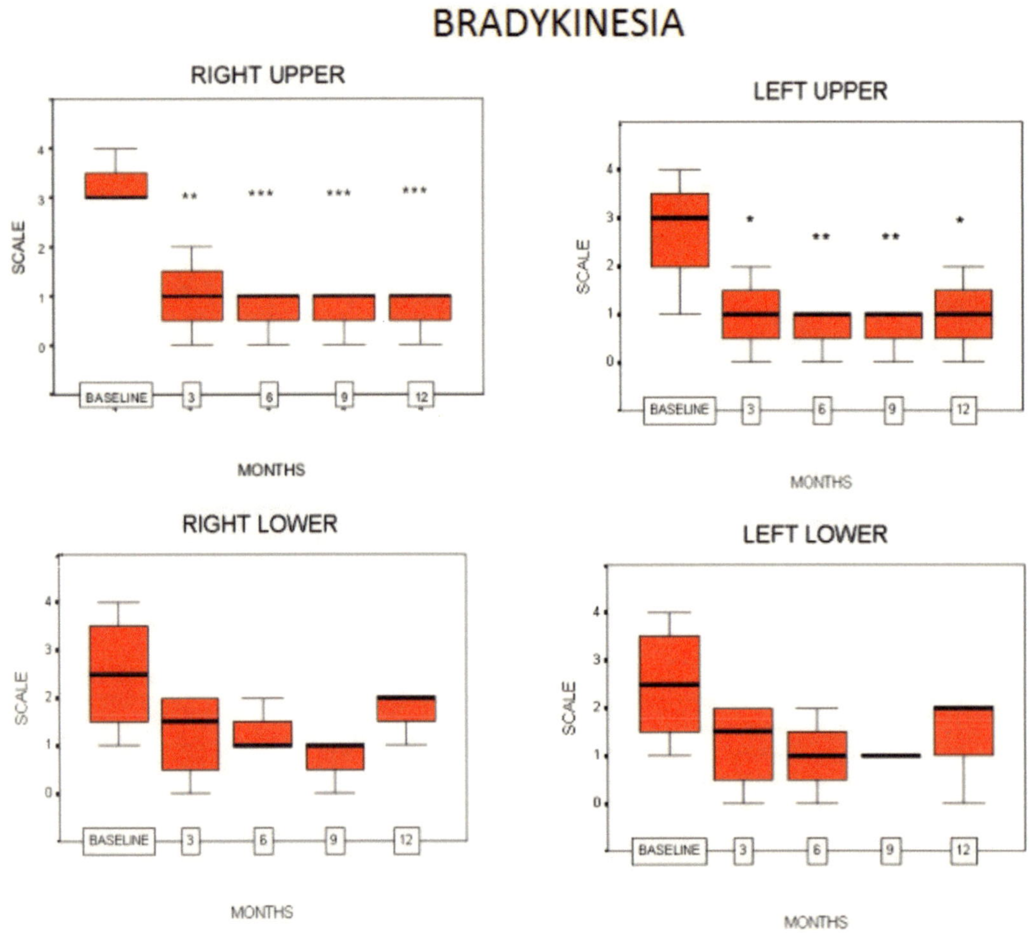

Fig. 15. Clinimetric evaluation uses for bradykinesia. Assessment of bradykinesia using subitem no. 32 of the UPDRS part III.The explanation is similar to figure 13 and 14 (Carrillo-Ruiz, 2003).

With respect to rigidity, Vim stimulation is not good (less than 40%), so it is not the best method to treat akinetic-rigid patients, this confirms the above that the tremor is more involved with the cerebellar pathway that the route of the basal ganglia. However, both the STN and the GPi are good targets for improved rigidity, but despite this, the percentage of Raprl has a greater efficiency.

Vim stimulation is not useful to improve the bradykinesia. The STN and Gpi alike improve these signs, being almost the same percentage held for the Raprl of about 65%.

In this sense the anatomical targets improve of gait, often the STN and GPi, as both through specific studies on the place have proven effective. The percentage is better than for Raprl, 50% vs. 45%, although the patients with Raprl are advanced (Hoeh & Yahr 5) and that STN patients have a varying degrees of Hoehn and Yahr, so no are fully comparable.

At last, the posture is a good example of improvement also mild level with the use of STN stimulation, but better than the Raprl neuromodulation. This may be due to connections with the brainstem to the STN and in the earliest stages of PD in these patients. The Vim and GPI are not good places to improve posture (Benabid et al, 1996 and 2000).

9. The future

The next point would be to establish what is the relationship of these findings with is currently known about the PD pathophysiology, both in animals and humans. If it refers to Alexander and DeLong classic diagram shows that none of the findings of this study fall in there. If it pays attention to the direct and indirect pathways have their starting point in the Gpi/ SNr and depending on their afferents may come from the putamen or the STN, respectively. However this scheme does not specify which routes are used from the STN or GPi. The pallidal and climbing pathways that reach the thalamus has been mentioned, are not Raprl as anatomically way is through the Forel´s fields that predate the site of interest, on the other side cannot be excluded that the fibers emanating from the STN may be added in the same Raprl but this is not contemplated in the scheme of Alexander (Alexander et al, 1986; Alexander & De Long, 1990).

It is relevant determinate exactly the anatomy of the white fibers, with the correlation to functional directions. In this effort, it is analyzing by different methods; tractography, potential unit neuron stimulation and other to determinate the role of brainstem with the subthalamus and basal ganglia.

10. Conclusions

Raprl neuromodulation in the treatment of PD is effective to improve tremor, rigidity and bradykinesia. The results over gait, posture and dyskinesia are less significant; results have been validated by different groups around the world.

11. References

[1] Adey W.R., Walter D.O., Lindsley D.F. Subthalamic lesions. Arch Neurol 6: 34-47, 1962.

[2] Alexander G.E., DeLong M.R., Strick P.L. Parallel organization of functionally segregated circuits linking basal ganglia and cortex. Annu Rev Neurosci 9:357-378, 1986.

[3] Alexander G.E., Crutchter M.D. Functional architecture of basal ganglia circuits: Neural substrates of parallel processing. Trends Neurosci 13:266-275, 1990.

[4] Andy OJ, Jurko MF, Sias FRJr. Subthalamotomy in treatment of parkinsonism tremor. J Neurosurg 20: 860-870, 1963.

[5] Barr K. Neuroanatomía Humana. 8ª ed. McGraw Hill, Mc Graw Hill ed, 2005.

[6] Benabid A.L., Pollak P., Gao D., Hoffmann D., Limousin P., Gay E., Payen I., Benazzouz A. Chronic electrical stimulation of the ventralis intermedius nucleus of the thalamus as a treatment of movement disorders. J Neurosurg 84:203-214, 1996.

[7] Benabid A.L., Koudsié A., Benazzouz A., Fraix V., Ashraf A., Le Bas J.F, Chabardes S., Pollak P. Subthalamic Stimulation for Parkinson´s Disease. Arch Med Res. 31, 3:282-289, 2000.

[8] Bertrand CM, Hardy J, Molina-Negro P, Martínez N: Optimum physiological target for the arrest of tremor, in Gillingham FJ, Donaldson ML (eds): *Third Symposium of Parkinson's Disease*. Edinburgh, E&S Livingston, 1969, pp 251–254.

[9] Bertrand C., Molina-Negro, P., Martínez, N., Velasco, F.: Stereotaxic surgery in Parkinson's disease. Progress in Neurological Surgery. Krayenbuhl, H., Maspes, P. And Sweet, W. (Eds.) Year Book Medical Publishers, Vol. V. 1974.
[10] Bertrand CM. Surgery of involuntary movements, particularly stereotactic surgery: reminiscences. Neurosurgery. 2004; 55(3):698-703.
[11] Birk P., Struppler A.: Functional neuroanatomy of the target area for the treatment of pathological tremor: an electrophysiological approach. Stereotact Funct Neurosurg 52:164-170, 1989.
[12] Bubnov AN [Neurosurgical anatomy of the zona incerta applicable to subthalamotomy]. Vopr Neirokhir. 1975; (1):36-40.
[13] Carrillo-Ruiz J., Velasco F., Jiménez F., Hernández-Silverio J.A., Arguëlles C. Bilateral Electrical Stimulation of Prelemniscal radiations in Advanced Parkinson´s disease. American Society for Stereotactic and Functional Neurosurgery 2003 Quadrennial Meeting, New York City, E.U.A., 18 to 21 of 2003. May 18 -21, 2003.
[14] Carrillo-Ruiz JD, Velasco F, Jiménez F, Velasco AL, Velasco M, Castro G. Neuromodulation of prelemniscal radiations in the treatment of Parkinson's disease. Acta Neurochir Suppl. 2007; 97(Pt 2):185-90.
[15] Carrillo-Ruiz JD, Velasco F, Jiménez F, Castro G, Velasco AL, Hernández JA, Ceballos J, Velasco M. Bilateral electrical stimulation of prelemniscal radiations in the treatment of advanced Parkinson's disease. Neurosurgery. 2008; 62 (2):347-57.
[16] Driollet R, Schvarcz JR, Orlando J. Optimum target for arrest tremor. Confin Neurol 36: 355, 1974.
[17] England MA and Wakely J. El cerebro y la médula espinal. Introducción a la neuroanatomía normal. Mosby Year Book, 1a ed., 1992.
[18] Espinosa J, Arango G, Fonseca M, Gálvez J, Atuesta J. Prelemniscal radiation deep brain stimulation: indications and results. In: Neuromodulation. Cukiert J (ed.) 2010: pp: 236-240.
[19] Espinosa J, Arango G. Surgical management of Parkinson's disease. Deep brain stimulation of the prelemniscal radiation. Movement disorders. 2005; 20 Suppl 10:S159-60.
[20] Forel A. Untersuchungen über die Haubenregion und thre oberen Verknüpfungen im Gehirne des Menschen und der Saugetiere, mit Beitrágen zu den Metoden der Gehirn-Untersuchung. Archiv für Psychiatrie und Nervenkrankheiten,Berlin 7(3). 393-495, 1877.
[21] Fytagoridis A, Bloomstedt P. Complications and side effects of deep brain stimulation in the posterior subthalamic area. Stereotact Funct Neurosurg. 2010; 88:88-93.
[22] Hamel W, Fietzek U, Morsnowski A, Schrader B, Herzog J, Weinert D, Pfister G, Müller D, Volkmann J, Deuschl G, Mehdorn HM. Deep brain stimulation of the subthalamic nucleus in Parkinson's disease: evaluation of active electrode contacts J Neurol Neurosurg Psychiatry. 2003; 74(8):1036-46.
[23] Hamel W, Herzog J, Kopper F, Pinsker M, Weinert D, Müller D, Krack P, Deuschl G, Mehdorn HM. Deep brain stimulation in the subthalamic area is more effective than nucleus ventralis intermedius stimulation for bilateral intention tremor. Acta Neurochir (Wien). 2007; 149(8):749-58.
[24] Hassler R, Mundinger F, Riechert T. Correlations between clinical and autoptic findings in stereotaxic operations of parkinsonism. Confin Neurol 26: 282-290, 1965.
[25] Herzog J, Hamel W, Wenzelburger R, Pötter M, Pinsker MO, Bartussek J, Morsnowski A, Steigerwald F, Deuschl G, Volkmann J. Kinematic analysis of thalamic versus

subthalamic neurostimulation in postural and intention tremor. Brain. 2007; 130 (Pt 6): 1608-25.

[26] Houdart R, Mamo H, Dondey M, Cophingnon J. Résultats des coagulations sous-thalamiques dans la maladie de Parkinson. Rev Neurol 112 (6): 521-529, 1965.

[27] Hullay J. Subthalamotomy in Parkinson's disease. Analysis of responses to electrostimulation. Acta Med Acad Sci Hung. 1971; 28(1):57-68.

[28] Ito Z. Stimulation and destruction of the pre-lemniscal radiations or its adjacent area in various extrapyramidal disorders. Confin Neurol, 37:41-48, 1975.

[29] Jasper, H.H., Bertrand C. Thalamic unit involved in somatic sensation and voluntary and involuntary movements in man. En: thalamus, Purpura D.P., y Yahr M.D. (eds) N.Y., Columbia University Press., pp 365-375, 1966.

[30] Jiménez F., Velasco F., Velasco M., Brito F., Morel C., Márquez I., Pérez M.L., Subthalamic prelemniscal radiation stimulation for the treatment of the Parkinson´s Disease: Electrophysiological characterization of the area. Arch Med Res 31, 3:270-281, 2000.

[31] Krack P, Batir A, Van Blercom N, Chabardes S, Fraix V, Ardouin C, Koudsie A, Limousin PD, Benazzouz A, LeBas JF, Benabid AL, Pollak P. Five-year follow-up of bilateral stimulation of the subthalamic nucleus in advanced Parkinson's disease. N Engl J Med 13; 349(20):1925-34, 2003.

[32] Kitagawa M, et al. Two-year follow-up of chronic stimulation of the posterior subthalamic white matter for tremor-dominant Parkinson's disease. Neurosurgery. 2005; 56:281-9.

[33] Momma H., Sabin H.I., Branston N.M.: Clinical evidence supporting origin of P15 wave of the somatosensory evoked potentials to median nerve stimulation. Electroenceph Clin Neurophysiol 67:134, 1980.

[34]Mundinger F. Stereotaxic interventions on the zona incerta area for treatment of extrapyramidal motor disturbances and their results. Confin Neurol 26:222-230, 1965.

[35] Murata J. Electrical stimulation of the posterior subthalamic area for the treatment of intractable proximal tremor. J Neurosurg. 2003; 99: 708-15.

[36] Murata J, Kitagawa M, Uesugi H, Saito H, Iwasaki Y, Kikuchi S, Sawamura Y. [Deep brain stimulation of the posterior subthalamic area (Zi/Raprl) for intractable tremor]. No Shinkei Geka. 2007 Apr;35(4):355-62.

[37]Nauta, W.J.H., Kuypers, H.G.: Some ascending pathways in the brain stem reticular formation. Henry Ford Hospital Symposium of Reticular Formation of the Brain. Jasper H.H., Proctor L.D., Knighton, R.S (Eds), Boston, Little Brown Co, 1958, pp 3 15.

[38] Nguyen JP, Degos JD. Thalamic stimulation and proximal tremor. A specific target in the nucleus ventrointermedius thalami. Arch Neurol 50:498-500, 1993.

[39]Luecking C.H., Struppler A., Erbel F., Reiss W.: Spontaneus and evoked potentials in human thalamus and subthalamus. Electrenceph. Clin Neurophysiol 31:351-2, 1971.

[40] Plaha P, Gill SS. Bilateral deep brain stimulation of the pedunculopontine nucleus for Parkinson's disease. Neuroreport 28; 16(17):1883-7, 2005.

[41] Plaha P, Ben-Shlomo Y, Patel NK, Gill SS. Stimulation of the caudal zona incerta is superior to stimulation of the subthalamic nucleus in improving contralateral parkinsonism. Brain 129(Pt 7):1732-47, 2006.

[42] Schaltenbrand G., Bailey P.: Introduction to stereotaxis with an atlas of the human brain. Sttutgart Verlag-Thieme, Vol IV, 1959.

[43] Tasker R.R. Surgical aspects: Symposium on extrapyramidal disease. Appl Ther 9: 454-462, 1967.

[44] Testut L. Tratado de Anatomía Humana. Segundo tomo: Angiología-Sistema Nervioso Central Ed. Salvat. pp: 875-1121, 1947.

[45] Velasco F, Molina-Negro P, Bertrand C, Hardy J. Further definition of the subthalamic target for arrest of tremor. J Neurosurg. 1972; 36(2):184-91.

[46] Velasco, F., Molina-Negro, P.: Electrophysiological topography of the human diencephalon. J. Neurosurg. 38:204-214, 1973.

[47] Velasco, M., Velasco, F., Maldonado, H., Machado, J.: Differential effect of thalamic and subthalamic lesions on early and late components of somatic evoked potentials in man. Electroenceph. Clin. Neurophysiol. 39:163-171, 1975.

[48] Velasco, M., Velasco, F., Maldonado, H., Machado, J.: Differential effect of thalamic and subthalamic lesions on early and late components of somatic evoked potentials in man. Electroenceph. Clin. Neurophysiol. 39:163-171, 1975.

[49] Velasco, F., Velasco, M. Maldonado, H.: Identificación y lesión de las radiaciones prelemniscales en el tratamiento quirúrgico del temblor. Arch. Invest. Méd. (Méx.) 7:29-42, 1976.

[50] Velasco, F. And Velasco, M.: A reticulo-thalamic system mediating propioceptive attention and tremor in man. Neurosurgery 4:30-36, 1979.

[51] Velasco, F., Velasco, M., Ogarrio, C.: Neglect induced by thalamotomy in man: a quantitative appraisal of the deficit. Neurosurgery 19:744-751, 1986.

[52]Velasco F, Jiménez F, Pérez ML, Carrillo-Ruiz JD, Velasco AL, Ceballos J, Velasco M. Electrical stimulation of the prelemniscal radiations in the treatment of Parkinson's disease: An old target revised with new techniques. Neurosurgery, 44:293-306, 2001.

[53] Velasco F, Palfi S, Jiménez F, Carrillo-Ruiz JD, Castro G, Keravel Y. Other targets to treat Parkinson's disease (Posterior subthalamic targets and motor cortex). In: Lozano AM, Gildenberg PL, Tasker RR. Textbook os Stereotactic and Functional Neurosurgery. 2nd Edition. Vol. 2. Berlin-Heidelberg, Springer-Verlag 2009, pp 1665-1678.

[54] Watson R.T., Heilman K.M., Miller B.D., King F.A.: Neglect after mesencephalic reticular formation lesions. Neurology 24: 294-298, 1974.

[55] Ward, A.A., Maculloch, V.S., Magoun, H.W. Production of alternating tremor in monkeys. J Neurophysiol 11:317-328, 1948.

[56] Yelnik J, Damier P, Demeret S, Gervais D, Bardinet E, Bejjani BP, François C, Houeto JL, Arnule I, Dormont D, Galanaud D, Pidoux B, Cornu P, Agid Y. Localization of stimulating electrodes in patients with Parkinson disease by using a three-dimensional atlas-magnetic resonance imaging coregistration method. J Neurosurg. 2003; 99(1):89-99.

[57] Yokoyama T, Sugiyama K, Nishizawa S, Yokota N, Ohta S, Akamine S, Namba H: The optimal stimulation site for chronic stimulation of the subthalamic nucleus in Parkinson's disease. Stereotact Funct Neurosurg 77:61–67, 2001.

Part 2

Neuromodulation Acting in Sensitive and Vascular System

5

Mechanisms of Spinal Cord Stimulation in Neuropathic Pain

Imre P. Krabbenbos, E.P.A. van Dongen, H.J.A. Nijhuis and A.L. Liem
Department of Anaesthesiology, Intensive Care and Pain Medicine
St. Antonius Hospital, Nieuwegein
The Netherlands

1. Introduction

The effects of electrical stimulation of the body or nervous system have been recognized for thousands of years in every culture. It is said that since circa 9000 BC, bracelets and necklaces of magnetite and amber were used to prevent headaches and arthritis (Schechter, 1971). The ancient Egyptians used electrical discharges of the Nile catfish to treat neuralgia, headaches and other painful disorders (Kane & Taub, 1975). The first documented attempt to use electricity for pain treatment appeared in circa 15 AD. A Roman physician, Scribonius Largus, observed torpedo fish shock relieved gout pain and subsequently recommended torpedo fish therapy as a general treatment of pain (Stillings, 1971). The first electrostatic generator was presented by the German engineer Otto von Guericke in 1672, almost a century before the Leyden yar was developed. From then, man was able to generate, store and discharge electricity at any time. It extended its application as physicians were able to provide on-demand electrotherapy in patients for the treatment of pain syndromes.

Since the 18th century, electro-analgesia therapy has been embedded in the armamentarium of physicians. Its clinical application in English hospitals was called 'Franklinism', after the American statesman and scientist Benjamin Franklin. He acquired fame after observing that lightening and electrostatic charge on a Leyden jar were identical. Moreover, he was the first to discriminate positive and negative electricity and investigated the effects of muscle contraction after the administration of electrical shocks. The 19th century, also called 'the golden age of medical electricity', commenced with the discovery of the electrochemical battery in 1800. Several years later, Michael Faraday exposed the principles of electromagnetic induction which was followed by the introduction of the electric generator in 1848 by Du Bois-Raymond. In those years electrical machines could be found in every doctors consulting room. However, the number of skeptics who depicted electrotherapy as 'medical quackery' grew. Eventually, the Flexner report led to the legally exclusion of electrotherapy from clinical practice in 1910 (Macklis, 1993). The association with 'quackery', growing influence of drug industry and the appearance of radiographic imaging contributed to the loss of interest of science in the phenomenon of electroanalgesia. A reawakened interest in the application of electricity for pain treatment was commenced, as Chaffee and Light presented a method for remote control of electrical stimulation of the nervous system in the early 1930s (Chaffee & Light, 1934). The contemporary evolution of cardiac pacing techniques contributed to the development of original neural stimulators. In the early years of the 20th century, the English neurologist Sir Henry Head postulated the conceptual basics for a theory of central inhibition of pain by non-painful stimuli. This concept was eventually presented as the Gate Control Theory by Melzack and Wall in 1965 (Melzack & Wall, 1965). The gate control theory, which is further explored in paragraph 2.4, states that stimulation of large primary afferent fibers 'close the gate' and inhibit nociceptive processes. After first stimulating their own infra-orbital nerves, Wall and Sweet initiated therapeutic stimulation of peripheral nerves clinically. The initial results were promising, as the first patients experienced partial or complete pain alleviation during stimulation (Wall & Sweet, 1967; Wall 1985). Shealy et al. documented the first clinical application of spinal cord stimulation (SCS) or dorsal column stimulation (DCS) in 1967 (Shealy, 1967a). It was then presented as a novel analgesic method to relieve pain in a variety of chronic pain syndromes. The mechanisms of action of SCS are actually a clinically outgrowth of the Gate Control Theory (Melzack & Wall, 1965). The supposed mechanisms of action of SCS were predominantly described in these 'gating terms'. Initially, evidence for the efficacy of SCS in exerting an significant analgesic effect in a broad spectrum of neuropathic pain syndromes was lacking. In the 70's and 80's several studies appeared with the aim to unravel the mechanisms of action of SCS (Handwerker et al., 1975). Numerous studies investigated the effects of SCS on noxious stimuli in healthy animals. SCS was administrated with current intensities that cannot be used in a clinical setting on patients who are awake. Thus, conclusions obtained from these studies cannot be translated 'from bench to bedside' without question. The development of an reliable animal model of neuropathic pain made it possible to investigate the mechanisms of SCS more thoroughly (Meyerson et al., 1994). As more studies appeared there was more convincing evidence that also supraspinal interactions have an eminent role in explaining mechanisms in which SCS exerts its analgesic-effects. The mechanisms of SCS-induced pain relief became elusive and complex. A significant part of the current knowledge is provided by a few prominent laboratories in this field (B. Linderoth M.D Ph.D. and B.A Meyerson M.D Ph.D., Department of Clinical Neuroscience, Karolinska Institute, Stockholm, Sweden, and Department of Neurosurgery, Karolinska University Hospital, Stockholm, Sweden. N.Saadé Ph.D., Professor, American University of Beirut, Beirut, Lebanon, and of R. Foreman, Ph.D., Professor and Chair, Department of Physiology, Oklahoma Health Sciences Center, Oklahoma, City, Oklahoma). It was not until recently that a reawakened interest in exploring the mechanisms of action of SCS was presented by Guan et al (Guan et al., 2010]. Over the years, much questions has been answered although certain details of the mechanisms of SCS are still controversial and require additional evidence. In the last two decennia, SCS is being increasingly used as an neuromodulation technique in a narrowing spectrum of pain diagnosis. It is estimated that, currently, more than 30,000 SCS systems are implanted every year worldwide (Linderoth & Meyerson, 2010).

2. Mechanisms of action

2.1 Physiological anatomy of the spinal cord

A thorough understanding of the mechanisms of spinal cord stimulation needs a thorough knowledge of the anatomy and neurophysiology of the spinal cord and related structures.

Furthermore, appreciation of the electrical characteristics of intraspinal structures is required. Primary afferent fibers have their cell bodies of the first order located in the dorsal root ganglia. Proximal to the dorsal root ganglion the afferent fibers form a single dorsal nerve root (Light, 1988). Dorsal root fibers have a curve shape and an average diameter of 15 µm. As these axons proceed towards the dorsal column they bifurcate into ascending and descending pathways. A segregation of innocuous and nociceptive afferents occurs as the axons approach the spinal cord. The angle of the fibers varies as they enter the spinal cord, which has major consequences on their excitation thresholds. The dorsal horn of the spinal cord encompasses the grey matter of the spinal cord located dorsal to the central canal. In the 1950s Rexed distinguished six more-or-less different laminae of the spinal grey matter, using cytoarchitectonic criteria (Rexed, 1952). However, based on cytoarchitecture, the spinal gray matter is currently divided into 10 laminae (Whitehouse et al., 1983). Collaterals of large-diameter fibers, which mediate tactile sense and proprioception, enter the dorsal horn and extent mainly to lamina III and IV (Light, 1988). The dorsal column refers to the area of white matter in the dorsomedial side of the spinal cord. Collaterals of large-diameters fibers occupies the largest part, about 85%, of the dorsal columns. Their averaged diameter diminishes from 12µm at the origin to 8µm a few segments rostrally (Barolat & Sharan, 2004). The fasciculus gracilis contains neurons of the dorsal column-medial lemniscus system, which carries primary afferents from the lower extremities, and synapse in the nucleus gracilis at the level of the foramen magnum. The fasciculus cuneatus is positioned more lateral in the dorsal column and carries primary afferent signals from the upper extremities (Barolat & Sharan, 2004). As the primary afferent fibers ascend, they gradually shift medially and dorsally. Therefore, the accessibility to dorsal medial-stimulating electrode changes as their location in the spinal cord varies. Posterior located ascending and descending pathways are most accessible at normal stimulation parameters (Oakley & Prager, 2002). Hence, the anatomy and physiology of the spinal cord is complex, but understanding is essential when discussing the issues around mechanisms of spinal cord stimulation.

2.2 Electrical stimulation

In spinal cord stimulation, a lead is positioned in the dorsal epidural space and connected to a subcutaneously implantable pulse generator (IPG). The rostrocaudal position of the lead, with multiple contacts, can be altered to enable electrical stimulation at several spinal levels. The cathode is positioned between the dorsal median sulcus and the dorsal root entry zone area. During a stimulation pulse, current flows from a negatively charged active electrode (cathode) to a positively charged electrode (anode). In principle, sufficiently high electrical stimulation can activate every neural structure in close proximity of the cathode (Holsheimer, 2002). However, current flow chooses the path of lowest resistance and is therefore directed through anatomic structures characterized by high electrical conductivity (*table 1*). Cerebrospinal fluid (CSF) obviously has the lowest electrical resistivity and therefore conduct approximately 90% of injected current, followed by longitudinal white matter. Because its anisotropic characteristics, transverse white matter is proven to be less conductive as is grey matter. Epidural fat and dura mater also demonstrates low conductivity. Vertebral bone is characterized by having the lowest electrical conductivity. Therefore it functions as an insulator and prevents surrounding tissues (e.g the heart and pelvic structures) from being stimulated (Oakley & Prager, 2002; Holsheimer 2002). Initially, it was thought that dorsomedial electrical stimulation first activated fibers in the dorsal column as the name 'dorsal column stimulation' implies (Shealy, 1967a; Struijk et al., 1993]. Coburn introduced the hypothesis that dorsal root fibers may be involved as well, based on a theoretical study which indicated that dorsal root fibers have lower stimulation thresholds than dorsal column fibers (Coburn, 1985). Moreover, the name 'dorsal column stimulation' has been proven physiologically simplistic. Despite the fact that the distance between electrodes and dorsal root fibers is higher compared to the dorsal column fibers, the activation threshold is predicted to be lower. Therefore, a correct position of the lead in the radiological midline is essential to prevent dorsal roots excitation. Several factors have been demonstrated to contribute to lower dorsal root activation threshold, including the curved shape and larger fiber diameter of dorsal root fibers. Dorsal root fibers are activated in the dorsal root entry zone (DREZ), where fibers enter the dorsal horn, because of its lowest activation threshold. Electrical activation of large fiber afferents in the dorsal root or dorsal column by configuration of cathodal and anodal contacts cause a tingling sensation, called paresthesia. Large fiber afferents are activated during stimulation within the usage range and can subsequently 'close the gate'. Excitation of dorsal root afferent fibers produces paresthesias in a few dermatomas, as only rootlets in close proximity of the cathode will be activated. Stimulation of one afferent Aβ fiber may elicit paresthesia in the whole corresponding dermatoma. Lemniscal dorsal column fiber stimulation generates an extensive area of paresthesia coverage, because all dorsal column fibers below the level of the electrode may potentially be activated. A prerequisite for effective pain management is to direct generated paresthesias to cover the whole painful area, which is often difficult to achieve because optimal lead positioning remains difficult. Several empirical and theoretical computer modeling studies were performed in order to obtain a more thorough understanding of factors determining optimal lead positioning (Law & Miller 1982; Coburn 1985). Holsheimer and collegues investigated whether the geometry of a rostrocaudal array of electrode contacts and contract combination changes the stimulation threshold ratio of dorsal column and dorsal root fibers. Monopolor stimulation with a large cathode favors activation of dorsal root fibers. Preferential activation of dorsal column fibers is effectuated by tripolar stimulation with small contacts and small contact spacings. The problem of optimal lead positioning can be solved by increasing the number of electrode contacts, which increases contact points and anode-cathode combinations and therefore the probability for generating effective paresthesias. The leads are positioned a few segments rostral to the level of where target dorsal roots enter the spinal cord (Barolat et al., 1991). Furthermore, several anatomical and technical factors have been described to determine the topographical area of induced paresthesias, including; pulse width, pulse amplitude, nerve fiber diameter, electrode-spinal cord distance, anode-cathode combination. Empirical studies showed that incomplete paresthesia coverage of the painful area can be compensated by increasing pulse width as the pulse amplitude extends caudally with increasing pulse width (Holsheimer et al., 2011). The therapeutic range of spinal cord stimulation is between the perception threshold (PT) and discomfort threshold (DT) (*figure 1*). The perception threshold is defined as the lowest stimulus amplitude needed to elicit paresthesia. The discomfort threshold is defined as the stimulation amplitude above which paresthesia become unendurable. DT is generally reached at a mean stimulus amplitude of 40-60% above perception threshold. The PT for eliciting paresthesia is related to the activation of dorsal root fibers, indicated by the observation of progressively decreased PT as the electrode deviates from the midline (Barolat et al., 1991). At cervical and low thoracic level it may occur that some dorsal column fibers are activated when the electrode-to-spinal distance is less than 2 mm. At mid-thoracic level (T4-T7) the electrode-to-spinal distance is largest in most patients. Therefore, it is unlikely that dorsal column fibers are stimulated within the therapeutic range, whereas paresthesiae get a segmentary distribution (Holsheimer & Wesselink, 1997). It is well known that the range of stimulation amplitude between PT and DT is narrow and therefore stimulation results regularly in incomplete paresthesia coverage of the painful area. Only large fiber afferents in the dorsal column and dorsal roots are activated during SCS at voltages within the therapeutic range. In the dorsal column only superficially oriented fibers (0.20-0.25mm depth) with a diameter > 9.4 μm are activated during SCS (Holzheimer, 2002). The mean diameter of large afferents in the dorsal root is 15μm. As voltage is increased to approximate DT, smaller fibers (±12μm) are excitated as well. These proprioceptive fibers elicit segmental motor effects and uncomfortable sensations, which is a major drawback of dorsal root stimulation. This prevents stimulation amplitude from being increased in order to recruit more dorsal column fibers. To increase SCS efficacy, recruitment of dorsal column fibers is maximized as it generally results in a broad paresthesia coverage of the painful area which is the main goal of SCS. Despite the fact that SCS techniques developed enormously over the past decennia, there are some major drawbacks in the application of SCS that needs to be solved (Holsheimer et al., 1997). Computer modeling provides a considerable contribution in

Compartment		Conductivity (S m^{-1})
Cerebrospinal fluid		1.7
White matter	(longitudinal)	0.60
	(transversal)	0.083
Grey matter		0.23
Epidural fat		0.04
Vertebral bone		0.04
Dura mater		0.03
Surrounding layer		0.004
Electrode insulation		0.001

Table 1. Conductivity of intraspinal structures. *Modified from [Holsheimer et al., 1995]*

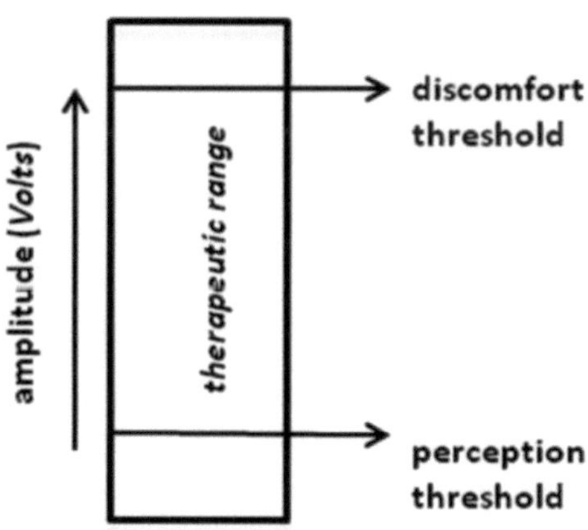

Fig. 1. Therapeutic range in Spinal Cord Stimulation

knowledge of the physiological effects of spinal cord stimulation. Most clinical phenomena observed in spinal cord stimulation are predicted by computer modeling studies, which emphasizes its usefulness. Because of the large intersubject variation in anatomical characteristics, a computer model remains a simplification of reality. Conclusions drawn from these studies needs to be questioned for their clinical relevance (Holsheimer et al., 1997). Close interdisciplinary collaboration is warranted in order to direct future research and provide a better understanding of the effects of electrical stimulation on spinal nerve fibers.

2.3 Animal models

At the time of the introduction of spinal cord stimulation in clinical medicine, insights in possible underlying mechanisms of action were sparse. Initially, there seemed to be little interest in the research community to explore the biological basis of the possible modulatory effects of SCS on neuropathic pain. In the beginning of the 1970s some first attempts were made in laboratories to explore the pathophysiological mechanisms of pain in animals. These studies concentrated on the acute behavioral and electrophysiological responses to a short-lived nociceptive (thermal or mechanical) stimulus. Clinical pain syndromes are mostly characterized by spontaneous pain and a hyperesthetic state (e.g. hyperalgesia and allodynia). Therefore, clinical relevancy of behavioral studies of intact animals subjected to acute nociceptive pain is questionable. Simultaneously, the first preclinical studies aimed at the elucidation of the effector mechanism of spinal cord stimulation appeared (Handwerker et al., 1975). The main shortcoming of these studies is that they used healthy anesthetized animals and applied only acute and noxious stimuli. Furthermore, spinal cord stimulation was only shortly applied at high current intensities which cannot be used clinically on conscious patients. Although these experiments are of limited clinical relevance, they gave direction to the design of more appropriate experiments. Of major importance was the recognition of distinct pathophysiological mechanisms elicited by peripheral nerve injury, which differed from that generated by an acute noxious stimulus (Wall & Gutnick, 1974). These findings were followed by numerous attempts to develop a preclinical neuropathic pain model, in which clinical pain states should adequately be mimicked. Since then, many animal models of peripheral nerve injury (trauma, disease, metabolic disorders, and toxins) have been described in literature. Until the chronic constriction model of Bennett was presented in 1988, none of them reported to produce disorders of pain sensations like those that accompany peripheral neuropathies in humans. The inability to produce these sensory disorders in laboratory animals has been a major obstacle to the experimental analysis of the problem (Bennett & Xie, 1988). In addition, the neuroma model, in which a peripheral nerve is transected completely, showed a limited spectrum of somatosensory disorders normally accompanying neuropathies. In particular hyperalgesia and allodynia were not seen after complete deafferentation and neuroma formation. Furthermore, high incidences of autonomy or self-mutilation were reported for rats with complete transections of the sciatic nerve (Wall et al., 1979; Sweet 1981). Bennett developed a model wherein painful peripheral mononeuropathy was produced by placing loosely tied constrictive ligatures around the common sciatic nerve (Bennett, 1988). A few years later, Selzer presented a slightly different behavioral model of neuropathic pain disorders in rats by a tight ligation of a part of the sciatic nerve (Selzer et al., 1990). Kim and Chung ligated an entire spinal segmental nerve in their experimental model for peripheral neuropathy (Kim & Chung, 1992). Decosterd and Woolf presented the 'spared nerve injury model' which comprises a partial lesion of the sciatic nerve as only the tibial and common peroneal nerves are ligated, leaving the remaining sural nerve intact (Decosterd & Woolf, 2000). This model differs from the previously mentioned preclinical neuropathic pain models as it allows behavioral testing of intact cutaneous areas adjacent to injured denervated regions (Decosterd & Woolf, 2000). In addition to these three extensively used models (the Bennett chronic constriction injury model, the Selzer partial sciatic nerve ligation model and the Chung spinal nerve ligation model), other animal models based on photochemically induced ischaemia in the spinal cord have been described (Watson et al., 1986; Hao et al., 1991; Gazelius et al., 1996). All preclinical pain models have been developed in order to mimick clinical pain states in humans as closely as possible. It was not until 1994 when a research group from the Karolinska Institute concentrated on the effects of spinal cord stimulation on neuropathic pain (Meyerson et al., 1994). They produced experimental models of neuropathic pain as described by Bennett and Selzer, implanted miniaturized electrodes in the awake animals and monitored the effects of stimulation during evoked pain (Bennett & Xie, 1988; Selzer et al., 1991; Meyerson et al., 1994). They applied SCS acutely of chronically with stimulation parameters similar to those used in patients. Since then, only a few experiments focused on the effects of spinal cords stimulation in patients.

From 'bench to bedside'. In general, preclinical pain models use a withdrawal response to noxious or innoculous stimulations as behavioral endpoint. In contrary, the numeric rating pain scale (NRS) or visual analog score (VAS) is commonly used in clinical research. This discrepancy makes results from preclinical studies difficult to interpreter, as different pain assessment methods focus on different aspects of pain (Mao, 2002). It is important to recognize the restraints of basic research as they can provide in guidelines for the development of clinically relevant studies. Translational pain research comprises a two-way direction. Equitably important as the translation from 'bench to bedside' is the translation from 'bedside to bench'. Guarantying a correct initial translation from 'bedside to bench' makes meaningful translation from 'bench to bedside' possible. Mao described some examples of structural weaknesses in the interpretation of results obtained in preclinical experiments, commonly incorrect generalized to prove their clinical relevancy (Mao, 2002). For example, chronic pain conditions are commonly characterized by the existence of spontaneous pain which is present without obvious stimulation. Prevention of thermal of mechanical stimuli is not sufficient to alleviate this pain. In the clinical setting, thermal stimulation is rarely followed by a persistent pain condition. A persistent pain condition is generally assessed in animal models using stimulus-induced nociception such as thermal hyperalgesia. Clinical significance of these unfiltered results obtained in animal models is doubtful, as thermal hyperalgesia is rarely present in the clinical setting. Furthermore, the understanding of how a chronic pain condition develops after a transient tissue injury is poor. For years clinicians are struggling to explain this phenomenon of central sensitization. In basic research most experiments focused on cellular and molecular changes shortly after nerve injury or inflammation. These observed changes during the early phase are thought to play a key role in explaining pathophysiological mechanisms in persistent pain states. However this is not necessarily true. Moreover, most observed cellular and molecular changes disappear before pain-like behavior does (Mao, 2002). It is important to acknowledge translation pain research as an essential contributor to increase the effectiveness and relevance of both preclinical and clinical research and for determining future research direction. Furthermore, there needs to be more attention for interaction between basic researchers and clinicians.

2.4 Neurophysiological mechanisms

The well-known Gate Control Theory (GCT) was proposed by Melzack and Wall in 1965 (*figure* 2). The theory describes in an elegant and concise way, that activation of afferent Aβ fibers attenuates spinal pain transmission (Melzack & Wall, 1965). The GCT hypothesizes that an excess of small fiber activity would 'open' and an excess of large fiber activity would 'close' the 'gate'. Moreover, large fibers have a lower activation threshold than small fibers for depolarization by an electrical field and they may be stimulated selectively. The GCT provided a framework for examining the interactions between local and distant excitatory and inhibitory systems in the dorsal horn (Dickenson, 2002). As formerly mentioned, spinal cord stimulation is actually a clinical outgrowth of the gate control theory. The exact mechanisms of spinal cord stimulation are still largely unknown, but the supposed mechanisms of actions are still predominantly described in these 'gating terms'. One would expect, based on the GCT, that spinal cord stimulation could alleviate nociceptive forms of pain. However, despite a few reports it is still very controversial whether spinal cord stimulation directly attenuates nociceptive pain components. Moreover, spinal cord stimulation is clinically most often administrated in specific neuropathic pain conditions. Flexion reflex thresholds of the lower limbs (RIII responses) has been reported to be lowered in neuropathic pain patients, which is in agreement with former experimental findings in rats (Garcia-Larrea et al., 1989). They also showed a close relationship between the threshold of flexor responses (RIII) and the subjective sensation of pain. Spinal cord stimulation induced an increase of these abnormally lowered withdrawal thresholds, which are mediated through alpha and beta fibers. These observations suggests SCS predominantly affects pain related to abnormal Aβ fiber function, as in allodynia (Handwerker et al., 1975; Carstens & Campbell, 1988; Garcia-Larrea et al., 1989; Meyerson et al., 1995; Oakley & Prager, 2002). Repetitive noxious stimulation of primary afferent fibers after peripheral nerve injury induces long-term changes of the excitability of spinal cord neurons (Rygh et al., 1999). These plastic neural changes involve increased spontaneous and evoked firing rate of wide dynamic range (WDR) neurons in the dorsal horn and contribute to the development of chronic pain. SCS may effectuate a normalization of the hyperexcitability of these wide dynamic range cells in de dorsal horn in response to innocuous stimuli (Yakhnitsa et al., 1999). Therefore, wide dynamic range neurons in the dorsal horn are thought to play a key role in spinal pain transmission and may play the integrative role of the 'transmission' (T) cells as described in the GCT (*figure* 2) (Woolf & Salter, 2000; Guan et al., 2006; Cervero, 2009; Guan et al., 2010). Since the 70's multiple studies suggested that the mechanisms of action of SCS could not solely be explained by interactions of neurons located in the dorsal horn and postulated the existence of supra spinal loops (Nyguist & Greenhoot, 1973; Bantli et al., 1975). In a series of studies Saadé and colleagues demonstrated the contribution of brainstem pain-modulating centres in inhibiting nociceptive processing (Saadé et al., 1985; Saadé et al., 1990; Saadé et al., 1999; El-Khoury et al., 2002). Roberts and Rees have shown that SCS in animals activates the anterior pretectal nucleus, which has descending pain inhibitory influences on lower segments (Roberts & Rees, 1994). Furthermore, SCS produces increased activity in the somatosensory cortex (SI and SII areas) and cingulated gyri. These brain areas activated by spinal cord stimulation correspond to pain pathways involved in processing of somatosensory (SI, SII) and affective components (cingulate gyri) of pain. Hence, during SCS both segmental and supraspinal (spinal-brainstem-spinal loops and thalamocortical systems) pathways are activated and contribute to the inhibition of neuropathic manifestations.

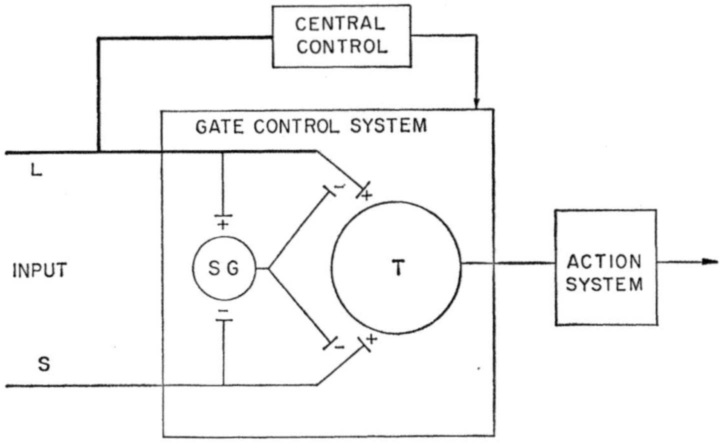

Fig. 2. **The Gate Control Theory**. Central transmission cell (T) cells, located in the dorsal horn of the spinal cord, receive a balanced input of large (Aβ) and small (Aδ and C) fiber activity in peripheral nerves. Inhibitory interneurons, located in the substantia gelatinosa (SG), can be activated by large (L) afferents and can modulate pain transmission via projection to small (S) fibers and central transmission cells. (Melzack & Wall, 1965).

2.5 Neurochemistry

Generally, patients use spinal cord stimulation intermittently to alleviate neuropathic pain. It is remarkable that pain-relieving activity continues for several hours after spinal cord stimulation has been switched off. These long-term effects are supposed to result from modulation of neural activity including neurotransmitter systems at the dorsal horn or supra-spinal levels. Little is known about which transmitter systems have a pivotal role in the pain-relieving effects of SCS in neuropathic pain. Only a few human studies have been performed and current knowledge is mainly based on data obtained from animal experiments. As previously mentioned, Meyerson described a suitable animal model comprising sciatic nerve injury and tactile allodynia for evaluating the mechanisms of SCS as treatment modality for neuropathic pain (Meyerson, 1994). Most of these experiments used a microdialysis technique in order to obtain fluid samples during SCS from areas involved. These microsamples have provided some insight into neurochemical mechanisms at the synaps level (Stiller et al., 1996; Oakley & Prager, 2002). There is evidence that substance-P (SP) and serotonin (5-HT) have a inhibitory role in nociceptive transmission in the spinal cord and recently the existence of a descending serotonergic pathways has been suggested (Song et al., 2009). There is evidence that a descending noradrenergic system is involved as well. Analysis of CSF dialysates in decerebrated and intact adult cats showed an elevation of the level of SP and 5-HT during SCS (Linderoth et al., 1992) (table 2). Whether these substances actually participate in the pain modulating effects of SCS in chronic neuropathic pain remains unclear, because most experimental studies investigated intact animals. Several behavioral studies appeared, aimed at elucidating the role of amino acids in exerting pain alleviation during SCS. The main inhibitory neurotransmitter in the central nervous system is gamma amino butyric acid (GABA). Preclinical neuropathic pain studies showed that GABA levels in the dorsal spinal cord of animals with allodynia are significantly lower in animals than GABA levels in nonallodynic nerve-lesioned and intact animals. It has been suggested that reduced GABA levels might result in hyperexcitability of other neurons involved in processing nociceptive information, in particular 'wide dynamic range' neurons. Experimental studies showed an increased release of GABA during spinal cord stimulation (table 2). Strikingly, increased GABA release was only observed in the so-called 'responders', the rats who showed behavior befitting symptom alleviation during SCS (Stiller et al., 1996). Thus, SCS normalized withdrawal response thresholds in these 'responders' by restoring normal GABA levels. This increased GABA release could be important for the suppression of tactile allodynia in humans. Similar mechanisms could also be involved in the SCS-induced alleviation of pain in patients with peripheral neuropathies (Stiller et al., 1996). In the 'non-responders' group, the rats who did not show behavior indicating symptom alleviation, they did not observe an increased GABA release. In these studies, alleviation of allodynia was defined as a significant increase in withdrawal threshold in response to innocuous stimulation using von Frey filaments administrated to the nerve-injured hindpaw. Cui et al. investigated mononeuropathic animals with allodynia, that did not respond to SCS (Cui et al., 1996). They showed that after intrathecal injection of baclofen, a $GABA_B$ receptor agonist, the animals showed increased withdrawal thresholds and thus potentiated the effect of SCS on allodynia. Actually, 'non-responders' transformed into 'responders' by manipulation of the GABA receptor with subclinical doses of baclofen. Furthermore, the administration of muscimol, a $GABA_A$ agonist, resulted in a significant but less obvious increase in withdrawal threshold (Cui et al., 1996). The action of $GABA_A$ and $GABA_B$ antagonists were also evaluated during the application of SCS. After the administration of a $GABA_B$ antagonist, 5-aminovalericacid (5-AVA), a significant reduction of the increased withdrawal threshold was observed during SCS. The intrathecal administration of the $GABA_A$ antagonist bicuculline had no significant effect. Thus, in particular the $GABA_B$-receptor system is likely to be linked to the effects of SCS. Allodynia and hyperalgesia characterizes peripheral hypersensitivity which in fact reflects underlying disturbances in GABA-mediated inhibition and increased levels of excitatory amino acids (Woolf & Doubell et al., 1994). The prime excitatory neurotransmitters, glutamate and aspartate, have a pivotal role in transmission of nociceptive information (table 2). Dorsal horn concentrations of excitatory amino acids have been shown to decrease during SCS, concurrently with antiallodynic effects (Cui et al., 1997). When a $GABA_B$ antagonist was administrated, the SCS-induced reduction of excitatory amino acids was abolished. Thus, SCS might exert its pain reducing effects, at least partially due to activation of GABAergic mechanisms which inhibit the release of excitatory amino acids which are already elevated in neuropathic pain conditions (Cui et al., 1997). Intravenous or intrathecal administration of the central neuromodulator adenosine seems to have potentiating effects comparable with selective $GABA_B$ agonists (e.g. baclofen). Therefore SCS is thought to exert its analgesic action by both $GABA_B$ and adenosine dependent systems (adenosine A-1 receptor). Some studies have showed that the cholinergic system is likely to be involved as well (table 2) (Schechtmann et al., 2004; Schechtmann et al., 2008). Subclinical intrathecal doses of clonidine enhanced the effect of SCS on tactile hypersensitivity in an animal model of neuropathic pain, when solitary SCS appeared to be ineffective. A synergistic effect was observed when electrical nerve stimulation and pharmacotherapy were combined. The way in which clonidine exerts its analgesic action is not fully understood. Clonidine, an $\alpha 2$-adrenoreceptor agonist, is thought to increase dorsal horn acetylcholine release and nitric oxide synthesis (Xu et al., 2000). Intrathecal administration of a selective muscarinic M_4 receptor antagonist completely abolished the analgesic action of SCS. Endogenous opioids are not likely to have a significant contribution to the pain alleviating effects of spinal cord stimulation (Linderoth & Foreman, 1999). Most convincing evidence is that effects of SCS are not blocked by the administration of naloxone, which is an opioid receptor antagonist. There are investigators who keep the door open for a potential role of the dynorphin system exerting its effect primarily through the κ-opioid receptor, which has a lower affinity for naloxone (Han et al., 1991). As already mentioned, most knowledge concerning neurochemistry is derived from animal experiments and its clinical significance needs to be explored. However, up to 40% of well selected neuropathic pain patients do not experience significant pain amelioration during SCS. Hence, adjunct pharmacological therapy can provide a major contribution in increasing efficacy of the application of SCS. Lind et al. illustrated the administration of intrathecal baclofen in patients increasing the effects of SCS in neuropathic pain of peripheral origin. These patients initially responded poorly to SCS however they experienced a satisfactory relief during SCS (Lind et al., 2004, Lind et al., 2008). A promising observation was that follow- up obviously demonstrated a sustained pain relieving effect. Most experiments have focused on segmental changes in transmitter systems (e.g. excitatory amino acids, adenosine) to explain the mode of action of SCS. However, 5-HT and noradrenalin might involve supra-spinal circuits and descending inhibitory pathways. The degree of contribution of descending inhibitory pathways compared to segmental mechanisms is currently under debate (Song et al., 2009).

Spinal transmitter	Influence of SCS
GABA	Increased
Serotonin (5-HT)	Increased
Substance-P (SP)	Increased
Norepinephrine	Increased
Acetylcholine (Ach)	Increased
Adenosine	Increased
Glutamate	Decreased
Asparate	Decreased

Table 2. Spinal transmitters possibly involved in alleviating neuropathic pain during Spinal Cord Stimulation (SCS). SCS may result in a decreased of increased release of a particular transmitter.

3. Spinal cord stimulators

3.1 Introduction

Shortly after the gate control theory was proposed by Melzack and Wall, pain research focused attention on the dorsal column as a target for pain management. First reports described they used a anesthetic needle, which was placed in the cerebrospinal fluid at the level of target nerve roots (Melzack & Wall, 1996). An electrode was advanced through the needle and positioned along the dorsal column. Patients experienced significant pain relief during short periods of gentle electrical stimulation (Wall & Sweet, 1967). After realizing electrical stimulation in the close proximity of sensory roots can alleviate chronic pain, more radical procedures were developed in order to allow chronic stimulation of the dorsal column (Shealy et al., 1967a). Shealy and colleagues first investigated the efficacy of dorsal column stimulation in cats in which electrodes were placed by cervical laminectomy. Shortly thereafter they reported the abolition of intractable pain in a patient suffering inoperable bronchiogenic carcinoma by electrical stimulation of the dorsal columns of the thoracic spinal cord (Shealy et al., 1967b). They placed an intradural electrode dorsal to the spinal cord. The circuit design was based on a modified Medtronic device (Medtronic, Inc, Minneapolis, MN, USA) for the stimulation of the carotid sinus to control angina and hypertension (Govolac, 2010). These procedures comprises major surgical interventions which were often complicated with equipment failure (lead breakage), cerebrospinal fluid leakage or infection. Furthermore, experienced pain relief appeared to be transient. These radicular methods of dorsal column stimulation were replaced in the mid 70's with percutaneously implantable flexible electrodes (Erickson, 1975). A 17G thin-walled Tuohy spinal needle allowed leads to be inserted in the spinal cord and positioned close to the dorsal columns. The development of percutaneous inserted flexible leads allowed a trial of stimulation which mimicks that of the permanent implantable device. During trial stimulation, candidate suitability for permanent implantation is determined. However, the technique of inserting electrodes into the spinal cord seemed inherent to several complications including spinal fluid leaks, postdural punction headache and infection (bacterial meningitis) (Erickson, 1975). It was realized that permanent implantation of stimulators over the dorsum of the spinal cord under the dura will ultimately fail (Cook, 1976). The technique of epidural electrode placement evolved, as complications like those seen after sub- or intradural electrode implantation, were less likely to occur.

3.2 Devices

Spinal cord stimulation systems consist of; trial or permanent (plate) electrodes, implantable pulse generators or radiofrequency (RF)-driven passive drivers. SCS systems have been produced by multiple manufactures; including Medtronic, Cordis, Advanced Neuromodulation Systems, and Boston Scientific. Initially, SCS systems used unipolar electrodes to deliver stimulation. Radiofrequency (RF)-driven passive drivers were nonprogrammable and could not be implantated. Because of the private industry contributions to the development of neuromodulatory systems, equipment improved enormously over the last 40 years. Moreover, progressive advances in cardiac pacemaker technology were utilized in the design and technology of the implantable pulse generators (IPG). Nowadays, systems are composed of complex electrodes arrays, and a implantable pulse generator (IPG) or radiofrequency (RF)-driven radio receiver. The basic goal of these connected components is to provide an isolated electrical pathway to the neural structures being activated. Several electrodes, either percutaneous or plate, with octapolar or even up to 16 electrodes are available. Contact spacing and contact points vary according to the therapeutic goal (e.g quadripolar electrodes for limb pain and octopolar electrodes for axial pain). Furthermore, multi-programmable and even rechargeable power units are available. Plate electrodes are implanted permanently and requires an open procedure and direct visualization for implantation. In the first phase of spinal cord stimulation, laminectomy was required to insert plate electrodes. Over the last years, thinner and more flexible plate electrodes were developed allowing insertion via smaller laminotomy.

3.3 Anesthetic management

Anesthetic management of spinal cord implantation comprises general anesthesia or local anesthetic techniques if necessary combined with sedation. When the procedure is performed using general anesthesia, it is difficult for the clinician to achieve optimal lead positioning. The clinician has to rely on radiographic positioning of the electrodes and/or somatosensory evoked potentials (SSEP). Moreover, it is difficult to assess whether uncomfortable motor effects occur during stimulation. It is well known that dermatomal coverage of paresthesia is a prerequisite for successful treatment, which is impossible to determine when a patient is anesthetized. In order to obtain immediate feedback of patients there are two options remaining; the electrodes are implanted using local anesthetic techniques (in combination with short acting sedatives), or waking up anesthetized patients in between. During the test phase the patient has to be alert and fully cooperative. Local anesthetics are used liberally in order to reduce the need for sedatives (propofol, benzodiazepines) and optimize patient comfort (Barolat & Sharan, 2004).

3.4 Spinal cord stimulator implantation

3.4.1 Percutaneous techniques

First of all it is important to emphasize the whole procedure of electrode placement is a sterile technique. Infection is potentially hazardous and requires re-operation and/or intravenous antibiotic therapy. Percutaneous placement is performed with the patient in prone position on a X-ray-compatible table with some pillows under the abdomen in order to create a kyphosis which facilitates electrode implantation. Prone position combined with sedation may complicate airway management. Some clinicians prefer the lateral decubitus position as it facilitates subcutaneous implantation of the pulse generator in de buttock or lateral abdominal wall. Moreover, positioning is important as rotation of the spine increases difficulty of electrode placement (Barolat & Sharan, 2004). The electrodes are placed under fluoroscopy guidance to allow anteroposterior and lateral views to ensure midline lead placement and appropriate entry into the epidural space. The insertion point of a 17G Tuohy needle is usually in the midline, although a paramedian approach may also be employed. Several methods have been used to identify the epidural space. Most clinicians use the loss-of-resistance technique. This technique comprises the use of a syringe filled with saline or air. When the needle is advanced through the ligamentum flavum, a sudden absence of resistance to injection is felt. There is no consensus as whether air or a liquid should be used for identifying the epidural space when using the loss-of-resistance technique. It has been hypothesized that the use of liquid expands the epidural space and therefore predisposes to lead migration. Furthermore, liquid flush may attenuate the uniformity of paresthesias (Brook et al., 2009). Alternative approaches to needle placement have been described as in specific circumstances (e.g congenital underdeveloped ligamentum flavum or defects of the ligamentum flavum after spinal surgery) the loss-of-resistance technique seems inappropriate. In these conditions identification of the epidural space using the loss-of-resistance technique is potentially difficult, because the level of resistance is unclear and the risk of false loss is present (Zhu et al., 2011). Zhu and colleagues described an approach for percutaneous lead placement which relies on lateral views of fluoroscopic landmarks to confirm when the needle tip enters the epidural space. When the epidural space is identified, electrodes are advanced rostrally under patient feedback in order to optimize their position. The lead is inserted at least a few centimeters into the epidural space to ascertain its position and prevent migration of the lead. After lead placement it is important to confirm its position in the epidural space as accidental subarachnoidal placement have been described in literature. Implantation of cervical electrodes is advisable below the cervical spine enlargement which extends from about C3 to Th2. For treatment of back and lower limb pain, identification of the epidural space at the level of Th12-L1, L1-2, or L2-3 is preferred (*figure 3*). Electrode insertion for upper extremity pain is recommended at the level of Th1-2 or Th2-3 (Barolat & Sharan, 2004; Brook et al., 2009). When optimal lead position is ascertained, for permanent stimulation the leads are anchored and sutured internally. Leads may then be tunneled subcutaneously a few centimeter laterally to the flank, where they may be externalized for trial stimulation or connected to an implanted pulse generator (*figure 3*) (North et al., 1977). The definite placement of a spinal cord stimulator is preceded by a trial stimulation phase of approximately 7 days. The introduction of a test phase and thorough preoperative screening increased success rates of the procedure. After the trial period, the patient will be asked whether the elicited paresthesias were effective in reducing the pain they experienced before the trial phase. A permanent system is implanted if trial stimulation reduces the patient's pain by more than 50%.

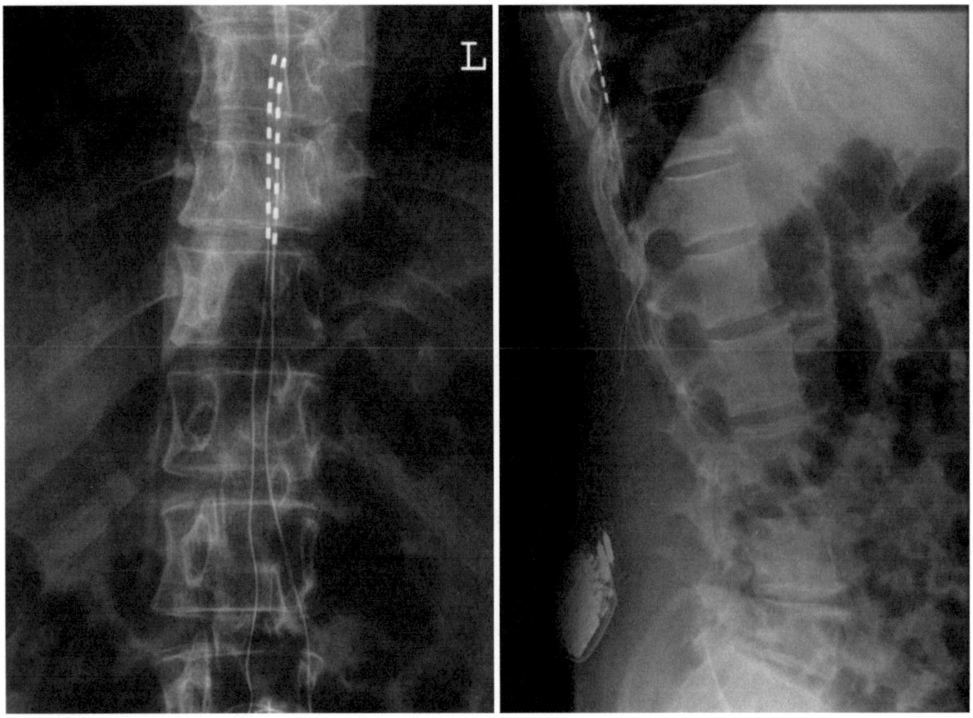

Fig. 3. Percutaneously inserted epidural electrodes including pulse generator

3.4.2 Surgical techniques

Most spinal cord leads are inserted percutaneously, as the technique is easier, less-invasive, and less-expensive compared to surgical methods. However, surgical lead placement may become a necessity when patients anatomy prevents leads from being implanted percutaneously; when lead breakage or dislodgement repeatedly requires lead revision; or when trial stimulation of percutaneous leads cannot suffice in adequate paresthesia coverage (Kumar et al., 2009). Surgical techniques comprises electrode positioning under direct vision, after a small laminotomy is performed. Under fluoroscopic guidance the plate electrode is introduced into the epidural space. Laminotomy, up to Th8-Th9, can be performed using spinal anesthesia (Lind et al., 2003). Moreover, during spinal anesthesia not all sensory transmission is blocked which enables intraoperative testing for proper lead positioning. However, laminotomy is generally performed using general anesthesia whereupon accurate lead positioning relies on radiographic imaging, somatosensory evoked potentials or patients feedback by waking them up in between. After paresthesia in elicited in the anatomic distribution of the patient's pain, a strain relief loop is placed in the epifascial plane and the lead is anchored (Kumar et al., 2009). There are some advantages of surgical leads compared to percutaneous leads; higher success rates (up to 80-90%); less long-term migration rates; and better long term survival have been described (Villavicencio et al., 2000; North et al., 2002). It has been suggested that increased effectiveness of stimulation and therefore higher success rates can be explained by the large sized plate electrodes which causes compression of the cerebrospinal fluid space and bringing electrodes into closer contact to the dorsal column of the spinal cord.

4. Clinical application of SCS in neuropathic pain syndromes

Neuropathic pain is often underdiagnosed and mistreated. Chronic neuropathic pain is regularly unresponsive to pharmacological and conventional treatment. Therefore, more treatment strategies such as neurostimulation techniques were assessed for efficacy in relieving neuropathic pain. Despite clear evidence for its efficacy was lacking, neurostimulation techniques were increasingly used by clinicians in a variety of neuropathic pain syndromes. The last decennia several studies appeared to provide comprehensive evidence for efficacy of SCS in specific neuropathic pain syndromes. An important development was the introduction of trial stimulation period. During a trial stimulation period the numeric rating pain scale (NRS) or visual analog score (VAS) can be used to document patients pain ratings. A trial period is considered to be successful when patient-reported pain relief was at least 50% at rest and during physical activity. Furthermore, patient satisfaction and potential reduction in analgesic consumption could be assessed. The most common painful neuropathies (Failed Back Surgery Syndrome and CRPS type I and II) for which SCS is clinically used will be discussed.

4.1 SCS for failed back surgery syndrome

Low back pain patients that fail to improve after (repeated) surgery are most commonly referred to as having 'failed back surgery syndrome'. Studies showed 10-40% of patients who underwent lumbosacral spinal surgery in order to alleviate neuropathic radicular pain experience persistent or recurrent pain. FBSS is thought to be an inaccurate term (Slipman et al., 2002). FBSS comprises a diverse group of disorders in which pain symptoms persists or recurs after lumbar surgery (Slipman et al., 2002). The etiology of FBSS is complex and encompasses multiple possible explanatory etiologies, which can be classified as surgical (e.g internal disc disruption, canal stenosis, epidural fibrosis) or non-surgical (e.g radiculopathy, degenerative disc, Facet syndrome). Pain in FBSS is most commonly considered to be of neuropathic origin. However, several studies showed that neuropathic and nociceptive pain are often concurrently present in FBSS patients and it is difficult to isolate the neuropathic component. The armamentarium of clinicians comprises pharmacological, physical, psychological and interventional techniques. In many FBSS patients pharmacological treatment is insufficient and the efficacy of interventional techniques is only modest. Neuropathic pain in the Failed Back Surgery Syndrome (FBSS) is the most common indication for the administration of SCS. Turner et al were the first to present a systematic literature synthesis to analyze the long-term risks and benefits of spinal cord stimulation for patients with failed back surgery syndrome (Turner et al., 1995). They concluded that approximately 50 to 60% of FBSS experienced a clinically significant pain relief of more than 50% during SCS treatment at long-term (mean, 16 months; range, 1-45 months) follow-up visits. Furthermore, North et al. presented some evidence in favor of SCS in relieving neuropathic pain compared to reoperation for FBSS, although results did not reach significance (North et al., 1994). SCS provides significant increased pain alleviation compared to conventional treatment when administrated in carefully selected FBSS patients suffering neuropathic pain. Furthermore, SCS provides improved functional status and quality of life (Kumar et al., 2007). It appears that SCS diminishes continuous and evoked pain (in particular tactile/thermal allodynia), while acute nociceptive pain is unaffected (Mailis-Gagnon et al., 2007). According to EFNS (European Federation of Neurological Societies) guidelines there is evidence that SCS is efficacious for failed back surgery syndrome (FBSS) (grade B recommendation) (Cruccu et al, 2007). The indicated evidence is Level II-1 or II-2 for long-term relief in managing patients with failed back surgery syndrome (Frey et al., 2009). However, a Cochrane review published in 2004 concluded there is limited evidence for the effectiveness of SCS in FBSS (and CRPS type I) and stated that more randomized clinical trial are needed to determine the effectiveness of SCS in specific neuropathic pain syndromes (Mailis-Gagnon et al., 2004).

4.2 SCS for complex regional pain syndrome

Evan introduced the name reflex sympathetic dystrophia (RSD) in 1946, formerly known as causalgia in the 19th century. Synonyms for RSD include; Sudeck's atrophy, posttraumatic pain syndrome, painful posttraumatic dystrophy, algodystrophia and algoneurodystrophia (Albazaz et al., 2008). RSD did not correctly reflected the symptoms the syndrome comprises and it assumes involvement of a sympathetically maintained reflex arc, which is controversial. Therefore, it was replaced with the name Complex Regional Pain Syndrome (CRPS) by the International Association for the Study of Pain (IASP). Symptoms and signs includes sensory, motor, autonomic dysfunction and trophic changes. CRPS can be divided into two categories: Type 1 (RSD), in which there is no evident nerve trunk injury but all the clinical features are present. Type 2 (causalgia), in which nerve trunk injury can be demonstrated. Additional differentiation is the distinction of 'sympathetically maintained pain syndrome' (SMPS) and 'sympathetically independent pain syndromes' (SIPS), based on the role of the sympathetic nerve system. SMPS is characterized by an augmented activity of the sympathetic nerve system which maintains neuropathic pain. SMPS can be differentiated from SIPS by the observation of pain alleviation following blockage of the sympathetic outflow tract. Several other factors, psychological, viral infections, peripheral nerve injury and systemic neuropathic processes, are important in maintaining neuropathic pain in SIPS. In 10% of the patients, possible maintaining factors remain unclear. CRPS is characterized by a minor injury (trauma of surgery) followed by severe pains which are disproportionate compared to the inciting event. The IASP developed explicit criteria to facilitate and demarcate the complex diagnosis of CRPS. However, the clinical diagnosis of CRPS remains difficult and is mainly based on the combination of a suggestive history and thorough physical examination. The pathophysiology of CRPS is largely unknown. Increased regional sympathetic tone was initially suggested to be of major importance in clarifying pathophysiological mechanisms. However, several alternative hypotheses have been presented based on current evidence. There is growing evidence that pathophysiological mechanisms of CRPS I are sited in central pathways, which is probably illustrated best by the presence of myoclonic activity (Sandroni et al., 1998). One hypothesis suggests the existence of a vicious circle, which is initiated by peripheral tissue injury leading to augmented afferent input to the dorsal horn. This increased activity is subsequently followed by increased sympathetic activity, which is thought to maintain augmented input of afferent signals to the dorsal horn. Another hypothesis suggests that activation of peripheral Aδ and C-fibers following tissue injury excites wide dynamic range (WDR) neurons, which subsequently become sensitized to afferent input (Roberts, 1986). Currently, there is no curative treatment for CRPS available. Numerous studies investigated the efficacy of pharmacological treatment (e.g. opioids, nonsteroidal inflammatory drugs, NMDA antagonists, antidepressants, antiepileptics, free radical scavengers and corticosteroids) in CRPS patients. Most pharmacological therapies are used to provide some analgesia during physical therapy, which is generally recommended as first-line treatment. Physical therapy can be helpful for reducing pain and improving active mobility in patients with CRPS I compared to occupational therapy (Oerlemans et al., 1999). Furthermore, several regional anesthesia techniques (e.g sympathetic blockade, sympathectomy) have been investigated. Patients who experience pain reduction after a diagnostic sympathetic blockade may be candidates for regional anesthetic blockade. Although evidence for its effectiveness is lacking, sympathetic blockade (e.g epidural infusion of anesthetics) is an important element in the armamentarium of clinicians. Invasive sympathectomy (chemical, surgical or radiofrequent) can provide long-term sympathetic blockage and long-term pain reduction in significant number of CRPS patients (Bandyk et al., 2002). However, recurrence of pain symptoms, possible due to regeneration of sympathetic chains, have also been described (Bandyk et al., 2002). However, because of its irreversibility and relative high complication rate (e.g. Horner syndrome, compensatory hyperhidrosis) it is generally considered as final therapeutic option. SCS can modulate neuropathic pain pathways and has therefore extensively been investigated for its efficacy in relieving pain in CRPS patients. Several attempts were made trying to elucidate the mechanisms by which SCS provides pain alleviation in CRPS patients. These possible mechanisms have been extensively described in preceding paragraphs. Several studies showed SCS to be effective in alleviating pain in CRPS patients in up to 80% and is a generally accepted treatment modality for CRPS (Bennet & Cameron, 2003; North et al., 2007). Kemler showed SCS in combination with physiotherapy provides a significant alleviation of neuropathic pain in CRPS patients at 6 months and 2 years compared to physiotherapy alone (Kemler et al., 2006). Ongoing research demonstrated SCS is also effective in the treatment of CRPS I in the medium-term. There is some recent evidence it also provides long-term efficacy, high percentages of patient satisfaction and the ability to improve functional status (Kumar et al., 2011). The first years of SCS treatment are more expensive compared to conventional therapies, mainly because of one-time purchasing the costly equipment and conducting a screening period. In life-time analysis showed favorable cost-effectiveness of SCS compared to conventional treatment modalities (Kemler et al, 2002). SCS is a safe, minimally invasive and reversible procedure. A major advantage is the possibility of patient selection during a trial stimulation period, before definite implantation is commenced. The majority of complications that occur are minor and correctable in which infection, lead breakage, battery failure and electrode migration were most common (Bennet & Cameron, 2003; Cameron, 2004). Its advantages compared to invasive sympathectomy are obvious. However, most studies have been retrospective or comprises small-cohorts with a limited follow-up period. There is some evidence in favor of SCS in CRPS type II patients. No firm recommendation can be made because literature comprises only class IV studies (Bennet & Cameron, 2003). Therefore, no clear-cut conclusion can be drawn at present and its application in CRPS I and II patients is still under debate.

4.3 Conclusion

In conclusion, most systematic reviews focused on the efficacy of SCS in failed back surgery syndrome and CRPS I. SCS has a grade B recommendation for administration in FBSS and CRPS I. However, the value of these systematic review is limited because of the heterogeneity of the literature. Several other specific neuropathic syndrome have not been extensively studied and more randomized clinical trials are urgently needed, before the use of SCS can be recommended without question in specific neuropathic pain syndromes. At present it is unclear at which point in treatment SCS must be considered, which patient factors can predict treatment successful and optimal stimulation parameter needs to be explored (Frey et al., 2009).

5. References

Albazaz R, Wong YT & Homer-Vanniasinkam S. Complex regional pain syndrome: a review. *Ann Vasc Surg* 2008;22:297-306

Bandyk DF, Johnson BL, Kirkpatrick AF, Novotney ML, Back MR & Schmacht DC. Surgical sympathectomy for reflex sympathetic dystrophy syndromes. *J Vasc Surg* 2002;35:269-277

Bantli H, Bloedel JR & Thienprasit P. Supraspinal interactions resulting from experimental dorsal column stimulation. *J Neurosurg* 1975;42:296-300

Barolat G, Zeme S, et al. Multifactorial analysis of epidural spinal cord stimulation. *Stereotact Funct Neurosurg* 56:77-103, 1991

Barolat G & Sharan AD. Spinal cord stimulation for chronic pain management. *Seminars in Neurosurgery* 2004;15:151-175

Bennett GJ & Xie YK. A peripheral mononeuropathy in rat produce disorders of pain sensation like those seen in man. *Pain* 1988;33:87-107

Bennett DS & Cameron TL. Spinal cord stimulation for complex regional pain syndromes. In: B.A. Simpson (ed.), *Electrical Stimulation and the Relief of Pain. Pain research and Clinical Management*, Vol 15. Amsterdam: Elsevier, 2003;111-129

Brook AL, Georgy BA, Olan WJ. Spinal Cord Stimulation: a basic approach. *Tech Vasc Interventional Rad* 2009;12:64-70

Buonocore M, Bonezzi C & Barolat G. Neurophysiological evidence of antidromic activation of large myelinated fibres in lower limbs during spinal cord stimulation. *Spine* 2008;33:90–93

Cameron T. Safety and efficacy of spinal cord stimulation for the treatment of chronic pain: a 20-year literature review. *J Neurosurg* 2004;100:254-67

Carstens E & Campbell IG. Parametric and pharmacological studies of midbrain suppression of the hind limb flexion withdrawal reflex in the rat. *Pain* 1988;33:201-213

Cervero F. Spinal cord hyperexcitability and its role in pain and hyperalgesia. *Exp Brain Res* 2009;196:129-137

Chaffee EL & Light RE. A method for remote control of electrical stimulation of the nervous system. *Yale J Biol Med* 1934;7:83-128

Coburn B. A theoretical study of epidural electrical stimulation of the spinal cord - part II: Effect on long myelinated fibers. *IEEE Trans Biomed Eng* 1985;32:978-986

Cook J. Percutaneous Trial for Implantable Stimulating Devices. *J Neurosurg* 1976;44:650-651

Cruccu H, Aziz TZ, et al. EFNS guidelines on neurostimulation therapy for neuropathic pain. *Eur J Neurol* 2007;14:952-70

Cui JG, Linderoth B & Meyerson BA. Effects of spinal cord stimulation on touch-evoked allodynia involve GABAergic mechanisms. An experimental study in the mononeuropathic rat. *Pain* 1996;66:287-95

Cui JG, O'Connor WT, Ungerstedt U, Linderoth B & Meyerson BA. Spinal cord stimulation attenuates augmented dorsal horn release of excitatory amino acids in mononeurpathy via a GABAergic mechanism. *Pain* 1997;73:87-95

Decosterd I & Woolf CJ. Spared nerve injury: an animal model of persistent peripheral neuropathic pain. *Pain* 2000;87:149-58

Dickenson AH. Gate Control Theory of pain stands the test of time. *BJA* 2002;88:755-57

El-Kouhry C, Hawwa N, Baliki M, Atweh SF, Jabbur SJ & Saadé NE. Attenuation of neuropathic pain by segmental and supraspinal activation of the dorsal column system in awake rats. *Neuroscience* 2002; 112:541-53

Erickson DL. Percutaneous trial of stimulation for patient selection for implantable stimulating devices. *J Neurosurg* 1975;43:440-444

Frey ME, Manchikanti L, Benyamin RM, Schultz DM, Smith HS & Cohen SP. Spinal Cord Stimulation for patients with failed back surgery syndrome: A systematic review. *Pain Physician* 2009;12:379-397

Garcia-Larrea L, Sindou M & Mauguière F. Nociceptive flexion reflexes during analgesic neurostimulation in man. Pain 1989;39:145-156

Gazelius B, Cui JG, Svensson M, Meyerson B & Linderoth B. Photochemically induced ischaemic lesion of the rat sciatic nerve. A novel method providing high incidence of mononeuropathy. *Neuroreport* 1996;7:2619-2623

Govolac S. Spinal Cord Stimulation: uses and applications *Neuroimag Clin N Am* 2010;20:243–254

Guan Y, Borzan J, Meyer RA & Raja SN. Windup in dorsal horn neurons is modulated by endogenous spinal mu-opioid mechanisms. *J Neurosci* 2006;26:4298-307

Guan Y, Wacnik PW, et al. Spinal cord stimulation-induced analgesia: Electrical stimulation of dorsal column and dorsal roots attenuates dorsal horn neuronal excitability in neuropathic rats. *Anesthesiology* 2010;113:1392-405

Han JS, Chen XH, et al. Effect of low and high-frequency TENS on Met-enkephalin-Arg-Phe and dynorphin A immunoreactivity in human lumbar CSF. *Pain* 1991;47:295-298

Handwerker HO, Iggo A & Zimmermann M. Segmental and supraspinal actions on dorsal horn neurons responding to noxious and nonnoxious skin stimuli. *Pain* 1975;1:147-165

Hao JX, Xu XJ, Aldskogius H, Seiger A & Wiesenfeld-Hallin Z. Allodynia-like effects in rat after ischaemic spinal cord injury photochemically induced by laser irradiation. *Pain* 1991;45:175-185

Holsheimer J, Struijk JJ & Tas NR. Effects of electrode geometry and combination on nerve fibre selectivity in spinal cord stimulation. *Med Biol Eng Comput* 1995;33:676-682

Holsheimer J. Effectiveness of Spinal Cord Stimulation in the management of chronic pain: analysis of technical drawbacks and solutions. *Neurosurgery* 1997;40:990-996

Holsheimer J & Wesselink WA. Effect of anode-cathode configuration on paresthesia coverage in spinal cord stimulation. *Neurosurgery* 1997;41:654-659

Holsheimer J. Which neuronal elements are activated directly by spinal cord stimulation. *Neuromodulation* 2002;5:25–31

Holsheimer J, Buitenweg JR, Das J, de Sutter P, Manola L & Nuttin B. The effect of pulse width and contact configuration on paresthesia coverage in spinal cord stimulation. *Neurosurgery* 2011;68:1452–1461

Kane K & Taub A. A history of local electrical analgesia. *Pain* 1975;1:125-138

Kemler MA, De Vet HC, Barendse GA, Van Den Wildenberg FA & Van Kleef M. Effect of spinal cord stimulation in patients with chronic reflex sympathetic dystrophy: two years' follow-up of the randomized controlled trial. *Ann Neurol* 2004;55:13-18

Kemler MA, De Vet HC, Barendse GA, van den Wildenberg FA & van Kleef M. Spinal cord stimulation for chronic reflex sympathetic dystrophy – five year follow-up. *N Eng J Med* 2006;354:2394-6

Kim SH & Chung JM. An experimental model for peripheral neuropathy produced by segmental spinal nerve ligation in the rat. *Pain* 1992;50:355-63

Kumar K, Taylor RS, et al. Spinal cord stimulation versus conventional medical management for neuropathic pain: a multicentre randomised controlled trial in patients with failed back surgery syndrome. *Pain* 2007;132:179-88

Kumar K, Lind G, et al. Spinal stimulation: Placement of surgical leads via laminectomy – techniques and benefits. In: E. Krames (ed.), *Neuromodulation,* Vol 2. Amsterdam: Elsevier, 2009:1005-1011

Kumar K, Rizvi S & Bishop S. Spinal cord stimulation is effective in management of complex regional pain syndrome (CRPS) I: Fact or Fiction. *Neurosurgery* 2011. Ahead of print.

Law JD & Miller LV. Importance and documentation of an epidural stimulating position. *Appl Neurophysiol* 1982;45:461-464

Light AR. Normal anatomy and physiology of the spinal cord dorsal horn. *Appl Neurophysiol* 1988;51:78-88

Lind G, Meyerson B.A, Winter J & Linderoth B. Implantation of laminectomy electrodes for spinal cord stimulation in spinal anesthesia with intra-operative dorsal column activation. *Neurosurgery* 2003;53:1150-1154

Lind G, Meyerson BA, Winter J & Linderoth B. Intrathecal baclofen as adjuvant therapy to enhance the effect of spinal cord stimulation in neuropathic pain: a pilot study. *Eur J Pain* 2004;8:377–383

Lind G, Schechtmann G, Winter J, Meyerson BA & Linderoth B. Baclofen-enhanced spinal cord stimulation and intrathecal baclofen alone for neuropathic pain: Long-term outcome of a pilot study. *Eur J Pain* 2008;12:132–136

Linderoth B, Grazelius B, Franck J & Brodin E. Dorsal column stimulation induces release of serotonin and substance P in the cat dorsal horn. *Neurosurgery* 1992;31:289-297

Linderoth B & Foreman RD. Physiology of Spinal Cord Stimulation: Review and Update. *Neuromodulation* 1999;2:150-64

Linderoth B & Meyerson BA. Spinal Cord Stimulation: Exploration of the physiological basis of a widely used therapy. *Anesthesiology* 2010;113:1265-7

Macklis RM. Magnetic healing, quackery, and the debate about the effects of electromagnetic fields. *Ann Intern Med* 1993;118:376-383

Mailis-Gagnon A, Furlan AD, Sandoval JA & Taylor R. Spinal cord stimulation for chronic pain. *Cochrane Database of Systemic Reviews* 2004, Issue 3. Art no. CD003783. DOI: 10.1002/14651858.CD003783.pub2.

Mao J. Translational pain research: bridging the gap between basic and clinical research. *Pain* 2002;97:183-187

Melzack R & Wall PD. Pain mechanisms: a new theory. *Science* 1965; 150:971-79

Melzack R & Wall PD. *The challenge of pain* 1996: 2nd edition. England, Penguin books ltd:234-235

Meyerson BA, Herregods P, Linderoth B & Ren B. An experimental animal model of spinal cord stimulation for pain. *Stereotact Funct Neurosurg* 1994;62:256-62

Meyerson BA, Ren B, Herregodts P & Linderoth B. Spinal cord stimulation in animal models of mononeuropathy: Effects on the withdrawal response and the flexor reflex. *Pain* 1995;61:229-243

North RB, Fischell TA & Long DM. Chronic dorsal column stimulation via percutaneous inserted electrodes. Preliminary results in 31 patients. *Appl Neurophysiol* 1977-1978;40:184-191

North RB, Kidd DH, et al. A prospective, randomized study of spinal cord stimulation versus reoperation for failed back surgery syndrome: initial results. *Stereotact Funct Neurosurg* 1994;62:267-72

North RB, Kidd DH, Lee MS & Piantodosi SA. Spinal cord stimulation electrode design: prospective, randomized, controlled trial comparing percutaneous and laminectomy electrodes - part 1: Technical outcomes. *Neurosurgery* 2002; 51:381-390

North R, Shipley J, et al. Practice parameters for the use of spinal cord stimulation in the treatment of chronic neuropathic pain. *Pain Med* 2007;8(Suppl 4):S200-S275

Nyguist JK & Greenhoot JH. Responses evoked from the thalamic centrum medianum by painful input: suppression by dorsal funiculus conditioning. *Exp Neurol* 1973;39:215-222

Oakley JC & Prager JP. Spinal Cord Stimulation: Mechanisms of action. *Spine* 2002;27:2574-83

Oerlemans HM, Oostendorp RA, de Boo T & Goris RJ. Pain and reduced mobility in complex regional pain syndrome I: outcome of a prospective randomized controlled clinical trial of adjuvant physical therapy versus occupational therapy. *Pain* 1999;83:77-83

Rexed B. The cytoarchitectomic organization of the spinal cord in the cat. *J Comp Neurol* 1952;96:414-495

Roberts WJ. A hypothesis on the physiological basis for causalgia and related pain. *Pain* 1986;24:297-311

Roberts MHT & Rees H. Physiological basis of spinal cord stimulation. *Pain Rev* 1994;1184-1198

Rygh LJ, Svendsen F, Hole K & Tjølsen A. Natural noxious stimulation can induce long-term increase of spinal nociceptive responses. *Pain* 1999;82:305–310.

Saadé NE, Tabet MS, Banna NR, Atweh SF & Jabbur SJ. Inhibition of nociceptive evoked activity in spinal neurons through a dorsal column-brainstem-spinal loop. *Brain Res* 1985;339:115-118

Saadé NE, Atweh SF, Jabbur SJ & Wall PD. Effects of lesions in the anterolateral columns and dorsolateral funiculi on self-mutilation behavior in rats. *Pain* 1990;42:313-321

Saadé NE, Atweh SF, Privat A & Jabbur SJ. Inhibitory effects from various types of dorsal column and raphe magnus stimulations on nociceptive withdrawal flexion reflexes. *Brain Res* 1999;846:72-86

Sandroni P, Low PA, Ferrer T, Opfer-Gehrking TL, Willner CL & Wilson PR. Complex regional pain syndrome I (CRPS I): prospective study and laboratory evaluation. *Clin J Pain* 1998;14:282-289

Schechter DC. Origins of electrotherapy. I. *N Y State J Med* 1971;71:1114–1124

Schechtmann G, Wallin J, Meyerson BA & Linderoth B. Intrathecal clonidine potentiates suppression of tactile hypersensitivity by spinal cord stimulation in a model of Neuropathy. *Anesth Analg* 2004;99:135–9

Schechtmann G, Song Z, Ultenius C, Meyerson BA & Linderoth B. Cholinergic mechanisms involved in the pain relieving effect of spinal cord stimulation in a model of neuropathy. *Pain* 2008;139:136–145

Selzer Z, Dubner T & Shir Y. A novel behavioral model of neuropathic pain disorders produced in rats by partial sciatic nerve injury. *Pain* 1990;43:205-18

Shealy CN, Mortimer JT & Reswick JB. Electrical inhibition of pain by stimulation of the dorsal columns: preliminary clinical report. *Anesth Anal* 1967a;46:489-91

Shealy CN, Taslitz N, Mortimer JT & Becker DP. Electrical inhibition of pain: experimental evaluation. *Anesth Analg* 1967b;46:299–305

Slipman CW, Shin CH, et al. Etiologies of Failed Back Surgery Syndrome. *Pain Med* 2002;3:200-214

Song Z, Ultenius C, Meyerson BA & Linderoth B. Pain relief by spinal cord stimulation involves serotonergic mechanisms: An experimental study in a rat model of mononeuropathy. *Pain* 2009;147:241-248

Stiller CO, Cui JG, O'Connor WT, Brodin E, Meyerson BA & Linderoth B. Release of gamma-aminobutyric acid in the dorsal horn and suppression of tactile allodynia by spinal cord stimulation in mononeuropathic rats. *Neurosurgery* 1996;39:367-75

Stillings D. The first use of electricity for pain treatment. *Medtronic Archive on Electro-Stimulation* 1971.

Struijk JJ, Holsheimer J & Boom HBK. Excitation of dorsal root fibers in spinal cords stimulation: a theoretical study. *IEEE Trans* 1993;40:632-639

Sweet WH. Animal models of chronic pain: their possible validation from human experience with posterior rhizotomy and congenital analgesia. *Pain* 1981;10:275-295

Turner JA, Loeser JD & Bell KG. Spinal cord stimulation for chronic low back pain. A systematic literature synthesis. *Neurosurgery* 1995; 37:1088-1096

Villavicencio AT, Leveque JC, Rubin L, Bulsara K & Gorecki JP. Laminectomy versus percutaneous electrode placement for spinal cord stimulation. *Neurosurgery* 2000;46:399-406

Wall PD & Sweet WH. Temporary abolition of pain in man. *Science* 1967;155:108–109

Wall PD & Gutnick M. Ongoing activity in peripheral nerves: the physiology and pharmacology of impulses originating from a neuroma. *Exp Neurol* 1974;43:580-593

Wall PD, Devor M, et al. Autotomy following peripheral nerve lesions: experimental anaesthesia dolorosa. *Pain* 1979;7:103-113

Wall P. The discovery of transcutaneous electrical nerve stimulation. *Physiotherapy* 1985;71:348-350

Watson BD, Prado R, Dietrich WD, Ginsberg MD & Green BA. Photochemically induced spinal cord injury in the rat. *Brain Res* 1986;367:296-300

Whitehouse PJ, Wamsley JK, et al. Amyotrophic lateral sclerosis: alterations in neurotransmitter receptors. *Ann Neurol* 1983;14:8-16

Woolf C & Doubell T. The pathophysiology of chronic pain-increased sensitivity to low threshold A-beta fiber inputs. *Curr Opin Neurobiol* 1994;4:525-34

Woolf CJ & Salter MW. Neuronal plasticity: increasing the gain in pain. *Science* 2000; 288:1765-1769

Xu Z, Chen S-R, Eisenach J & Pan HL. Role of muscarinic and nicotinic receptors in clonidine-induced nitric oxide release in a rat model of neuropathic pain. *Brain Res* 2000;861:390–8

Yakhnitsa V, Linderoth B & Meyerson BA. Spinal cord stimulation attenuates dorsal horn neuronal hyperexcitability in a rat model of mononeuropathy. *Pain* 1999;79:223-233

Zhu J, Falco F, et al. Alternative approach to needle placement in spinal cord stimulator insertion. *Pain Physician* 2011;14:195-210

6

Intrathecal Drug Administration for the Treatment of Cancer and Non-Cancer Chronic Pain

William Raffaeli[2], Francesco Magnani[1],
Jessica Andruccioli[1] and Donatella Sarti[1]
[1]*Department of Pain Therapy and Pallitive Care – Infermi Hospital- Rimini*
[2]*Pain Clinic, Institute for Research on Pain "Fondazione Isal", Torrepedrera*
Italy

1. Introduction

1.1 Pain classification

Pain is nowadays one of the major reasons for medical consultation worldwide. Pain is always a subjective experience, which is often verbally non-communicable. Sometimes it starts as acute pain arising from a disease (such as cancer), an injury (such as a road accident), or a post-surgical intervention; then it persists and becomes a disease itself (1-3). The International Association for the Study of Pain (IASP) definition of pain is accordingly the following: "an unpleasant sensory and emotional experience associated with actual or potential tissue damage, or described in terms of such damage" (1). Many people, however, report pain also in absence of tissue damage or any likely pathophysiological cause; usually this is due to psychological factors. For this reason pain has two components: a perceptive component, nociception, sensorial reception of the potential harmful stimulus to the central nervous system, and experiential component, individual, which is the psychological perception of an unpleasant sensation.

In relationship to the duration of painful perception, pain can be acute, or chronic. Acute pain has a short duration, and usually has a clear cause/effect, and disappear when the damage is repaired. Chronic pain is defined as pain persisting for more than 3 months, it has no prevention treatments, persists for several months or years and often does not have a single or identifiable cause.

As concerning the pathological classification of pain, there are different types of chronic pain, according to the tissues involved. Neuropathic pain, for example, is defined by IASP as "Pain caused by a lesion or disease of the somatosensory nervous system", and can be central, if "Pain is caused by a lesion or disease of the central somatosensory nervous system" or peripheral if "Pain caused by a lesion or disease of the peripheral somatosensory nervous system", including visceral organs (1). Trigeminal neuralgia, and postherpetic neuralgia are examples of neuropathic pain.

Nociceptive pain, on the contrary, is defined by IASP as "Pain that arises from actual or threatened damage to non-neural tissue and is due to the activation of nociceptors", which are high-threshold sensory receptor of the peripheral somatosensory nervous system that is capable of transducing and encoding noxious stimuli (1). This type of pain can be somatic or visceral, according to the localizartion of tissues involved; it usually indicates a damage occurred in non-neural tissues, hence in presence of a normally functioning somatosensory nervous system to contrast with the abnormal function seen in neuropathic pain.

The two types of pain may also coexist in the same patient, in this case pain can be identified as mixed neuropatic and nociceptive.

1.2 Cancer pain

Pain may also be secondary to cancer, in this case is defined as cancer pain. Chronic cancer pain represents the third largest health problem in the world, and involves around 30% of the world's population (4). The World Health Organization (WHO) has stated that inadequate treatment of cancer pain represents a serious problem for public health all over the world (5). It is calculated that there are 10 million new cases of cancer and 6 million deaths from this illness worldwide. It is estimated that the incidence of cancer, currently greater in developed countries, will become more significant in developing countries as a result of the better prevention strategies being adopted in the former. The WHO program on the control of cancer has estimated that by the year 2020, around 70% of the 20 million new cases of tumours will be in the developing world, where most patients are diagnosed when the disease is already in the last stages.

More than 50% of cancer patients do not undergo adequate pain treatment (6). The pain prevents patients from carrying out normal daily activities and influences appetite, mood, self-esteem, relationships with others and mobility. In some countries it is seen that untreated pain leads to a desire for death, euthanasia or assisted suicide (4). Pain relief improves the quality of life (7).

Unfortunately, cancer pain is often not treated or is treated inadequately. The WHO have demonstrated that most, if not all, cases of cancer pain, could be treated successfully, if existing medical knowledge and suitable therapies were put into practice. There exists a lacuna in the treatment that is represented by the difference between what could be done and what is actually done in the fight against cancer pain. Training, informing health workers and facilitating access to analgesic treatments and palliative care can close this gap (5).

The WHO Expert Committee on Cancer Pain Relief and Active Supportive Care (8), stated in 1990 that "freedom from pain should be considered a right of every cancer patient and access to pain therapy as a measure of respect for this right".

In 1986, the World Health Organization, in an effort to optimize cancer pain therapy, suggested a simple three point analgesic ladder (figure 1) for the use of opioids for the treatment of cancer pain (6).

Although adoption of the therapies suggested by this analgesic ladder improves pain management in the majority of patients, it is estimated that from 5% to 15% of patients with cancer pain are unable to adequately control their pain, following these guidelines (9-11). In addition there are pains classified as "breakthrough pains" (12) which are difficult to manage and contain, both because they are unpredictable and because there is a lack of suitable drugs. In order to tackle this need, new drug formulations have been developed such as immediate release morphine, transmucosal fentanyl (13) and indications for invasive treatments with analgesic infusion in the liquor.

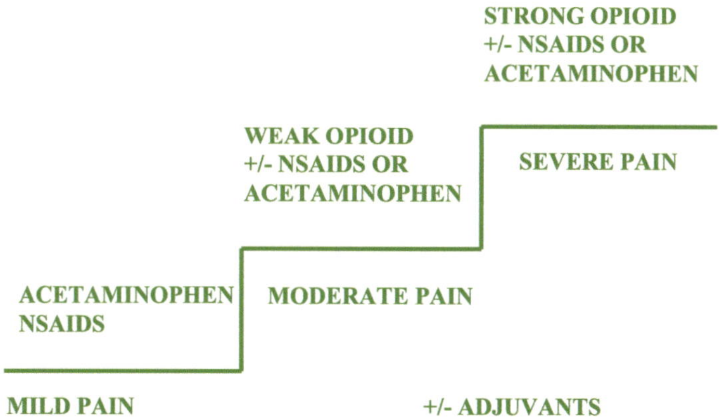

NSAID—nonsteroidal anti-inflammatory drug

Fig. 1. The World Health Organization analgesic ladder for treating cancer pain

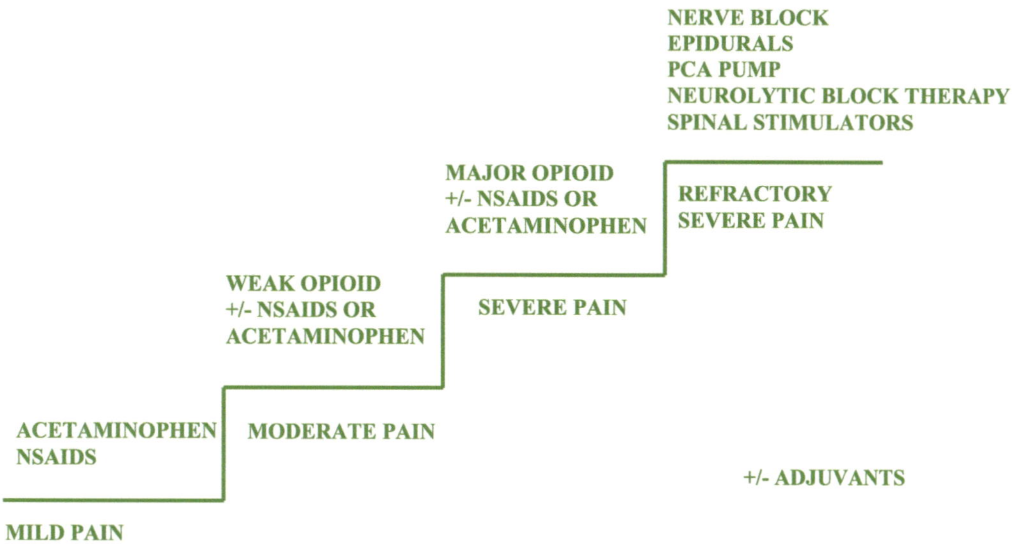

NSAID—nonsteroidal anti-inflammatory drug, PCA—patient-controlled analgesia

Fig. 2. Adaptation of the WHO ladder

Therefore, in 1997, the WHO, according to the model described by Catala, proposed a change in the analgesic ladder, adding a fourth step dedicated to intrathecal (IT) drug administration (14, 15) (figure 2). They suggested that intrathecal therapy is indicated in patients who are unable to control painful symptoms with traditional method of administration or in those who cannot tolerate high doses of oral opioids because of systemic side-effects.

However, while this practice has been known for a while (16-18), it has still not yet become sufficiently widespread as to define its role. When it should be used, for what pain types it is most effective and what effect it has on the biological homeostasis of the patient (18) and the development of their primary pathology.

2. Intrathecal administration

2.1 History of infusion pumps

Intratecal (IT) delivery systems for opioid infusion have been introduced in the later 1980s for the treatment of chronic pain, because of their several advantages: opioid-related systemic effects are reduced, lower opioid dosages are required, and opioid receptors are directly reached (19).

The first models of spinal analgesia were experimented in rats by Yaksh and Rudy in 1976 (19). They used morphine administered via a chronically inserted catheter, and observed that opioids elevated the analgesic threshold when the infusion was performed into the subarachnoid space. This effect was antagonized by naloxone, and had onset and duration variable according to the type of opioid used. Fentanyl onset was 2-3 minutes and expired in 20-30 minutes, whereas morphine required twice as long to start its effect, but it lasted longer, up to 2 hours.

IT therapy is a key therapeutic option for patients who have failed all other treatment avenues, require high enteral or parenteral dosages, or have unbearable opioid related-side effects (20).

The study of the spinal pathways in patients with non-malignant pain is still being developed, as there are many obstacles which prevent its widespread application. Anyway the long-term intrathecal administration with totally implantable systems has been recommended for the treatment of noncancer pain, both by a consensus of specialists from the United States in 1997 (21) and by the International Consensus Conference in Brussels in 1998 (22). Experts believe that it should be used in pathologies characterized by the presence of long-term persistent pain, where other therapeutic strategies have been judged to be ineffective or inapplicable because of serious adverse effects (23).

2.2 IT drugs

There are five main classes of IT drugs: opioids, including morphine, hydromorphone, sufentanil, fentanyl, methadone, and ,meperidine; local anaestetics, such as bupivacaine, ropivacaine, and tetracaine; adrenergic agonist: clonidine and tiazinidine; N-methyl-D-aspartate (NMDA) antagonist, including dextrorphan, dextromethorphan, mematine and ketamine; other agents, such as baclophen, ziconotide, midazolam, neostigminie, aspirin, and droperidol (24).

Opioids are a heterogeneous group of synthetic and semisynthetic opium derivates, their analgesic effect and therapeutic use is lost in time. The power of an opioid depends on several factors: affinity with their receptor, specific pharmacological potency, or the ability to express the desired effect. The amount and type of receptors in a tissue affects the response to opioids in terms of both quality and quantity (intensity and duration of effect).

Intratecal infusion of major opioids is increasingly used for the treatment of chronic pain, and morphine is the gold standard (25). Morphine delivered IT, and its metabolites, especially morphine-6-glicuronide (M-6-G) (26), can provide prolonged analgesic because there is a slow replacement of the cerebrospinal fluid (CSF) over time, and it is approximately ten time more potent than the same amount administered systemically or epidurally (27-29). In the chronic infusion, M-6-G plays a larger role; it enters the CSF from the plasma, but can also be created in situ by the brain (30-32).

Hydromorphone administered intratecally has been less applied, and few studies are present in the literature. It is known to be 5 times more potent than morphine, but the adverse events profile is equivalent or better than that of morphine (33).

Bupivacaine belongs to the amino amide group; it is known to act synergistically with the opioids for the treatment of pain (34-36) allowing the administration of lower doses of morphine to achieve the same analgesic effect (37). The use of IT bupivacaine has been shown to be free of bone marrow toxicity and to have positive synergy with opioids (35, 36). Despite the excellent results obtained with morphine and bupivacaine, there still remains difficulty in treating all pains, particularly the pains of neuropathic origin.

Clonidine has been shown to be helpful in difficult to treat cases. It has been reported that the spinal administration of clonidine not only acts synergistically when administered with opioids, increasing the analgesic power and reducing side-effects (38), but it is also a powerful analgesic agent when used alone, especially for the treatment of neuropathic pain (39-41).

Local anesthetics and opioids work on differing analgesic systems, so low doses of these agents, when added to each other IT, provide analgesic synergy (42). Moreover, the use of a low dose of bupivacaine when added to IT morphine allows for a low dose of morphine thereby reducing the incidence of opioid-related side-effects (43). Although morphine is the gold standard agent used for IT therapy, experts in the field of IT therapy today use a variety of drug combinations, such as morphine/bupivacaine, hydromorphone, and morphine/clonidine (32, 44).

An interdisciplinary expert panel of both physicians and non-physicians in the field of intrathecal therapies met in 2007 at the Polyanalgesic Consensus Conference, in order to update previous recommendations/guidelines for the management of pain by IDDS (45). They suggested the following classification and drug dosages (table.1).

Morphine and ziconotide are approved by the Food and Drug Administration of the United States for intrathecal analgesic use and are recommended for first line therapy for nociceptive, mixed, and neuropathic pain. Hydromorphone is recommended based on clinical widespread usage and apparent safety. Fentanyl is a line 2 agent and is reccommended by the consensus conference when the use of the more hydrophilic agents of line 1 (morphine, ziconotide) result in intractable supraspinal side effects (table 2).

IT drug type	Maximum dose/day (mg)
Morphine	15
Hydromorphone	4
Fentanyl	Unknown upper limit
Sufentanil	Unknown upper limit
Bupivacaine	30
Clonidine	1.5
Ziconotide	19.2 mcg

Table 1. IT drug doses as recommended by the polyanalgesic consensus 2007.

Line	IT drug
1	a) morphine b) hydromorphone c) ziconotide
2	d) fentanyl e) morphine/hydromorphone + ziconotide f) morphine/hydromorphone + bupivacaine/clonidine
3	g) clonidine **h)** morphine/hydromorphone/fentanyl + bupivacaine + clonidine + ziconotide
4	i) sufentanil j) sufentanil +bupivacaine + clonidine + ziconotide
5	k) ropivacaine, buprenorphine, midazolam meperidine, ketorolac
6	l) Experimental Drugs: gabapentin, octreotide, conopeptide, Neostigmine, Adenosine, XEN2174, AM336, XEN, ZGX 160

Table 2. Recommended algorithm for intrathecal polyanalgesic therapies, 2007.

Combinations of opioid/ziconotide or opioid/bupivacaine or clonidine are recommended for mixed and neuropathic pain and may be used interchangeably. Clonidine alone or in combination with opioids such as morphine/ hydromorphone /fentanyl; bupivacaine and/or clonidine mixed with ziconotide are line 3 agents, and may be used when agents in line 2 fail to provide analgesia or side effects occur when these agents are used. Sufentanil alone or mixed with bupivacaine and/or clonidine plus ziconotide (suggested for neuropathic pain) is recommended in line 4. Midazolam and octreotide are line 5, and should be tried when all other agents in lines 1-4 have failed in end-of-life patients. Experimental agents are line 6, and must only be used experimentally and with appropriate Independent Review Board (IRB) approved protocols (45).

IT drug administration can be performed through bolus or continuos infusion. Bolus administration may result in better distribution of anesthetic solution compared with continuous infusion of the same anesthetic solution. Automated methods of bolus injection, moreover, may combine the advantages of manual boluses and continuous infusion, while sparing on drug consumption.

The constant infusion, however, is the most diffused method of IT drug administration, and the comparison between bolus and constant-flow pumps shows no difference as concerning efficacy and safety in non-cancer pain (46, 47) and cancer pain (48).

2.3 Opioid receptor

Opioid action is mediated by the activation of opioid receptors. The receptors are several and the major are called μ, k and δ, are responsible for both the positive effects (analgesia), but also of opioid related side effects (respiratory depression, itching, vomiting etc.) (table 3).

Opioid receptor type	Function	Endogenous peptides	Agonist	Antagonist
μ	Subtype μ1: analgesia Subtype μ2: adverse events (Sedation, vomiting, respiratory depression, pruritus, euphoria, anorexia, urinary retention) and physical dependence	Enkephalins β-Endorphin Dynorphin A	Morphine Codeine Fentanyl Meperidine Methadone	Naloxone (Weak) Naltrexone
δ	Analgesia, spinal analgesia	Enkephalins β-Endorphin	Codeine (weak) Meperidine	Naloxone (Weak) Naltrexone (Weak)
κ	Analgesia, sedation, dyspnea, psychomimetic effects, miosis, respiratory depression, euphoria, dysphoria, dyspnea	Dynorphin A	Morphine (Weak)	Naloxone Naltrexone

Modified from ref. 49

Table 3. Major Opioid receptors

The opioid receptor is a macromolecule that includes an extracellular N terminus, 7 transmembrane helical twists, 3 extracellular and intracellular loops, and an intracellular C-terminus (49) (Fig. 3). Once the receptor is activated, it releases the inhibitory G protein, which diffuses within the membrane and activates a cascade of biochemical reactions leading to the decrease of cAMP intracellular. The final result is the neuronal inhibition, blocking the release of excitatory neurotransmitters (Fig. 4). This block is obtained inducing changes (inhibition) of calcium channels activity in pre-synaptic neurones and alterations of hyperpolarization (activation of potassium channels) in postsynaptic neurones (terenius).

The binding sites of the various opioid receptors are sufficiently flexible to accommodate structurally different ligands and to allow selectivity in the activation. (table 3).

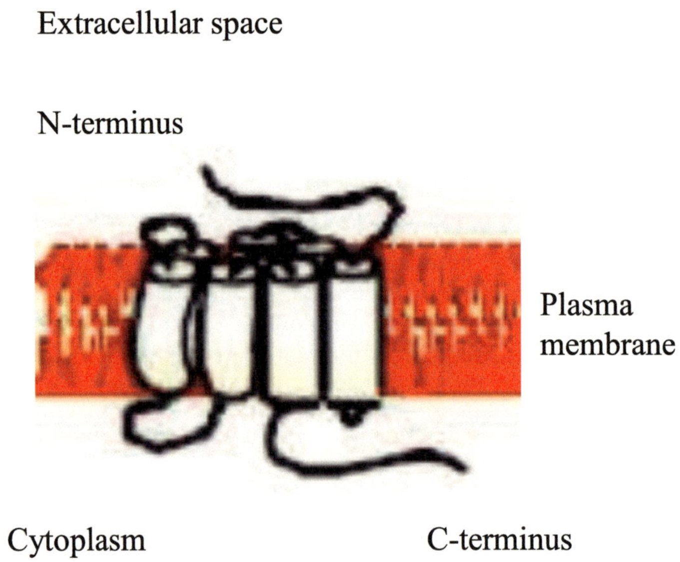

Fig. 3. Opioid Receptors structure

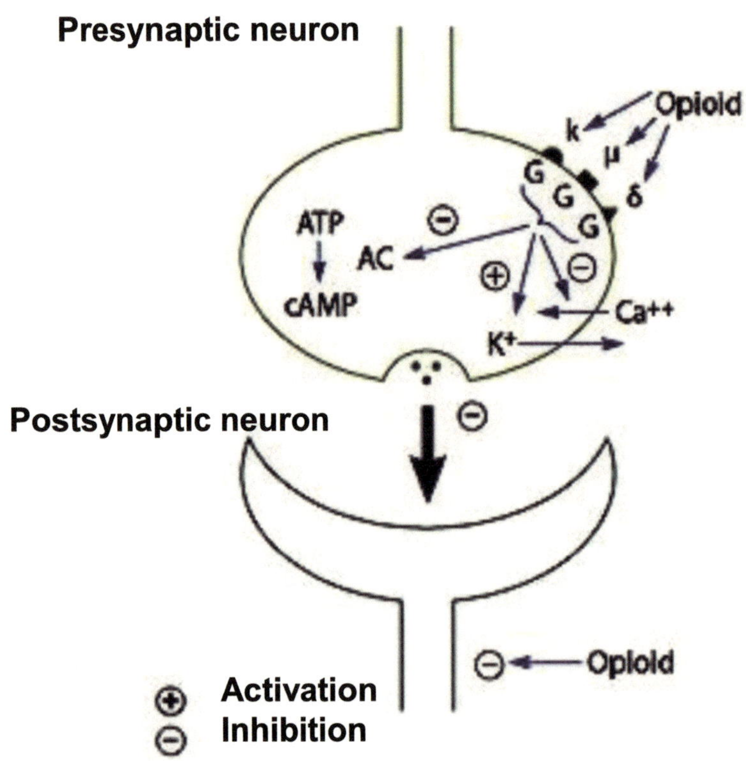

Fig. 4. Opioid Receptor signalling (Modified from ref. 49)

Most of the common opioids, such as morphine, codeine and fentanyl, are agonists of opioid receptors, and act by stimulating them with different intensity and efficacy.

Opioid receptor partial agonists, such as buprenorphine, on the contrary, bind with high affinity, but low efficacy at the mu receptor (partial effect). These agents can be used as analgesics, but have a ceiling to their analgesic effect, and increasing the dose beyond a certain threshold will not result in a corresponding increase in efficacy, but only in greater side effects (49).

Opioid receptor Agonists-Antagonists, such as pentazocine, nalbuphine, and butorphanol, have poor mu opioid receptor efficacy, acting as functional antagonist, and kappa agonistic properties, causing undesired dysesthesias. As the partial agonist, they have a partial or a complete ceiling to their analgesic effect. (49).

The opioid receptor antagonists, naloxone and naltrexone, are competitive antagonists at the mu, kappa, and delta receptors, in particular, with a high affinity for the mu receptor, but lacking any mu receptor efficacy, hence they do not activate the opioid cascade. (49).

2.4 Biological consequences of long-term intrathecal administration of opioids

In the last years data have been accumulated on the biological effects of systemic administration of morphine (50-52). Less is known about the effects of spinaly administered opioids on various body systems which are not purely nociceptive.

Biological systems are characterized by an accurate mechanism of auto-control. Indeed, we call homeostasis the tendency to uniformity or stability in the normal body states (internal environment or fluid matrix) of the organism. This tendency aims at maintaining the organism under optimal physiological condition (53). Whenever a biological system is altered, a congruent cascade of physiological response is activated to eliminate the perturbation factor and to circumscribe the effects of the biological answer to that perturbation. Examples for such behaviour are the immune and the endocrine system. The homeostatic regulation of these systems normally occurs through a feedback mechanism, driven by their own products. Moreover, it is known that many regulatory molecules may exert their effect, directly or indirectly, on more than one system. Cytokines, the principle mediators of the immune system, are a known example for such regulatory molecules. Homeostasis fails when the feedback mechanism is overwhelmed by the perturbation factor or when a positive feedback occurs and the biological answer is perpetuated, not being counterbalanced by a suitable reaction in the opposite sense.

A growing body of evidence suggests that exogenous and endogenous opioids influence both the endocrine and the immune systems and that they share many properties of the cytokines (54). This concept is of an extreme clinical relevance. Indeed, as opioids are shown to have a regulation role of the above mentioned systems, a careful insight is needed to understand the biological impact of their utilization in long term pain treatments.

2.5 Opioid Immunomodulation

Exogenous opioids are known to mediate immunosuppression, while endogenous opiates enhance immune function (54). *In vitro*, the augmentation of natural killer (NK) cell activity by endogenous opiates is antagonized by naloxone (55). These findings are consistent with the notion that opioid receptors are expressed by immunocytes. Administration of opioids has been associated with increased vulnerability to infections in humans and with reduced survival in animals bearing tumours. In fact, administration of opioids inhibits NK cell activity, immune response, cytokine expression and phagocytosis.

Both central and peripheral mechanisms are implied in the exogenous opioids immunosuppression. Central mechanism may involve both the hypothalamic-pituitary-adrenal pathway and the autonomic nervous system. It is believed that the latter is implied during acute administration of morphine whereas the former during chronic administration. It is noteworthy that in the periphery, cytokines may induce endogenous opioids secretion from immunocytes and influence both analgesia and inflammation. On the other hand, exogenous opioids may induce the secretion and the expression of inflammatory cytokines in peripheral immunocytes. Thus opioids may be considered as an important inflammation and immune regulatory molecules.

Modulation of immune response by central opioid receptors has been described (56-60). It has been reported that such modulation involves the delayed-type hypersensitivity reactions and humoral immune responses. Moreover, it appears that central immune modulation is influenced by the type of the activated opioid receptor, as well as by the source and nature of the opioid agonist. Indeed, different endogenous opioid effect differentially humoral and cell mediated immune responses by differentially activating brain μ, δ and κ opioid receptors. Permissive central immunomodulatory action of endogenous opioids seems to be mediated by the μ and δ receptors while suppression by the κ receptor (54). Further, acute administration of morphine seems to alter immune response through the activation of the sympathetic system while long term morphine administration decreases lymphocyte proliferation and NK cell activity by the modulation of the hypothalamic-pituitary-adrenal axis (61). Moreover there is a direct correlation with the way of administration and that the intraspinally way cause an important immunosupressive effect on NK and lymphokine activated killer (LAK) cells cytotoxic activity via a second messenger probably prolactin (PRL) mediated (15) and an interfrence on u-receptor expression (62).

So, opiates widely influence the immune system and may be considered as cytokines. Opioid receptors that mediate immunomodulation are located in the central nervous system, peripheral sensory neurons, and immunocytes. Activation of these receptors exerts direct or indirect immunomodulation in a complex fashion. Exogenous opioids tend to suppress cell-mediated immune function especially when administered systemically. Hence, the route of exogenous opioid administration may play an important role in preventing immunosuppression. Indeed, theoretically, the intrathecal route may avoid central and peripheral opioid receptors and hence reduce the likelihood of opioid immunosuppression (54).

2.6 Opioid and the endocrine system

Opioids are known to interfere with the neuroendocrine function (63). Animals and humans studies have explored both the acute and the chronic neuroendocrine effects of opiates and different opioid peptides. Acute administration of opioids in humans increases the secretion of PRL, growth hormone (GH), thyroid-stimulating hormone (TSH), and adrenocorticotropic hormone (ACTH) while it inhibits the release of luteinizing hormone (LH) (64, 52). It has been argued that the inhibition of LH release is mediated through central inhibition of hypothalamic GnRH secretion (65). Opioids influence on endocrine pathways and products is mediated by endogenous opioid legands. It has been reported that PRL and TSH secretion is probably modulated by the ε and μ receptors, respectively while ACTH secretion by δ or κ receptors; ε receptors are thought to be involved in the inhibitory control of LH (66, 67). The receptors involved in GH modulation have not been established yet.

Endocrine response to chronic administration of opioids differs from that of acute administration. In fact, the increased secretion of PRL, seen in the acute setting is increased only by systemic administration and not by intraspinally administration. No change in the TSH and β-endorphin secretion has been reported (62). Exogenous opioids are known to exert an inhibitory effect on the concomitant release of β-endorphin and ACTH through a feedback mechanism. Such mechanism may explain the suppression of ACTH release in long term opioid administration (68).

It has been reported recently that long term intrathecal opioid therapy induces hypogonadotropic hypogonadism (69) and that altered sexual function and low testosterone levels may be observed in individuals addicted to opioids or on methadone maintenance or in males with chronic non-cancer pain treated with intrathecal opioids (70, 71).

In conclusion, chronic opioid administration influence multiple endocrine functions. Data on this issue are scantly regarded in the literature. Yet, the advent of endocrine effects of opioid therapy cannot be ignored as it has no doubt an extraordinary clinical relevance especially in young adults. Particular attention should be paid to wether the administration route of chronic opioid therapy has any influence on the endocrine response to long term opioid therapy.

2.7 Indications and contraindication for IT therapy

Intrathecal analgesia is a key pain therapy for patients who have failed other treatment routes as well as patients with adequate analgesia on high dose enteral or parenteral therapy but with unacceptable side effects. The current body of literature supports the use of intrathecal agents for the treatment of moderate or severe pain related to cancer and non-cancer origins (72).

It emerges, in particular, that the evidence for opioid intrathecal infusion efficacy was strong for short-term improvement in pain of malignancy or neuropathic pain (73). The evidence was moderate for long-term management of persistent pain, and reasonably strong for long-term therapy of cancer pain. The evidence supporting long-term efficacy in persistent non-cancer pain is however less convincing (73).

As concerning more specifically the type of pain responding to IT morphine, it is effective for long-term treatment of neuropathic-nociceptive, peripheral neuropathic, deafferentation and nociceptive pain, resulting in significant improvement over baseline levels of visual analog scale pain (74). Other types of pain indicated for IDDS are failed back syndrome, axial spinal pain, complex regional pain syndrome, widespread pain, central pain, pain non-responding to spinal cord stimulation (SCS), arachnoiditis, central neuropathic pain (post-stroke, spinal cord).

Intrathecal delivery systems (IDDSs) have also short-term clinical success in pain control, reduce significantly common drug toxicities, and improved survival in patients with refractory cancer pain (75).

The most important authors use and results on cancer and non cancer pain are reported in tables 4 and 5.

Authors	Patients	Pain intensity before treatment	Treatment	Length of treatment	Results
Van Dongen et al., 1999 (110)	20 patients, mean age 55 years	I. NRS 5-9/10 II. NRS 6-10/10	I. IT morphine II. IT morphine/ bupivacaine.	I. 51-191 days (mean 85) II. 22-154 days (mean 58)	The group with morphine/bupivacaine showed a slower increase rate in the IT morphine dose (r=0.0003) compared to the group with morphine alone (r=0.005). I. NRS 2-4/10 II. NRS 1-4/10
Smith et al., 2002 (111)	101 patients mean age 56.2 _ 13.2 100 comprehensive medical management (CMM)	VAS 7.57/10	48 with morphine, 2 morphine/clonidine, 36 with hydromorphone, 15 hydromorphone/bupivacaine	4 weeks	71 IDDS patients (84.5%) achieved clinical success, 52% pain reduction, and 37.2% of the CMM group
Rauck et al., 2003 (112)	119 patients, mean age 60.6 ±13.5 years	VAS 6.1/10	IT morphine sulphate (initial dose 1.8 mg/day and 5.2 mg/day at 4 months).	13 months	Excellent results ≥50% reduction in NAS, in the use of systemic opioids or in the opioid complication severity index) observed in 83%, 90%, 85% and 91% of patients at 1, 2, 3, 4 months respectively.
Smith et al 2005 (113)	52 patients average age 56.2 ± 13.2; 45 comprehensive medical management (CMM) average age 57.8 ± 13.7	VAS 7.44 /10 and 7.59/10, respectively	Morphine oral equivalent dose (mg/day) 260 and 280 respectively	12 weeks	82.5% of IDDS patients had clinical success compared with 77.8% of comprehensive medical management (CMM)

Modified from ref. 109

Table 4. Intraspinal therapy: cancer pain

Authors	Patients	Pain intensity before treatment	Treatment	Length of treatment	Results
Willis e Doleys, 1999 (114)	29 patients, mean age 57.79 years	VAS 8.91/10	Intraspinal therapy	31 months	VAS 5.03/10. Improvement in pain (63.4%), in level of activity (45.5%), in performing activity (53.8%). 86% of patients reported good or excellent results. 50% of patients reported side effects.
Brown et al., 1999 (115)	38 patients, mean age 48.84 years (lower back pain)		IT opioids (3.23 ± 0.54 mg meq./d in the first 6 months and 18.58 ± 2.93 mg meq./d at 48-54 months	Mean 50 months	Patients reported a reduction in pain of 64% and both they and their families were satisfied with the treatment. Despite these benefits, there was substantial weakening in physical functionality and a high number of side effects.
Roberts et al., 2001 (116)	88 patients, mean age 53.4 years		IT morphine (9.95 ± 1.49 mg/day at 6 months and 15.26 ± 2.52 mg/day at 36 months)	36.2 months	Mean pain reduction of 60% in the 74% of patients who report an increase in level of activity. 88% of patients are satisfied.
Franco Gay, 2002 (117)	39 patients, mean age 63.4 years	VAS 5-10/10	IT morphine (initial dose 0.5 and final dose 2 mg/day)/ bupivacaine, clonidine.	36 months - 6.5 years (mean 2.2 years)	55.6% reported excellent results, 22.2% good. Level of activity: 30.5% good, 61% fair, 3% poor, 5.5% no change. 91% of patients were satisfied with the treatment.
Grider et al 2011 (118)	22 patients	VAS 7.3 ± 1.9/10	IT morphine, average dosage 335 mcg/day	12 months	Average pain VAS reduction of 53.4%

Modified from ref. 109

Table 5. Intraspinal therapy :non-cancer pain

The implantation of IDDS is contraindicated (surgical contraindication) in every case of serious cardiovascular disease, coagulation disorders, anatomical abnormalities of the spine and/or bone infections, in place, CSF fistulas, abnormal CSF flow, anatomical malformations that impede the creation of a pocket for the pump accommodation. There are also opioid-related contraindications, including severe respiratory failure, intolerance to opiates, and opioid non-responsiveness as emerged from pre-implant spinal test.

2.8 IT devices

Intrathecal drug administration is usually provided by a programmable Infusion Pump, a small machine implanted in patients' bodies (fig. 5) which allow IT infusion of drug stored in their reservoir (fig. 6). Their electronic and mechanic devices work with precision and reliability and allow liquid infusion for some hours to few months' periods, during that time a strict control of the amount infused is essential. In this way pump therapy allows drug administration only when it's required, keeping drug amount between prescribed limits. The benefits of an infusion pump are summarised in table (6).

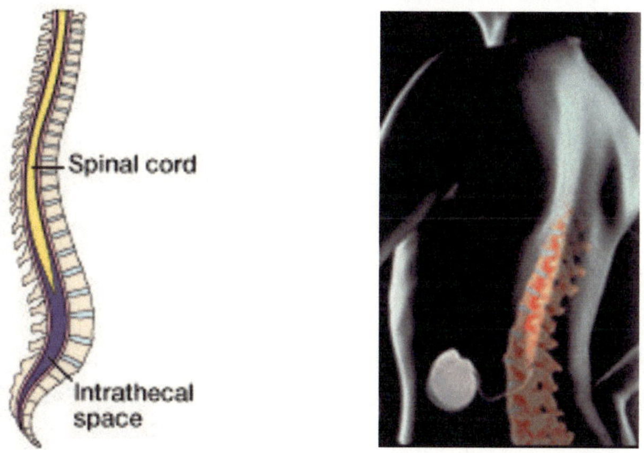

Fig. 5. Spinal Space and localization of the Infusion pump

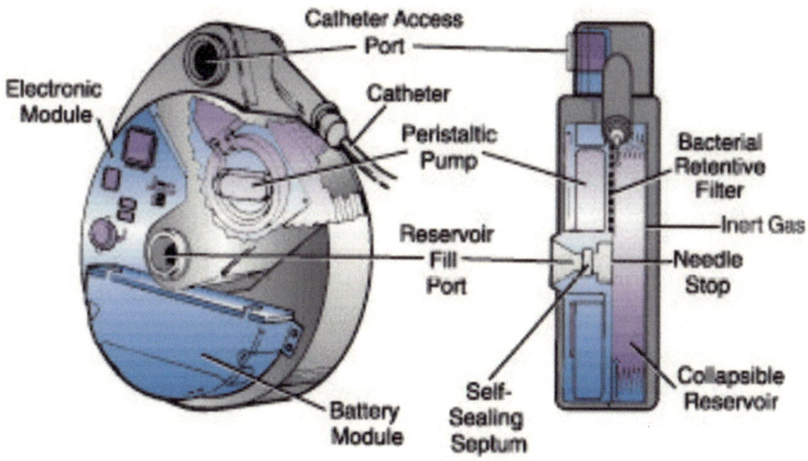

Fig. 6. Characteristics of infusion pump

Benefits of infusion pump
The pump is programmed to administer the drug at times and in amounts determined by the physician in the area of the body where it is most effective in order to better respond to patient needs.
Effect optimal with dosages of drugs extremely reduced, even 1/400 or 1/1000 compared to parenteral administration.
Easy variation of the amount of drug administered by acting directly with the programmer without having to modify the concentration of the solution contained in the reservoir.
The patient should undergo frequent drug injections. The injection is needed only for the periodic refilling of the pump.
Absence or low incidence of side effects.
Improving the quality of life of the patient.
Decrease in infections.
Administration of the drug according to the scheme more appropriate for the patient.
Different modes of injection: a single bolus term, discrete boluses at specific intervals, continues.

Table 6. Benefits of infusion pump

All systems of infusion are constituted by two implanted components: a pump and a catheter. The pump has a central reservoir where it stores and delivers the drug daily basis the amount prescribed. This reservoir has a filling port, which is used for the refilling. The pump is provided with an antibacterial filter and of a point of secondary access, which allows a direct access to the catheter and consequently to the space where this ends, that the doctor may use to administer drugs or solutions directly in the catheter, skipping the pump. The catheter is a flexible tube connected to a port of the pump, and brings the drug to the area of the body designated.

A surgical operation is required for the implantation of a programmable pump and a catheter in the body. The potential risks correlated with the implantation are: infection to the point of implantation; displacement, blockage or entanglement of the catheter; run out of the pump internal battery; breakage of device components, requiring a pump replacement.

The core of the infusion system, which is commonly called pump, is a metal disc with a diameter of 7 cm and a thickness of 3 cm (weight 180 gr.), which is made entirely of titanium and silicon (highly bio-compatible materials). The pump is provided with an antibacterial filter and of a point of secondary access, which allows a direct access to the catheter (a small tube a few millimeters in diameter and 20 to 30 cm long silicone). Each type of pump has its specific catheter, which are sold together.

The pump includes 3 sealed chambers: one containing the propellant of the reservoir, the second a hybrid electronic module and the battery and the third contains a peristaltic pump and reservoir for the drug (fig. 6). The peristaltic pump pushes the drug through an elastomeric connector, from the reservoir to a catheter, and then up to the site of administration.

The electronic circuits control the pump function, while the valve of the prevents the further introduction of fluid into the reservoir once it reaches its full capacity. This type of pump is reliable and more secure compared to other systems with gas propellants, as it is not affected by variations in temperature or pressure, ensuring an accurate control of the amount to be infused.

The reservoir for the drug has a capacity of 18-20 ml (Isomed and Syncromed) or 40 ml (Archimedes), and is made of titanium. The electronic circuit is composed of: a lithium thionyl chloride battery, with 44 months of autonomy to a continuous flow of 0.5-1 ml / day (Isomed, Archimedes respectively) or less in case of the syncromed model; an antenna allowing the contact with the operator.

The electronic module is the system memory, where are stored all the data such as the drug concentration, residual quantity, unit of measurement and data relative to the infusion programme (amount and timing).

It is possible to perform rest periods, filling the pump with saline solution thus allowing for a continuous washing of the catheter, as a prevention of the risk of occlusion resulting from the return of blood, in the case the catheter remains empty for a long time.

Refilling operations are limited to the puncture (fig. 7), through the skin with a Huber needle, of the self-sealing septum, which can be localized with palpation by the physician.

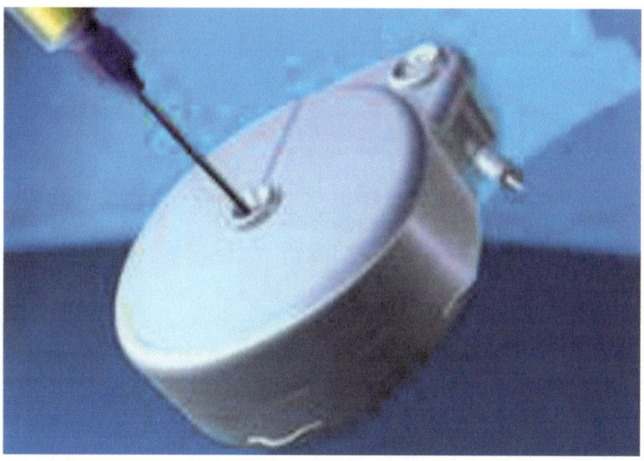

Fig. 7. Refilling procedure

A programmer interacts with the pump by establishing a contact in radiofrequency (fig. 8) thanks to which you can get a report of the programming parameters and of the prescription of medication (quantity and time of infusion). There are different models of pump, but can be divided into 2 types: fixed flux and electronic pumps, which are fully programmable via an external computer with telemetry head, they are battery powered and can last from 5 to 7 years of life, the most popular model is the Synchromed (fig. 9).

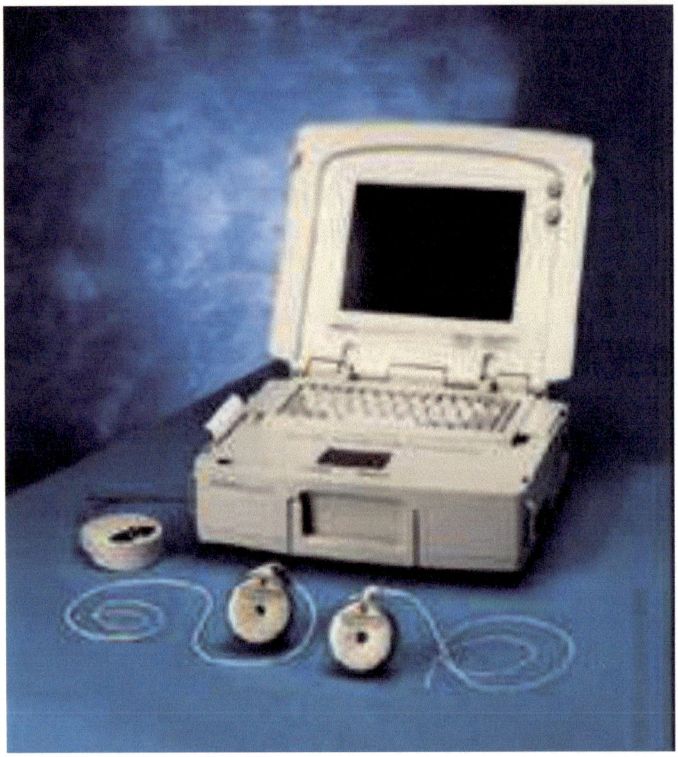

Fig. 8. Pump programer

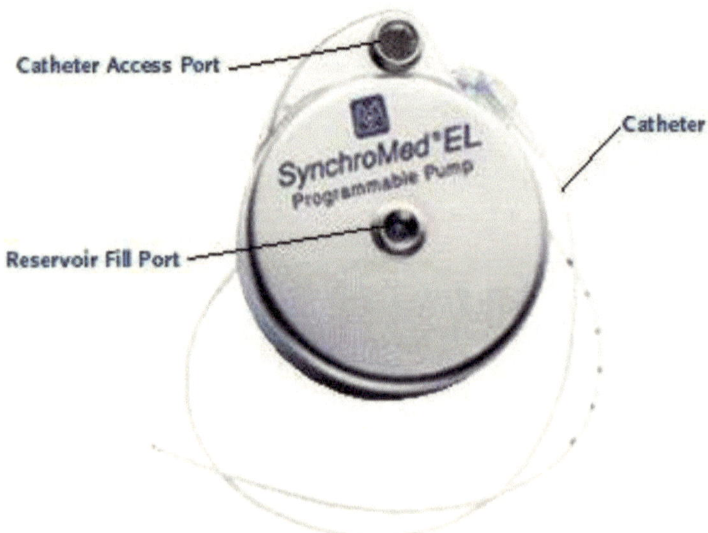

Fig. 9. Programmable infusion pump

The programmable parameters for Syncromed type of pumps are the following: date and time of refilling; identification of the patient, name and concentration of the drug; mode of infusion, dosage of the drug and rate of administration; volume of the reservoir and low alarm setting reservoir; low battery alarm control (acoustic).

The Syncromed (Medtronic Italia, S.p.A., Rome, Italy) pumps are, moreover, supplied of acoustic alarm systems, which signal: drug in exhaustion (falls below the level of reserves); battery in exhaustion; memory alterations programming.

Isomed (Medtronic Italia, S.p.A., Rome, Italy) and Archimedes (Anschütz, Kiel, Germany) models are at constant flux (fig. 10), and hence at the refilling the daily concentration is attained modulating the refilling solution concentration, taking into account the daily flux (0,5 or 1 ml/day).

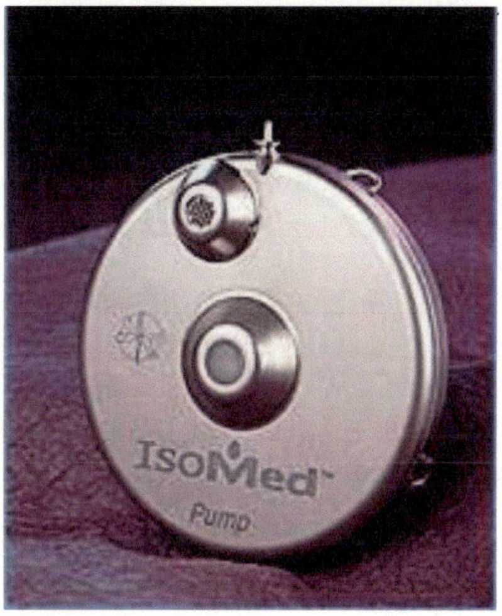

Fig. 10. Fixed flux infusion pump

Fixed flow pumps have a longer life by virtue of the absence of batteries, but are less precise than in the selection of the dose and can not afford the infusion of doses differentiated throughout the day, but for the change of dosage is required the emptying of the pump and filling with a new solution, to the dosage selected.

3. Patient selection

Careful patient selection is a fundamental factor for the positive outcome to the treatment. Intrathecal administration should be considered in patients who are unresponsive to treatment with oral opiates due to ineffective therapy or to intolerable side effects, who have good circulation of the cerebrospinal fluid and who possess a life expectancy of at least three months as diagnosed by the pain specialist and the oncologist.

Before beginning treatment, patients must pass a screening test which can be epidural or intrathecal. The intrathecal test is performed with single intrathecal injections of drug at L2-3 via a 27 Gauge Whitacre spinal needle (Becton Dickinson Caribe LTD. Juncos, PR), while patients is in prone position with a pillow under the chest, to keep the spine stretched. Agents used for this trial included either morphine 0,1 mg and isobaric-bupivacaine (0,5%) 0,125 mg, or saline solution (2ml) for the placebo test (3). This trial for efficacy and safety lasts usually 7 days. Placebo or morphine/bupivacaine IT injections are administered to patients on days 1, 3 and 7 of the trial. Patients are considered to be positive responders to IT analgesia if they have pain relief > 70% after administration of morphine and bupivacaine, and <30% after injection of the placebo. The dosage of morphine/bupivacaine that provided relief of pain during the trial is the initial dose used after implantation.

If a patient does not respond optimally to the morphine, another test is carried out using a different opioid (e.g. hydromorphone, fentanyl, sufentanil); ziconotide or, depending on the type of pain, a combination of opiates + local anaesthetic (e.g. bupivacaine) or clonidine.

Patients responding positively to the test, the are programmed for implantation of the infusion system. Firstly a temporary implant is used, which includes a catheter implanted that is connected to an external pump CADD (Smiths-Medical Italia, S.r.l., Latina, Italy), which is programmable.

IT drug titration is performed as follows: the initial morphine dose is 0.1 mg/day, in order to limit side effects, during the post-operative period, if the pain is not adequately controlled (Visual analogue scale, VAS 0-10 reduction <3 points), the dosage is increased of 20% after 3-5 days. Then increments of 10% to 20% are used until pain is attenuated or intolerable side effects appear. When morphine dose is 0.5mg/day, then 0.5mg/day of bupivacaine is added to morphine infusion, if pain is still not controlled. The bupivacaine dose is then increased of 0.25mgs/day until a pain reduction =3 points in VAS (fig. 11). After two increases of bupivacaine dosage, if the VAS reduction is still < 3 points, then the dosage of morphine is increased (max dosage 1.0mg/day) (76).

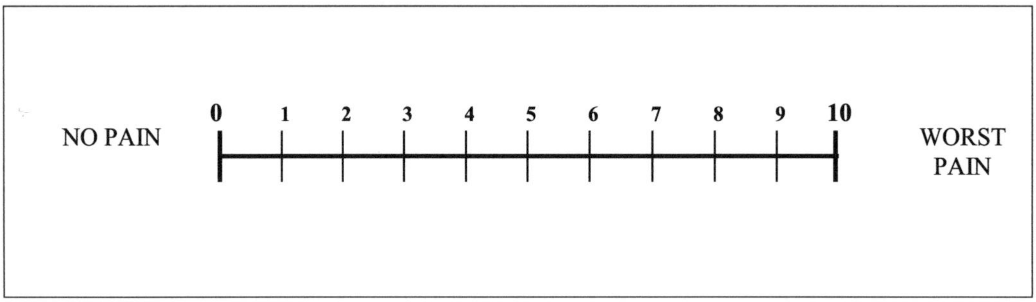

Fig. 11. VAS scale

When a optimal response is obtained (usually after 1-2 months), the permanent pump is implanted: after a precise preventive antibiotic therapy, and local anesthesia, the catheter, previously implanted, is connected to a pump that is inserted into a pocket under the skin, generally in the abdomen. The totally implanted pump is not visible outside and allows the subject to be free to move and make a normal life.

Management of patients throughout the various stages of the treatment should be based on a multidisciplinary approach involving psychologists, nurses, physiotherapists, social workers and spiritual advisors.

The selection criteria which characterize patients with cancer pain or non-malignant pain are similar. However, patients with non-malignant pain require a more comprehensive psycho-social assessment.

Regarding the cost-effectiveness of intrathecal therapy for the treatment of pain, even though initial costs, associated with the surgical implant of an intrathecal pump, appear to be substantial; moreover the maintenance costs of intrathecal administration are significantly lower over time compared to other methods of delivery. In this way the overall cost of the therapy is reduced in the long term (21). Cost analysis of alternative methods (including oral) for the administration of opiates indicates that intrathecal treatment is more cost-effective in patients who require long-term management of cancer pain (≥ 3-6 months) or non-malignant pain (≥ 11-22 months).

4. Risk associated with intrathecal administration

Intrathecal administration of analgesic agents have some risks: specific drug-related side-effects, medical complications (surgery), and technical complications related to the infusion device (77) (table 7, 8). Extremely dangerous are the complications related to pump delivery malfunctions, which may cause high dosage infusion or acute withdrawal (table 7), resulting in life-threatening side effects, such as coma or death.

Postoperative complications	Instrumental Complications
- Infection of the pocket, the subcutaneous tunnel and the CSF space - CSF fistula, can be identified by the following symptoms: headache gravitational, exacerbated the assumption of the upright, sometimes associated with nausea, vertigo, tinnitus and, rarely, diplopia due to the interest of the sixth cranial nerve. The most serious complication of CSF fistulas is represented by meningitis. - Spinal tumors (granuloma), due to the retention of the catheter into the subarachnoid space; - Development of inflammatory mass at the tip of catheter, which can cause serious neurological damage, including paralysis. Symptoms: spinal cord compression, change in intensity or type pain or contractions, onset of pain at the tip of the catheter, need for continuous increases in dose, which give only temporary relief. - Hygroma of the pocket or a reflux of CSF resulting in loosening and widening of the pocket - Bruising, bleeding, swelling, serous pocket - Headache due to loss of CSF during surgery - Paralysis	- Occlusion of the catheter or angolamento - Stoppage due to malfunction or depletion of usable life - Twisting movements of the pump in the pocket on its longitudinal axis with possible displacemnt of the catheter, or on the transversal axis with impossibility to reach the points of injection for the filling of the reservoir - Loss, breakage or disconnection of the catheter, resulting in delivery of the drug along in its path, or implanted under the skin where the pump

Table 7. Complications of infusion pump

Withdrawal syndrome can also be observed if refilling is not performed inside the correct range of time, for this reason it is extremely important to refill the pump at least 2-3 days before the emptying of the reservoir. In any case of withdrawal a substitutive oral opioid therapy must be promptly started, while technical problems are solved.

Moreover, regarding cancer pain, there is a hesitancy to use invasive techniques by palliative care physicians in cancer patients at the end of life because their patients are often weak and suffering from frequent changes in painful pathology. In addition, there also is a low level of awareness of the procedures involved and a lack of professionals who are expert in the field.

Opioid Overdose Symptoms	Opioids Withdrawal symptoms
- Respiratory depression - bradycardia - Point miosis ("pinheads" pupil) - Coma.	- yawn - runny nose - piloerection - Sweating - tearing - tremor - mydriasis - Hot flashes - Chills - restlessness - vomiting - Muscle spasms - Abdominal cramps - anxiety

Table 8. Drug-related complications of infusion pump

Anyway it is believed that the benefits of this method (table 6) could greatly outweigh the possible risks of implanting these devices and that prevention, early identification, and rapid management of the adverse effects, could allow for an optimal clinical outcome for the patients (77).

Intraoperative complications are extremely rare, and may be related to perforation of the dura mater that, given the calibre of the needle, can cause clinically significant CSF loss during the perioperative period, and require treatment with blood-patch and normal therapies indicated in such situations. Another complication is the bleeding into the epidural space, which can occur only if the patient has severe bleeding disorder, which is why blood tests are performed pre-operatively, to exclude patients with such problems. As concerning post operative complications, they are summarised in table 7.

Sometimes experts in this spinal procedure dedicate insufficient attention to the interference between drugs (opioids) given and its effects on biological functions. Today, failure to understand the side-effects of intrathecal therapy by a implanting physician might be considered negligence, because it has been known for a long time that the use of opioids, for both acute and chronic pain, modifies the release of hypopituitary hormones and the activity of immune cells (62, 50). We believe that this spinal procedure should include clinical risk management and monitoring of hormonal function in all individuals (52).

4.1 Drug-related side-effects

The side effects associated with intrathecal administration of opiates or other analgesics are similar to those produced by systemic administration, but the delivery of extremely low doses means that the most important side effects (table 9), such as respiratory depression, are avoided or lessened (78).

Short-term Opioid Adverse effects	Long-term Opioid Adverse effects
- Itching, - Nausea, - Vomiting, - Diarrhea, - Constipation, - Drowsiness, - Loss of appetite, - Dry mouth, - Dizziness, - Hyperhidrosis, - Urinary retention, - Respiratory depression.	- Nausea, - Vomiting, - Drowsiness, - Dry mouth, - Constipation, - Impotence, - Urinary retention, - Immunosuppression, - Interference with hormone levels (prolactin, growth hormone, thyroid hormone, adrenocorticotropic hormone and luteinizing hormone, testosterone), - Inhibition of the nociceptin, - Onset of tolerance (increased doses of opioids continuously).

Table 9. Opioid related adverse events

The most serious risk associated with intrathecal morphine was the development of respiratory depression, even if it is extremely rare, appearing in only 1% of cases. It can arise in the 3 to 16 hours following infusion. For this reason, patients need to be carefully monitored, above all in the 24 hours following infusion or a dose increase. Hyperalgesia, myoclonus, urinary retention, nausea, vomiting and itching are other side effects associated with the use of spinal opiates, above all in patients which require higher dosages.

Slow titration of the dosage, suitable prophylactic co-treatment and careful patient screening mean many of the side effects can be avoided. Management of the side effects associated with intrathecal administration of opiates involves reducing opiate doses, administering adjuvant drugs or, in serious cases, an opiate receptor antagonist. The side effects can be reduced by changing to another opiate (e.g. hydromorphone), or by combining bupivacaine or clonidine to a smaller dose of morphine.

There are dose-related effects to the use of bupivacaine. Side-effects such as paresthesia, motorsensory block, arterial hypotension, and urinary retention are associated with the anesthetic effects of bupivacaine at spinal levels, usually linked to daily doses above 45 mg / day (79). The delivery of lower doses of bupivacaine means that these side-effects can be avoided or lessened.

Slow titration of a given dose, suitable prophylactic pre-treatment and careful patient screening may mitigate many of these side-effects. Management of the side-effects associated with intrathecal administration of opioids involves reducing opioid-doses, administering adjuvant medications or, in serious cases, an opioid-receptor antagonist. The side-effects also can be reduced by changing to another opioid as in opioid rotation (e.g., hydromorphone), or by combining bupivacaine or clonidine to a smaller dose of the opioid infused.

4.2 Opioid: Addiction and tolerance

One of the worst risks associated to the opioid use is the rise of tolerance and addiction. Drug addiction is a constant psychological and physical craving for legal or illegal substances, even in the face of adverse consequences, according to the National Institute on Drug Abuse. Drug addiction is a disease, because drug abuse causes changes in brain chemistry that make it difficult to function without the substance of choice; however, like diabetes and heart disease, it can be managed with proper intervention. Biology, genetic development and living environment may all play a role in why some people become addicts and other users do not.

The term "addiction" is often applied to two phenomena, one psychological, the other physical, which must be clearly distinguished from each other (80, 81). On one hand there is the irresistible urge to take the drug, on the other the sudden deprivation syndrome, both depending by the drug intake in the organism. The neuro-anatomical substrates of these two phenomena appear distinct. Bulbar and mesencephalic structures, particularly the Locus Coeruleus, the Raphe Nucleus and Periaqueductal gray matter, are involved in the event of the withdrawal syndrome. Limbic territories (Ventral Nidbrain, Ventral Striatum, Hippocampus, Amygdala, etc) are involved mainly in the persistent desire for opioids and in the mechanism of addiction that they generate. The mesolimbic dopaminergic system plays a central role, as it is involved in both the euphoric effects of opioids, both in the modulation of neuronal circuits, which are directly responsible of the withdrawal symptom (82).

Repeated administration of opioids can result in the development of tolerance, which can be defined as the rightward shift of the dose response curve for a substance. The associative tolerance is related to conditioning, while the so-called pharmacological tolerance is due to the mechanism of action of the drug. The pharmacological tolerance may be due to constitutional factors, changes in pharmacokinetic or, more frequently, due to decreased pharmacodynamic effects of analgesic related to some process of neural adaptation.

These processes are characterized by great variability intra- and interpatient. Tolerance to different effects of opioids develops at different speeds and can occur quickly after acute administration or develop more gradually as the recurrence of the hiring (83, 84). Development of tolerance can be maintained during long-term administration or appear and progress quickly in the first phase of treatment.

Opioids exert their actions via membrane receptors which are coupled to their effectors by G protein. Scientist tried to find out whether these alterations are involved in the different elements of tolerance and dependence. Probably changes in the number and/or affinity of opioid receptors for their ligands are mechanisms that are not involved. In fact, when these changes are eventually found, tolerance and dependence have already developed; therefore, alterations of receptors would rather be the consequences and not the cause of tolerance and dependence. On the other hand, a functional coupling between opioid receptors and their effectors is probably one of the mechanisms involved in the development of tolerance to morphinomimetics, despite the interaction mechanism is still not clearly established (83).

Recently an imbalance between the excitatory and inhibitory effects of opioids was suggested. In fact, in addition to classical receptors responsible for the actions of opioids, whose stimulation causes inhibitory effects that result in a hyperpolarization of neurons and a reduction of the release of neurotransmitters, there are opioid receptors whose stimulation has the opposite excitatory effect. Agonists have a much greater affinity for these excitatory receptors than for the inhibitory ones (85). In other words, the effect of the stimulation on opioid receptors, including their analgesic action (86), it would be the result of: the exciter action connected to the involvement of higher-affinity receptors for the agonists; and of the inhibitory action due to lower-affinity receptors stimulation (87). Chronic treatment with opioids results in a reduction of its inhibitory influence and a hypersensitivity to its action exciter (88,89). It is believed that these alterations may be involved in the development of tolerance to the inhibitory effects of opioids and in the manifestations of withdrawal syndrome.

The morphinomimetics influence the activity of neurons that have opioid receptors and a number of neurons networks are involved in a given pharmacological effect of these substances. Many neuronal central regions and almost all neurotransmitters, such as dopamine, norepinephrine, serotonin, acetylcholine and GABA (90), are implicated in the onset or expression of different manifestations of tolerance and/or morphine addiction. Recently the role of excitatory amino acids (EAA) was emphasised, in fact, blocking some EAA receptors (NMDA) inhibits the development of tolerance to the analgesic effects of morphine (80).

Some of the target neurons of morphinomimetics could be part of a homeostatic system that tends to reduce the action of opioids. Thus opioids would activate neurons which would release neuropeptides, that act as antagonists of endogenous opioids. The hyperactivity of neurons to cholecystokinin-8 (CCK-8) and to neuropeptide FF (NPFF), induced by prolonged administration of morphine, is partly the cause of drug tolerance and addiction (91).

The different hypotheses are not mutually exclusive; it is likely that these different mechanisms contribute to the appearance of tolerance and dependence in different ways and degrees. Tolerance develops as a result of spinal administration of opioids, although it seems to grow more slowly and in a reduced way than the use of systemic opioids (92).

5. Guidelines to threat patiens intrathecally

Management of patients throughout the various stages of the diagnosis and treatment of pain should be based on multidisciplinary expertise. Careful patient selection is the one fundamental factor accounting for positive outcomes to treatment.

These are the suggested criteria for patients receiving intrathecal therapy:

- Intrathecal administration should be reserved for patients who are unresponsive or poorly responsive to treatment with oral /transdermal opioids, either because of the development of tolerance, in spite of sequential drug trialing, or because of the development of dose-specific side-effects.

- The selection criteria for patients with cancer pain or noncancer pain are similar. However, patients with noncancer pain, because of their life expectancy, should require a more comprehensive sychosocial assessment.
- A psychosocial evaluation should explore:

1. patients' expectations of their therapy,
2. analyze the quality of the patient's pain and the meaning of the pain to the patient,
3. the presence of psychologic disease that might prevent adequate outcomes to the therapy, and
4. barriers to patient and family compliance to the use of the pump system.

- No pathology on cerebrospinal fluid found.
- Informed consent to the procedure.

Step no. 1

A temporary trial of spinal opioid therapy should be performed to assess the potential benefits of this approach before implantation. In order to be considered an ideal candidate for intrathecal administration, a patient must demonstrate a reduction in pain of at least 50% with the observable absence of intolerable side-effects from the agent tested. Morphine should be the first agent trialed because more is known about morphine than any other agent. If a patient does not respond optimally to morphine, an another agent should be trialed such as hydromorphone, fentanyl, sufentanil, or, depending on the type of pain, as in neuropahtic pain, a combination of opioids and local anesthetic (e.g., bupivacaine). Many differing methods for this trial have been reported, such as the continuous epidural or intrathecal infusion of agents or single shot injections of these agents, either epidural or intrathecal (93, 94).

Step no. 2

After a successful trial and once the pump has been implanted, the initial daily dose of morphine or agent found to be the best at trial should be that dose that gave the most efficacious response at the time of trial. In an effort to limit side-effects during the initial postoperative therapy period, an intrathecal morphine dose, that is 20% lower than the screening test dose, should be used. The initial dose should be increased, if necessary, by 20% every 3–5 days until the dose used at trial is reached. After that dose has been reached, increases in dose should be by increments of no more that 10% to 20% until pain control is reached or until intolerable side-effects appear.

Monitoring

Patients with implanted drug delivery systems must be monitored at regular intervals of time. Monitoring for efficacy and side-effects, especially those due to perturbations of the endocrine system, is good medicine and standard of care.

Anyway a clear standard for the correlation of a specific combination of drugs to the treatment of a specific type of pain is still lacking. An effective dose of opioids is variable and individual to the needs of each and every patient; however, the effective dose of any one opioid often reaches high levels for various reasons including syndromespecific opioid resistance, receptor phenotype-determined resistance, and/or tolerance to the opioid delivered. Appropriate patients are selected for Intrathecal Drug Delivery System using IT / epidural trials either by single shot injection or titration through an implanted catheter until effective dosage is reached (33).

6. IT in geriatric population

The IT administration of low-dose agents for the attainment of satisfactory pain control is particularly important for the geriatric population. Nowadays, the number of elderly people and the average age of the population are increasing. The elderly often suffer from age-related diseases such as vascular cardiopathies, cerebrovascular diseases, osteoporosis, and arthrosis, which are, in-ofthemselves, themselves allergenic (95) and from pneumonias, diabetes, peripheral arterial diseases, and fractures, which generate further pain (96). These diseases result in serious disabilities and limitation of patients' physical, cognitive, and social activities, resulting in loss of the autonomy and worsening of their quality of life. For this reason, it is of primary importance to find an efficient analgesic therapy for the elderly that avoids pharmacologic interactions with other medications used by patients for the treatment of their comorbid diseases that result in unwanted effects and adverse events. It is also well established that the elderly (older than 64 years) need lower doses of drugs to achieve the same level of efficacy that younger patients need. The aging process, indeed, involves a series of metabolic modifications that result in important alterations of the pharmacokinetics and dynamics of a drug (97). In particular, the reduction of body water level results in a reduced distribution of hydrophilic drugs, such as morphine. Similarly, the agerelated reduction of plasma proteins causes an increase in the concentration of active drug and, hence, a reduction in drug dosage needed. Moreover, the decrease of renal and hepatic output requires an adjustment of drug dosages given to the elderly (98, 99).

7. Future work

Intrathecal pump implantation has its advantages and its advantages; the main concern is if the elimination of systemic side-effects justifies an invasive procedure with its own potential serious complications. The costs of the device is high, however, it is cost-effective in the long term in patients responding to this treatment (100).

From the literature, actually, there is no solid outcome evidence that supports intrathecal therapy use, indeed, randomized studies are still scarce, and in several studies the number of patients is low.

Despite the fact that opioids and morphine in particular are the most used intrathecal drug, ziconotide is increasingly used for intrathecal therapy. It has also been recently indicated as first line IT drug by the Polyanalgesic Consensus Conference (45), thanks to its property and efficacy (101-104), and it is extremely useful also for patients intolerant or refractory to the common IT drugs (such as morphine).

Our recent work shows that ziconotide has good levels of efficacy and long-term safety, which can be attained at stable doses with a constant pain relief, suggesting the absence of tolerance effects (104). This suggests, moreover, that, once the early side effects are overcome, the responders are not exposed to long-term risks

We believe that this drug has a great potential for future IT therapy, in order to reduce common long-term opioid related adverse events: immunomodulation, influence on the endocrine system and tolerance.

IT therapy, moreover is useful also for the treatment of spasticity: baclofen is widely applied for this purpose (105-108), alone or in association with ziconotide, or local anesthetics, in cases of spasticity associated with pain (73, 108).

8. Conclusion

Intrathecal administration of drugs by qualified personnel significantly enhances pain relief and improves the quality of life in patients who fail conservative therapies with oral or transdermal delivery of analgesics, while reducing the risk of adverse effects and complications. According to indications suggested by the International Consensus Conference (17), that took place in Belgium in 1998, the fundamental prerequisite for the correct application of intrathecal therapy with opioids is appropriate professional training regarding: catheter and pump implant procedures; knowledge of the anatomy, physiology, and neuropharmacology of the neuromodulatory centers of the spinal cord and the brain; knowledge of systemic complications; a multidisciplinary approach to care.

However, because the literature is bereft of good clinical science that pertains to intrathecal therapy and is full of anecdotal material, we believe that long-term prospective and randomized studies are necessary to fully evaluate the safety and efficacy of the intrathecal administration of opioids and nonopioids alike for pain relief. It is important that these prospective, randomized, controlled trials identify not only the efficacy of intrathecal to provide pain management, but also the biological impact that the route of administration of analgesics (systemic vs. intrathecal) has on the general health and well-being of the patient.

9. References

[1] Merskey H, Bogduk N. Classification of Chronic Pain. Seattle: IASP Press; 1994:210.
[2] Shaladi AM, Saltari MR, Crestani F, Piva B. Post-surgical neuropathic pain. Recenti Prog Med 2009;100(7-8):371-9.
[3] Raffaeli W, Marconi G, Fanelli G, Taddei S, Borghi GB, Casati A. Opioid-related side-effects after intrathecal morphine: a prospective, randomized, double-blind dose-responce study. European Journal of Anaesthesiology 2006, 23: 605-610.
[4] Hassenbusch SJ, Paice JA, Patt RB, Bedder MD, Bell GK. Clinical realities and conomic considerations: efficacy of intrathecal pain therapy. J Pain Symptom Manage 1997;14 (Suppl.):S14–S26.
[5] World Health Organization Programme on Cancer Control. Developing a global strategy for cancer. Editor: Karol Sikora, March 1998.
[6] World Health Organization. Cancer pain relief. Geneva, Switzerland: WHO, 1986.
[7] World Health Organization. Achieving balance in national opioids control policy: guidelines for assessment. Geneva, Switzerland: WHO, 2000.
[8] World Health Organization. Cancer pain relief and palliative care: Report of a WHO expert committee (Technical Report Series 804). Geneva, Switzerland: WHO, 1990.
[9] Foley KM. Controversies in cancer pain: medical perspectives. Cancer 1989;63:2257–2265.
[10] Schug SA, Zech D, Don U. Cancer pain management according to WHO analgesic guidelines. J Pain Symptom Manage 1990;5:27–32.
[11] Zech DFJ, Grond S, Lynch J, Hertel D, Lehmann KA. Validation of World Health Organization Guidelines for cancer pain relief: a 10-year prospective study. Pain 1995;63:65–76.
[12] Mercadante S et al. Episodic (breakthrough) pain. Consensus Conference of an expert working group of the European Association for Palliative Care. Cancer 2002.
[13] Gardner-Nix J. Oral transmucosal fentanyl and sufentanyl for incident pain. J Pain Symptom Manage 2001;22:627.

[14] Catala E. Intrathecal administration of opioids in cancer patients. Paper presented at a satellite symposium of the European Federation of IASP Chapters Second Congress, September 22–23, 1997, Barcelona, Spain.
[15] Vargas-Schaffer G. Is the WHO analgesic ladder still valid? Twenty-four years of experience. Can Fam Physician;56(6):514-7, e202-5.
[16] Wang JF, Nauss LA, Thomas JE. Pain relief by intrathecally applied morphine in man. Anesthesiology 1979;50:149-151.
[17] Coombs DW, Saunders RL, Gaylor MS, Pageau MG, Leith MG, Schaiberger C. Continuous epidural analgesia via implanted morphine reservoir. Lancet 1981; 2: 425-426.
[18] Kwan JW. Use of infusion devices for epidural or intrathecal administration of spinal opioids. Am J Hosp Pharm 1990;47 (Suppl. 1):S18-S23.
[19] Yaksh TL, Rudy TA. Analgesia mediated by a direct spinal action of narcotics. Science 1976;192(4246):1357-8.
[20] Smith HS, Deer TR, Staats PS, Singh V, Sehgal N, Cordner H. Intrathecal drug delivery. Pain Physician 2008;11(2 Suppl):S89-S104.
[21] Portenoy RK. Clinical realities and economic considerations: introduction. J Pain Symptom Manage 1997;14 (Suppl.):SI–S2.
[22] Task Force of the European Federation of IASP Chapters (EFIC). Neuromodulation of pain: a consensus statement prepared in Brussels 16–18 January. Eur J Pain 1998;2:203–209.
[23] Krames ES, Olson K. Clinical realities and economic considerations: patient selection in intrathecal therapy. J Pain Symptom Manage 1997;14 (Suppl.): S3-S13.
[24] Bennett G, Serafini M, Burchiel K, Buchser E, Classen A, Deer T, et al. Evidence-based review of the literature on intrathecal delivery of pain medication. J Pain Symptom Manage 2000;20(2):S12-36.
[25] Deer T, Winkelmuller W, Erdine S, Bedder M, Burchiel K. Intrathecal therapy for cancer and nonmalignant pain: patient selection and patient management. Neuromodulation 1999;2(2):55-66.
[26] Stain F, Barjavel MJ, Sandouk P, Plotkine M, Scherrmann JM, Bhargava HN. Analgesic response and plasma and brain extracellular fluid pharmacokinetics of morphine and morphine-6-beta-D-glucuronide in the rat. J Pharmacol Exp Ther 1995;274(2):852-7.
[27] Krames E. The chronic intraspinal use of opioid and local anesthetic mixtures for the relief of intractable pain: when all else fails! Pain 1993;55:1–4.
[28] Nordberg G, Hedner T, Mellstrand T, Dahlstrom B. Pharmacokinetic aspects of intrathecal morphine analgesia. Anesthesiology 1984;60:448–454.
[29] Sullivan ARF, McQuay HJ, Bailey D, Dickenson AH. The spinal antinociceptive actions of morphine metabolites: morphine-6-glucuronide and normorphine in the rat. Brain Res 1989; 482:219–224.
[30] Sandouk P, Serrie A, Scherrmann JM, Langlade A, Bourre JM. Presence of morphine metabolites in human cerebrospinal fluid after intracerebroventricular administration of morphine. Eur J Drug Metab Pharmacokinet 1991;Spec No 3:166-71.
[31] McQuay HJ, Sullivan AF, Smallman K, Dickenson AH. Intrathecal opioids, potency and lipophilicity. Pain 1989;36(1):111-5.

[32] Sullivan AF, McQuay HJ, Bailey D, Dickenson AH. The spinal antinociceptive actions of morphine metabolites morphine-6-glucuronide and normorphine in the rat. Brain Res 1989;482(2):219-2
[33] Georges P, Lavand'homme P. Intrathecal hydromorphone instead of the old intrathecal morphine: the best is the enemy of the good? Eur J Anaesthesiol;2012, 29(1):3-4.
[34] Wallace M, Yaksh TL. Long-term spinal analgesic delivery: a review of the preclinical and clinical literature. Reg Anesth Pain Med 2000;25:117–157.
[35] Li DF, Bahar M, Cole G, Rosen M. Neurological toxicity of the subarachnoid infusion of bupivacaine, lignocaine or 2-chloroprocaine in the rat. Br J Anaesth 1985;57:424–429.
[36] Dahm P, Nitescu P, Appelgren L, Curelaru I. Efficacy and technical complications of long-term continuous intraspinal infusions of opioid and/or bupivacaine in refractory nonmalignant pain: a comparison between the epidural and the intrathecal approach with externalized or implanted catheters and infusion pumps. Clin J Pain 1998;14:4–16.
[37] Van Dongen RT, Crul BJ, van Egmond J. Intrathecal coadministration of bupivacaine diminishes morphine dose progression during long-term intrathecal infusion in cancer patients. Clin J Pain 1999;15:166–172.
[38] Franco Gay ML. Spinal morphine in nonmalignant chronic pain: a retrospective study in 39 patients. Neuromodulation 2002;5:150–159.
[39] Eisenach J, DuPen S, Dubois M, Miguel R, Allin D. Epidural clonidine analgesia for intractable cancer pain. Pain 1995;61:391–399.
[40] Yaksh T. Pharmacology of spinal adrenergic systems which modulate spinal nociceptive processing. Pharmacol Biochem Behav 1985;22:845–858.
[41] Levy R, Leiphart J, Dills C. Analgesic action of acute and chronic intraspinally administered opioid and alph6 agonists in chronic neuropathic pain. Stereotact Funct Neurosurg 1994;62:279–289.
[42] Krames ES, Lanning RM. Intrathecal infusional analgesia for nonmalignant pain: analgesic efficacy of intrathecal opioid with or without bupivacaine. J Pain Symptom Manage 1993;8:539–548.
[43] Sjoberg M, Appelgreen L, Einarsson S et al. Long-term intrathecal morphine and bupivacaine in refractory cancer pain. I. Results from the first series of 52 patients. Acta Anaesthesiol Scand 1991;35:30–43.
[44] Hassenbusch SJ, Portenoy RK. Current practices in intraspinal therapy – a survey of clinical trends and decision making. J Pain Symptom Manage 2000;20:4–11.
[45] Deer T, Krames ES, Hassenbusch SJ, Burton A, Caraway D, Dupen S, Eisenach J, Erdek M, Grigsby E, Kim P, Levy R, McDowell G, Mekhail N, Panchal S, Prager J, Rauck R, Saulino M, Sitzman, T, Staats P, Stanton-Hicks M, Stearns L, Willis KD, Witt W, Follett K, Huntoon M, Liem L, Rathmell J, Wallace M, Buchser. E, Cousins M, Ver Donck A. Polyanalgesic consensus conference 2007: recommendations for the management of pain by intrathecal (intraspinal) drug delivery: report of an interdisciplinary expert panel. Neuromodulation 2007;10(4):300-28.
[46] Lara NA, Jr., Teixeira MJ, Fonoff ET. Long term intrathecal infusion of opiates for treatment of failed back surgery syndrome. Acta Neurochir Suppl; 2011,108:41-7.
[47] Brazenor GA. Long term intrathecal administration of morphine: a comparison of bolus injection via reservoir with continuous infusion by implanted pump. Neurosurgery 1987;21(4):484-91.

[48] Gourlay GK, Plummer JL, Cherry DA, Onley MM, Parish KA, Wood MM, et al. Comparison of intermittent bolus with continuous infusion of epidural morphine in the treatment of severe cancer pain. Pain 1991;47(2):135-40.
[49] Trescot AM, Datta S, Lee M, Hansen H. Opioid pharmacology. Pain Physician 2008;11(2 Suppl):S133-53.
[50] Raffaelli W, Salmosky-Dekel BG. Biological consequences of long-term intrathecal administration of opioids. Minerva Anestesiol 2005;71(7-8):475-8.
[51] Campana G, Sarti D, Spampinato S, Raffaeli W. Long-term intrathecal morphine and bupivacaine upregulate MOR gene expression in lymphocytes. Int Immunopharmacol; 2010,10(9):1149-52.
[52] Raffaeli W, Salmosky-Dekel B.G, Rita M, Righetti D, Caminiti A, Balestri M, Sarti D, Fanelli G. Long-term intrathecal morphine influence on major compounds of the endocrine system in elderly population. Eur J of Pain Suppl,2009;3:71–76
[53] Kellum JA. The modern concept of homeostasis. Minerva Anestesiol 2002;68:3-11.
[54] Vallejo R, Leon-Casasola O, Benyamin R. Opioid therapy and immunosuppression: a review. Am J Ther 2004;11:354-65.
[55] Mathews PM, Froelich CJ, Sibbitt WL Jr, Bankhurst AD. Enhancement of natural cytotoxicity by beta-endorphin. J Immunol 1983;130:1658-62.
[56] Dimitrijevic M, Stanojevic S, Kovacevic-Jovanovic V, Miletic T, Vujic-Redzic V, Radulovic J. Modulation of humoral immune responses in the rat by centrally applied Met-Enk and opioid receptor antagonists: functional interactions of brain OP1, OP2 and OP3 receptors. Immunopharmacology 2000;49:255-62.
[57] Jankovic BD, Veljic J, Pesic G, Maric D. Enkephalinaseinhibitors modulate immune responses. Int J Neurosci 1991;59:45-51.
[58] Radulovic J, Jankovic BD. Opposing activities of brain opioid receptors in the regulation of humoral and cellmediated immune responses in the rat. Brain Res 1994;661:189-95.
[59] Radulovic J, Miljevic C, Djergovic D, Vujic V, Antic J, Von Horsten S, et al. Opioid receptor-mediated suppression of humoral immune response in vivo and in vitro: involvement of kappa opioid receptors. J Neuroimmunol 1995;57:55-62.
[60] Veljic J, Ranin J, Maric D, Jankovic BD. Modulation of cutaneous immune reactions by centrally applied methionine-enkephalin. Ann N Y Acad Sci 1992;650:51-5.
[61] Mellon RD, Bayer BM. Evidence for central opioid receptors in the immunomodulatory effects of morphine: review of potential mechanism(s) of action. J Neuroimmunol 1998;83:19-28.
[62] Provinciali M, Raffaeli W. Evaluation of NK and LAK cell activities in neoplastic patients during treatment with morphine. Intern J Neuroscience 1991;59:127-33.
[63] Morley JE. The endocrinology of the opiates and opioid peptides. Metabolism 1981;30:195-209.
[64] Su CF, Liu MY, Lin MT. Intraventricular morphine produces pain relief, hypothermia, hyperglycaemia and increased prolactin and growth hormone levels in patients with cancer pain. J Neurol 1987;235:105-8.
[65] Rasmussen DD, Liu JH, Wolf PL, Yen SS. Endogenous opioid regulation of gonadotropin-releasing hormone release from the human fetal hypothalamus in vitro. J Clin Endocrinol Metab 1983;57:881-4.
[66] Delitala G, Devilla L, Musso NR. On the role of dopamine receptors in the naloxone-induced hormonal changes in man. J Clin Endocrinol Metab 1983;56:181-4.

[67] Grossman A, Moult PJ, Cunnah D, Besser M. Different opioid mechanisms are involved in the modulation of ACTH and gonadotrophin release in man. Neuroendocrinology 1986;42:357-60.
[68] Gold PW, Extein I, Pickar D, Rebar R, Ross R, Goodwin FK. Supression of plasma cortisol in depressed patients by acute intravenous methadone infusion. Am J Psychiatry 1980;137:862-3.
[69] Abs R, Verhelst J, Maeyaert J, Van Buyten JP, Opsoner F, Adriaensen H, et al. Endocrine consequences of long-term intrathecal administration of opioids. J Clin Endocrinol Metab 2000;85:2215-22.
[70] Paice JA, Penn RD, Ryan WG. Altered sexual function and decreased testosterone in patients receiving intraspinal opioids. J Pain Symptom Manage 1994;9:126-31.
[71] Roberts LJ, Finch PM, Pullan PT, Bhagat CI, Price LM. Sex hormone suppression by intrathecal opioids: a prospective study. Clin J Pain 2002;18:144-8.
[72] Patel VB, Manchikanti L, Singh V, Schultz DM, Hayek SM, Smith HS. Systematic review of intrathecal infusion systems for long-term management of chronic non-cancer pain. Pain Physician 2009;12(2):345-60.
[73] Smith HS, Deer TR, Staats PS, Singh V, Sehgal N, Cordner H. Intrathecal drug delivery. Pain Physician 2008;11(2 Suppl):S89-S104.
[74] Anderson VC, Burchiel KJ. A prospective study of long-term intrathecal morphine in the management of chronic nonmalignant pain. Neurosurgery 1999;44(2):289-300; discussion 300-1.
[75] Smith TJ, Staats PS, Deer T, Stearns LJ, Rauck RL, Boortz-Marx RL, et al. Randomized clinical trial of an implantable drug delivery system compared with comprehensive medical management for refractory cancer pain: impact on pain, drug-related toxicity, and survival. J Clin Oncol 2002;20(19):4040-9.
[76] Raffaeli W, Righetti D, Caminiti A, Ingardia A, Balestri M, Pambianco L, Fanelli G, Facondini F, Pantazopoulos P. Implantable Intrathecal Pumps for the Treatment of Noncancer Chronic Pain in Elderly Population: Drug Dose and Clinical Efficacy. Neuromodulation 2008; 11 (1): 33-39.
[77] Naumann C, Erdine S, Koulousakis A, Van Buyten JP, Schuchard M. Drug adverse events and systemic complications of intrathecal opioid delivery for pain: origins, detection, manifestations, and management. Neuromodulation 1999;2(2):92–107.
[78] Lamer TJ. Treatment of cancer-related pain: when orally administered medications fail. Mayo Clin Proc 1994;69:473-480.
[79] Sjöberg M, Nitescu P, Appelgren L, Curelaru I. Long-term intrathecal morphine and bupivacaine in patients with refractory cancer pain: results from a morphine: bupivacaine dose regimen of 0.5: 4.75 mg/mL. Anesthesiology 1994; 80:284–297.
[80] Trujillo KA, Akil H. Opiate tolerance and dependence: recent findings and synthesis. New Biologist 1991;3:915-923.
[81] Stolerman I. Drugs of abuse: behavioural principles, methods and terms. Trends Pharmacol Sci 1992;13:170-176.
[82] Harris GC, Aston-Jones G. Involvement of D2 dopamine receptors in the nucleus accumbens in the opiate withdrawal syndrome. Nature 1994;371:155-7.
[83] Collin E, Cesselin F. Neurobiological mechanisms of opioid tolerance and dependence. Clin Pharmacol 1991;14:465-488.
[84] Portenoy RK. Tolerance to opioid analgesics: clinical aspects. Cancer Surveys 1995;21:49-65.

[85] Crain SM, Shen KF. Opioids can evoke direct receptor-mediate excitatory effects on sensory neurons. Trends Pharmacol Sci 1990;11:77-81.
[86] Shen KF, Crain SM. Antagonists at excitatory opioid receptors on sensory neurons in culture increase potency and specificity of opiate analgesics and attenuate development of tolerance/dependence. Brain Res. 1994 Feb 14;636(2):286-97.
[87] Cruciani RA, Dvorkin B, Morris SA, Crain SM, Makman MH. Direct coupling of opioid receptors to both stimulatory and inhibitory guanine nucleotide-binding proteins in F-11 neuroblastoma-sensory neuron hybrid cells. Proc Natl Acad Sci U S A. 1993 Apr 1;90(7):3019-23.
[88] Crain SM, Shen KF, Chalazonitis A. Opioids excite rather than inhibit sensory neurons after chronic opioid exposure of spinal cord-ganglion cultures. Brain Res. 1988 Jul 5;455(1):99-109.
[89] Gintzler AR, Chan WC, Glass J. Evoked release of methionine enkephalin from tolerant/dependent enteric ganglia: paradoxical dependence on morphine. Proc Natl Acad Sci U S A. 1987 Apr;84(8):2537-9.
[90] Redmond DE Jr, Krystal JH. Multiple mechanisms of withdrawal from opioid drugs. Annu Rev Neurosci. 1984;7:443-78.
[91] Cesselin F. Opioid and anti-opioid peptides. Fundam Clin Pharmacol. 1995;9(5):409-33.
[92] Sabbe MB, Yaksh TL. Pharmacology of spinal opioids. J Pain Symptom Manage. 1990 Jun;5(3):191-203.
[93] Krames ES. Intraspinal opioid therapy for chronic nonmalignant pain: current practice and clinical guidelines. J Pain Symptom Manage 1996;11:333–352.
[94] Krames ES. Intrathecal infusional therapies for intractable pain: patient management guidelines.J Pain Symptom Manage 1993;8:36-46.
[95] Brody JA, Schneider EL. Age dependent and age related disease. J Chronic Dis 1956;39:11–871.
[96] Chodosh J, Solomon D, Roth OP. The quality of medical care provided to vulnerable older patients with chronic pain. J Am Geriatr Soc 2004;52:756–771.
[97] Holford NHG, Sheiner LB. Pharmacokinetic and dynamic modelling in vivo. CRC Crit Rev Bioeng 1981;5:273–322.
[98] Moffat JA, Milne B. pharmacokinetics in anaesthesia. Can Anaesth Soc J 1983;30:300–307.
[99] Hilgenberg JC. Inhalation and intravenous drugs in the elderly patient. Semin Anesth 1986;5:44–53.
[100] Anderson VC, Cooke B, Burchiel KJ. Intrathecal hydromorphone for chronic nonmalignant pain: a retrospective study. Pain Med. 2001;2:287-97.
[101] Staats PS, Yearwood T, Charapata SG, et al. Intrathecal ziconotide in the treatment of refractory pain in patients with cancer or AIDS: a randomized controlled trial. JAMA. 2004;291:63-70
[102] Wallace MS, Charapata SG, Fisher R, et al. Intrathecal ziconotide in the treatment of chronic nonmalignant pain: a randomized, double-blind, placebo-controlled clinical trial. Neuromodulation. 2006;9:75-86
[103] Rauck RL, Wallace MS, Leong MS, et al. A randomized, double-blind, placebo-controlled study of intrathecal ziconotide in adults with severe chronic pain. J Pain Symptom Manage. 2006;31:393-406

[104] Raffaeli W, Sarti D, Demartini L, Sotgiu A, Bonezzi C; Italian Ziconotide Group. Italian registry on long-term intrathecal ziconotide treatment. Pain Physician. 2011 Jan-Feb;14(1):15-24.

[105] Ucar T, Kazan S, Turgut U, Samanci NK. Outcomes of intrathecal baclofen (ITB) therapy in spacticity. Turk Neurosurg. 2011 Jan;21(1):59-65.

[106] Haranhalli N, Anand D, Wisoff JH, Harter DH, Weiner HL, Blate M, Roth J. Intrathecal baclofen therapy: complication avoidance and management. Childs Nerv Syst. 2011;27(3):421-7.

[107] Saval A, Chiodo AE. Intrathecal baclofen for spasticity management: a comparative analysis of spasticity of spinal vs cortical origin. J Spinal Cord Med. 2010;33(1):16

[108] Carrillo-Ruiz JD, Andrade P, Godínez-Cubillos N, Montes-Castillo ML, Jiménez F, Velasco AL, Castro G, Velasco F. Coupled obturator neurotomies and lidocaine intrathecal infusion to treat bilateral adductor spasticity and drug-refractory pain. J Neurosurg. 2010;113(3):528-31.

[109] Raffaeli W, Andruccioli J, Righetti D, Caminiti A, Balestri M. Intraspinal therapy for the treatment of chronic pain: a review of the literature between 1990 and 2005 and suggested protocol for its rational and safe use. Neuromodulation. 2006;9(4):290-308.

[110] Van Dongen RTM et al. Intrathecal coadministration of bupivacaine diminishes morphine dose progression during long-term intrathecal infusion in cancer patients. The Clinical Journal of Pain 1999;15:166-172.

[111] Smith TJ, Staats PS, Deer T, Stearns LJ, Rauck RL, Boortz-Marx RL, Buchser E, Catala E, Bryce DA, Coyne PJ, Pool GE. Randomized clinical trial of an implantable drug delivery system compared with comprehensive medical management for refractory cancer pain: impact on pain, drug-related toxicity, and survival. J Clin Oncol 2002;20(19):4040-9.

[112] Rauck RL, Cherry D, Boyer MF, Kosek P, Dunn J, Alo K. Long-term intrathecal opioid therapy with a patient-activated, implanted delivery system for the treatment of refractory cancer pain. J Pain 2003;4(8):441-7.

[113] Smith TJ, Coyne PJ, Staats PS, Deer T, Stearns LJ, Rauck RL, et al. An implantable drug delivery system (IDDS) for refractory cancer pain provides sustained pain control, less drug-related toxicity, and possibly better survival compared with comprehensive medical management (CMM). Ann Oncol 2005;16(5):825-33.

[114] Willis KD, Doleys DM. The effects of long-term intraspinal infusion therapy with non-cancer pain patients: evaluation of patients, significant-other and clinic staff appraisals. Neuromodulation 1999;2:241-253.

[115] Brown J, Klapow J, Doleys D, Lowery D, Tutak U. Disease-specific and generic health outcomes: a model for the evaluation of long-term intrathecal opioid therapy in noncancer low back pain patients. Clin J Pain 1999;15(2)122-31.

[116] Roberts LJ, Finch PM, Goucke CR, Price LM. Outcome of intrathecal opioids in chronic non-cancer pain. Eur J Pain 2001;5(4):353-61.

[117] Franco Gay ML. Spinal morphine in nonmalignant chronic pain: a retrospective study in 39 patients. Neuromodulation 2002;5(3):150-159.

[118] Grider JS, Harned ME, Etscheidt MA. Patient selection and outcomes using a low-dose intrathecal opioid trialing method for chronic nonmalignant pain. Pain Physician;14(4):343-51.

7

Electrical Neuromodulation and the Heart with Special Emphasis on Myocardial Ischemia

Mike J.L. DeJongste
Department of Cardiology, Thoraxcenter, University Medical Center Groningen and University of Groningen, Groningen
The Netherlands

1. Introduction

To describe the relation between the nervous system and the heart Natelson, among others, coined the term 'neurocardiology' in the eighties of the previous century.[1] In the nineties, the scope of neurocardiology was broadened by researchers from a largely neuroanatomical point of view to a focus that was more directed onto interaction between heart and nervous system from an integrative physiology focus. Finally, the center of attention of neurocardiology also shifted onto experimental science and technology at the neural interface of the heart. More specifically, the clinical interest became directed towards basic science through studying (modulation of) recruited neuro-humoral, neuro-inflammatory and neural pathways, in the presence or absence of angina pectoris, resulting from myocardial ischemia.[2]

In this respect, the chapter briefly highlights the available conventional therapies for ischemic heart diseases, followed by a discussion on efficacy and underlying neurocardiological mechanisms of available electrical neuromodulation therapies. In addition, a systematic and detailed review is offered on the antiischemic effects of electrical neuromodulation in patients with end-stage coronary artery disease.

2. Ischemic cardiovascular diseases

The average life span of the Western population has doubled over the last century as a consequence of major progress made in developments in socio-economic policies and improvements in hygiene. Further, advancements have been accomplished in preventive procedures and in the improvement of an armamentarium of therapeutic strategies to treat (infectious) diseases. Subsequently, to date in the Western world, civilians are no longer subjected to the deleterious menaces of infectious diseases and life expectancy is largely determined by atherosclerotic diseases and cancer, each presently representing $^1/_3$ of all deaths.

With respect to cardiovascular diseases, as a consequence of preventive measures such as life style changes (among others: stopping smoking, increasing physical exercise, eating healthy food, reducing stress and treating risk factors), pharmacotherapeutics (nitroglycerin, beta-blockers, calcium-antagonists, renin-angiotensin-aldosteron system blockers, lipid lowering drugs, anticoagulants) and revascularization procedures (percutaneous coronary interventions [PCI] and coronary artery bypass surgery [CABS]), mortality from cardiovascular diseases has declined significantly during the last four decades. As a consequence, more patients will survive their heart disease for a longer period. Moreover, since the population is graying and therapies have been improved, it is to be expected that the number of patients suffering from ischemic heart disease will increase. Ischemic heart disease is most often the consequence of atherosclerotic narrowing of one or more coronary arteries. During exercise, when the heart muscle demands more oxygen, the shortage in oxygen supply, due to the narrowed coronary arteries, provokes chest discomfort, so-called angina pectoris.

2.1 Angina pectoris

Stable angina is considered as a clinical syndrome, characterized by indistinctly distributed chest distress, described as sensations of tightness, pressure, heaviness, squeezing, burning, or choking provoked during exercise. The occurrence of angina and its emotional components have been brilliantly expressed by Heberden in 1772.[3] In acute cardiovascular syndromes a coronary artery is closed up and chest discomforts occur at rest, while angina is not relieved by nitroglycerin use. Specifically in acute syndromes these symptoms are often escorted with vaso-vegetative and emotional sensations such as nausea, transpiration, anxiety or thoughts of an impending death.

To examine the neural pathways, involved in ischemia-induced angina, the heart-brain axis is the subject of many years' thoughtful research on the nervous involvement in cardiac control. Following the development of a model for angina, we and others have injected analgesic substances, such as bradykinin and capsaicin,[4] to study the involved nervous pathways, by means of the early gene c-fos.[5] Exploration of this neurocardiological field of interest has also been focus of behavioral aspects of angina [6] and made the participation of the transient receptor potential vanilloid-1 (TRPV-1), at the heart likely.[7] Virus tracing studies executed by means of a pseudo-rabies virus, injected into the myocardium, made it possible to visualize the stained recruited pathways.[8,9] See for an overview of our studies on neurocardiology reference [10].

2.2 Chronic refractory angina

In spite of many innovative developments in pharmacotherapeutic and surgical treatment strategies, which have significantly improved life expectancy of patients suffering from ischemic heart disease, an increasing number of patients are resistant to all conventional opportunities. These patients remain severely disabled and suffer from chest discomfort during minimal exercise, or sometimes even at rest. They typically have become refractory to maximal tolerated standard anti-ischemic medication and are no longer candidates for revascularization procedures, such as PCI and CABS.[11] The presence of myocardial ischemia should be clinically established to be the cause of symptoms.[12] Patients enduring this condition are usually characterized by a long history of artery disease, have received at least one revascularization(s) procedure(s), are between sixty and seventy years of age, of the male gender, experienced one or more myocardial infarction, however, have maintained the left ventricular ejection fraction.[13] Furthermore, due to progress of their coronary disease, these patients most often experience life threatening events such as an acute coronary syndrome and therefore the need of hospital admission.[14] The patients have become an increasing medical and psychosocial problem resulting from their devastating chest discomforts. The impact of the severe complaints of angina on social life and quality of life of these patients is often underestimated.[15] Whether this is a syndrome that differs from the chronic angina patients is doubtful.

Life expectancy of these patients varies in the literature between 5-8% which may be considered as fairly favorable. In this regard, these patients may be considered as survivors of their coronary artery disease. It is estimated that the incidence is about 1:10,000 the prevalence is 1:30,000 and the total number in the Western World is over 200,000.[16] Since more patients survive their disease, perceived quality of life issues become more important for these patients. Because the patients are severely hindered by their severe angina and because conventional treatment options are lacking, the patients have unmet medical needs. As a consequence, therapies relieving their angina, without adversely influencing their prognosis are imperative. From this point of view, exploration of newer therapies has to be promoted with the emphasis on a reduction of both ischemic burden and angina, so that the patients may subsequently harvest an improved quality of life. During the last decade for patients with surgically and pharmacologically uncontrollable chronic angina, several additional therapies have become available,[17] of which electrical neuromodulation may be considered to be one of the safest, most effective and best evaluated strategies in the current therapeutic arsenal, currently available for these patients.[18,19] In this regard, electrical neuromodulation has become accepted as an adjunct therapy for refractory angina pectoris in the ACC/AHA guidelines since 2002.[20]

3. Myocardial ischemia (see Fig 1)

To enhance the metabolism of the muscles during exercise, sufficient oxygen is required. The heart receives oxygenated blood from the lungs and exchanges the oxygen for CO_2 at the muscular level, more specifically via the mitochondrial membrane of the muscle cell. However, the heart muscle itself also needs oxygen to perform its contracting force. The heart muscle receives its oxygen through the coronary arteries. At rest, the heart subtracts about 95% of the oxygen from the coronary arteries. The only option the heart muscle has to subtract more oxygen from the coronary arteries is to dilate its coronary artery vascular tree. Subsequently, the cardiac oxygen supply can increase five fold to meet the increased oxygen demand. In a normal situation, exercise is limited through a shift from aerobic to anaerobic metabolism. As a result of this metabolic change more effluents (lactate, potassium etc) are produced. These effluents activate chemical and mechanical receptors in the heart (among others TRPV1), conveying signals to the brain which result in withholding exercise, most often because of fatigue and dyspnea (vide infra). However, in the presence of coronary artery disease, the atherosclerotic plaque reduces the dilatory facilities of the coronary artery and so the aerobic threshold is reached much sooner. The (exercise) induced discrepancy between oxygen supply and demand is called myocardial ischemia. Stable angina comprises that the complaints of angina are induced during exercise. The heart muscle (myocardium) becomes 'ischemic' at the aerobic threshold at which the critical balance between oxygen (O_2) supply and demand is perturbed (Figure 1). The metabolic demand of the heart is determined mainly by contraction force -build upon the amount of ATP energy storage- and the product of heart rate and systolic blood pressure, the so-called rate pressure product (RPP) or double product. The increase in O_2 demand, as is required during cardiac stress, is proportional to the increase in the RPP.[21]

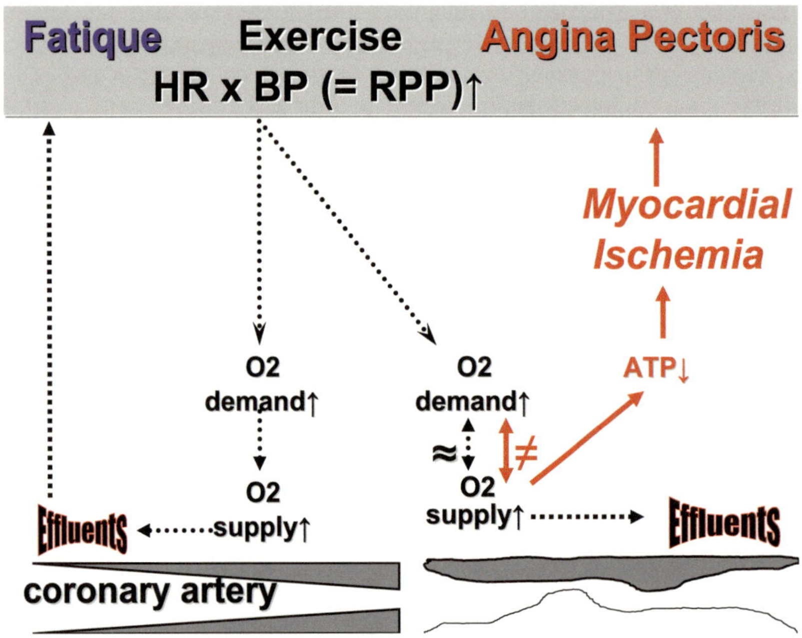

≠ =mismatch. HR= heart rate. RPP=rate pressure product; BP = blood pressure; ATP = adenosine triphosphate.

Fig. 1. See text for details

3.1 Ischemic heart disease

The most common manifestation of ischemic coronary artery disease (CAD), the leading cause of death in the United States, is angina pectoris. In a substantial proportion (~10.2 million) of the estimated 17.6 million affected American patients with obstructive CAD, angina has become the main clinical symptom.

Many strategies have been developed to improve the ischemic capacity through reducing the demand (by means of, for instance, β-blocking agents) or by improving the supply (by means of, for example, revascularization). Novel approaches are required to improve clinical outcomes in patients with coronary heart disease. To date the focus of antiischemic therapies is also on making the heart, i.e. the myocyte, more resistant to ischemic challenges by enhancing the ischemic threshold, which is determined by both collateral flow and preconditioning. These two alternatives improve the ischemic tolerance and will be discussed further.

3.2 Cardiac microcirculation

A pluriform array of mechanisms, including metabolic, neural and myogenic systems are involved in regulating blood flow within the coronary vascular tree; increases in blood flow involve corresponding increases in vessel diameter at the level of the small vessels and arterioles. In the heart, diminished oxygen delivery in response to myocardial ischemia is countered by an increase in regional blood flow and functional capillary density within the microcirculation. Under resting conditions only a small number of coronary capillary vessels in the heart are open for blood flow; during exercise (increased oxygen demand) additional capillary vessels are opened (i.e., recruited). Understanding the various factors that control post-ischemic coronary capillary blood flow across the myocardial wall remains an important challenge. In the setting of coronary artery disease, maldistribution of blood flow is attributed to dysfunction of specific components of the vessel wall, in particular the endothelium.

Of fundamental importance for post-ischemic tissue viability in the heart is the delivery of oxygen and nutrients, either via pre-existing coronary vascular or collateral networks or via promotion of new vessel growth (i.e., vasculogenesis or neovascularization). In a canine preparation of chronic myocardial ischemia, Kersten and co-workers documented that coronary collateral development in response to repeated coronary occlusions requires an extended timeframe for coronary collateral growth.[22] These findings confirmed earlier results that coronary collateral conductance improved over time and was associated with increased transmural distribution of blood flow in the heart after brief coronary occlusion in the canine.

Remodeling of existing small vessels by addition of vascular smooth muscle cells and extracellular matrix around a larger diameter may be important in formation of collateral vessels. There is ample reference to coronary collateral recruitment at onset of ischemia in the scientific literature. It would be more reasonable to use the terminology of microvessel or capillary recruitment (as suggested initially by Krogh in his capillary-tissue exchange cylinder model). He reported that opening of coronary collateral channels occurs in man during coronary occlusion.[23a,b,c] More recently ischemic adaptation to collateral channel opening was observed during ischemic preconditioning, which is thought to play an important role in the development of ischemic tolerance.[24] In animal experiments "opening" of coronary collateral channels has not been documented;[25] this would suggest that augmented blood flow to ischemic myocardium in animals via capillary vessels does not play a role in the cardioprotective actions induced by preconditioning. Consequently, experimental studies may not provide sufficient evidence to elucidate the underlying mechanisms of action of electrical neuromodulation in humans.

3.3 Ischemic preconditioning (IPC) and postconditioning

In their recent report on ischemic conditioning, described as "the practice of applying brief episodes of nonlethal ischemia and reperfusion to confer protection against a sustained episode of lethal ischemia and reperfusion injury", the authors discuss this potentially therapeutic strategy.[28] They noted that the protective stimulus can be applied before ischemic preconditioning (IPC), during the onset of sustained episodes of lethal ischemia (ischemic conditioning), or at the onset of myocardial reperfusion (ischemic post-conditioning)." In brief, IPC is an intrinsic process, usually induced by repeated short periods of ischemia, most often performed through a temporary occlusion of a vessel, through pharmacological substances, or through exercise stress to protect the myocardium against a subsequent ischemic insult. The phenomenon was described first by Murry *et al,* in 1986, exposing anesthetised dogs to 5 minutes of coronary artery occlusions, followed by a 5 minute period of reperfusion and finally to a 40 minute continuous occlusion. In controls ischemic preconditioning was withheld. The control animals experienced larger infarct sizes, compared to the preconditioned dogs.[26] IPC was initially thought to be the result of slower ATP-energy depletion, later interference with effectors of cell death, free radicals, attenuation of mitochondrial permeability and involvement of adenosine, opioid receptors and connexin 43.[27] Ischemic postconditioning, a series of mechanical interruptions of reperfusion after ischemia, is performed immediately after reperfusion, for protection of myocardium against infarction, secondary to ischemia and reperfusion damage.[28] Albeit that basic evidence of conditioning is abundant, its clinical effect remains debatable since mechanism of action remain partly unraveled, making translation to patients still difficult.

4. Methods of electrical neuromodulation for refractory angina

4.1 A brief history of electrical neuromodulation methods

The encouraging effects of electrical current for all kind of ailments have been in use since the pharaohs, Greeks and later the Romans. In ancient history physicians were aware of the power of electrical current, provided for instance by the electric eel, to heal discomforts, like headache and gout.[29] In the early nineteenth century stimulation of nerves to reduce pain was termed electro-analgesia or electro-narcosis.[30] In 1965 the landmark study by Melzack and Wall was published. They proposed the model of the gate control,[31] implying that electrical current applied to the myelinated, relatively fast conducting, thicker A-fibers, modulates the pain processing in the non-myelinated slower conducting C-fibers via interneurons in the dorsal horn, and so affects pain. Although the theory still stands, it is not tenable in all its aspects anymore. In higher brain centers, it was shown with positron emission tomography (PET) that angina affects areas involved in cardiovascular control.[32] In patients with angina, active neuromodulation was unable to suppress the conduction of cardiac pain signals to the cerebrum, during cardiac distress.[33] Comparison of these two studies demonstrated activation of the same cardiovascular control centers during active neuromodulation as were recruited following angina. At the cardiac level the intra-cardiac neurons (ICN) are considered as the final common pathway, integrating the peripheral nervous system with the heart. These ICN are hidden in the fatty patches on the heart, controlling cardiac function. The more central superimposed neural hierarchy, controlling the ICN, has been described in relation to the presence of myocardial ischemia, in detail.[34]

The presence of this neural environment does not make an involved placebo unlikely in the field of electrical neuromodulation. In this regard, in the 1930s, Beecher coined and described nicely the placebo effect of, among others, surgical procedures in relation to intrinsic and extrinsic factors.[35] Specifically for therapies like electrical neuromodulation, with a not entirely unraveled mechanism of action, it is important to note that the therapy is conspicious for placebo. To exclude placebo as the one and only factor explaining the effect of electrical neuromodulation, unraveling of mechanisms and performing well designed studies, such as randomized control studies, are of paramount importance. Though all therapies encounter a certain percentage of placebo, since the effects of electrical neuromodulation often last for years (vide infra) and since randomized control studies (RCT) also demonstrate beneficial outcomes, it is unlikely that a placebo is the only explanation for the favorable effects of electrical neuromodulation. Further, several studies have shown clear evidence of somatic cardiovascular responses resulting from spinal cord stimulation, such as, among others, alterations in activity of spinothalamic tract cells[36] and of intra cardiac neurons[37] and changes in blood pressure.[38]

Over the last 50 years a number of techniques to produce electro-analgesia have been reported. We will briefly review these methods.

4.2 Stellate ganglion stimulation

Dr Braunwald, a brilliant pioneer in cardiology and his late wife, a thoracic surgeon, modified a pacemaker device to stimulate the stellate ganglion. Already in 1967 they reported an anti-angina effect using this method of electrical neuromodulation.[39] In addition, they coincidently observed in a patient experiencing an acute coronary event, normalization of the ST-T segment, following active stimulation. However, in spite of the initial encouraging results, this method of neuromodulation was discarded in the beginning of the seventies, because coronary artery bypass grafting became widely available.[40] In some centers, blocking of the stellate ganglion, by means of anesthetics, is still in vogue in specific circumstances.[41]

4.3 Transcutaneous Electrical Nerve Stimulation (TENS)

Since not all patients turned out to be suitable candidates for revascularization, a decade later clinicians started to use newer forms of electrical neuromodulation, such as TENS, to deal with the chest discomfort of patients. Neurostimulation for angina pectoris is usually performed by either Transcutaneous Electrical Nervous Stimulation (TENS) or by an implantable Spinal Cord Stimulator (SCS). Since 1982 TENS is considered as an effective method in the treatment of chronically disabled patients through reducing frequency and severity of the angina attacks and subsequently the necessity for the intake of short acting nitrates.[42] In addition, to the improvement in quality of life, TENS also improved exercise capacity, and lactate production (vide infra).[43] However, the drawback of TENS is that the plasters on the chest may induce ortho-ergic reactions (contact dermatitis) in 20-30% of the patients, come off during sweating and are difficult to attach on hairy chests or females with large mamma.[44,45] So, these shortcomings often necessitate a withdrawn from TENS therapy.

4.4 Spinal Cord Stimulation

The story of electro-analgesia goes on with the introduction of dorsal column stimulation in 1967,[46] which later was renamed epidural spinal cord stimulation (ESES) and today is known as spinal cord stimulation (SCS). However, taking into account the surgical procedure, with respect to TENS, SCS seems to be more effective with more pronounced and sustained effects, long-term.[47] In 1987, in the first report on the antianginal effect of SCS in patients with refractory angina, a reduction in both the frequency and severity of angina attacks was found, in conjunction with a reduction in sublingual intake of nitrogen tablets.[48] Later many authors advocated SCS as an effective strategy for patients with severe refractory angina. In addition, in patients with a high surgical risk, SCS is even considered as a substitute for coronary artery bypass surgery.[65]

The implantation procedure of this reversible non-destructive therapy is comparable to the implantation of a pacemaker, though the electrodes are placed epidurally and not in the heart. The success of SCS depends, among others, on the correct positioning of the stimulating electrode(s) in the dorsal epidural space. It is still considered mandatory that the paresthesias induced by the stimulator correspond with the area where most of the patients experience their angina. When the tip of the electrode of the SCS device is properly placed at C7-T2, the lead is anchored and connected to the implanted pulse generator (IPG). The IPG is positioned into a subcutaneously created pocket, in the chest, comparable with the placement of a pacemaker, or in the lower upper abdominal wall. The patient can (in)activate the IPG through a patient programmer or by application of a magnet.

The question was recently posed whether paresthesias are necessary for the beneficial effects of SCS. In this respect two studies have addressed this paradigm by randomizing patients to subthreshold stimulation and stimulation with induced paresthesias. The results were contradictory. In one study the investigators argued no difference between paresthesia induced stimulation and subthreshold, however the authors observed a significant difference with very low stimulation.[49] In another recent study this observation could not be demonstrated in naive patients.[50]

4.5 Subcutaneous Electrical Nerve Stimulation (SENS)

Subcutaneously electrical neurostimulation (SENS), also called among others SubQ, subcutaneous target stimulation, peripheral nerve or peripheral field stimulation is a promising method.[51] Recently, we and others have reported on the use of subcutaneous placed leads, implicating positioning of electrodes just underneath the thoracic skin, together with a subcutaneously implanted device. This method seems to be effective in the treatment of patients with therapeutically refractory angina.[52,53] Patients with severe coronary artery disease, in which withholding anti-thrombotic pharmacotherapeutics is not feasible, may be excellent candidates for both subcutaneously implanted device and leads. Other drawbacks of the SCS treatment are that electrode placement into the epidural space is rather critical when compared to epidural placement. Furthermore, a physician with neuromodulation skills is needed for placement of the electrodes under fluoroscopy, though sometimes even then an unsuitable anatomy of the spinal area makes positioning of the electrodes impossible. So, theoretically SENS may be unifying the "best of two worlds", including the better convenience in use (and efficacy?) of SCS over TENS and an implantation procedure which is more simple (cardiologists can do it themselves), possibly safer (considering the procedure) and, maybe at less cost (shorter operation procedure and lower thresholds), when compared to SCS.

5. Electrical neuromodulation and angina

To optimize and to tailor adjunct treatments for patients suffering from chronic refractory angina, a 'care pathway' for 'patient-centered guiding' has been developed.[54] The experts propose to start with less invasive methods, such as rehabilitation and TENS, later followed by more invasive but reversible methods, such as SCS or SENS. Ultimately, destructive methods such as ablation of nerves may be carried out.

Since the first publications, abundant articles have testified that electrical neuromodulation gained credentials in efficacy as an adjuvant therapy for in patients with severe refractory angina, irrespective of whether the method is applied at the skin of the chest,[42,43] cervically[55] at the T1-4 thoracic level,[56,57] or subcutaneously.[52,55] To assess the efficacy of electrical neuromodulation among patients with refractory angina receiving the various forms of electrical neuromodulation, comparative randomized control studies are warranted. The studies ought to have a placebo controlled design.[35] However, unfortunately the studies can not be blinded since the physician notifies the stimulation artifacts on the ECG and the patients are aware whether or not stimulation is present. These comparative studies have not yet been executed. However, there is scarce literature in open retrospective studies that SCS may be more effective than TENS.[58] The results show that SCS is effective in 80% of the patients after a period of 4 years. After that same period, TENS is effective in about 60% of the patients. On the other hand to improve the outcome, it is important to develop the screening before application of neuromodulation is started, since about 20% of the patients do not show improvement in quality of life following SCS implantation.

Many observational (long-term) studies on electrical neuromodulation have consistently observed a reduction in angina complaints and use of short acting nitrates [59,61,62,] with a subsequent improvement in exercise capacity [59,60,61,62] and quality of life.[15,63,64] Quality of life measure, in this severely disabled group of patients, is usually executed by way of questionnaires (Nottingham health profile; Short Form-20 and RAND-36) and diaries (to score the daily number of angina attacks and number of NTG intake). These findings have been substantiated by observational studies and RCTs showing that the improvements may last for up to 10 years.[60,61,63,64,65] These measures are, however, not taken co-morbidity and personality, which factors may affect outcome parameters, into account.[66,67]

The major flaw of many of the clinical studies on electrical neuromodulation is the inborn weakness of all open observational designs, implicating one does not know how much bias is found in outcome parameters. On the other hand observation studies are very useful in presenting the 'real world', instead of reporting a limited number of highly selected patients, as is the case in randomized studies.[68] Unfortunately, the greater part of studies regarding the subject of electro-neuromodulation for angina, are carried out with a limited number of patients. In this regard, two recent meta-analysis on randomized controlled trials (RCT) have been executed, showing significant improvements in both quality of life (Fig 2) and exercise duration (Fig 3). [69,70]

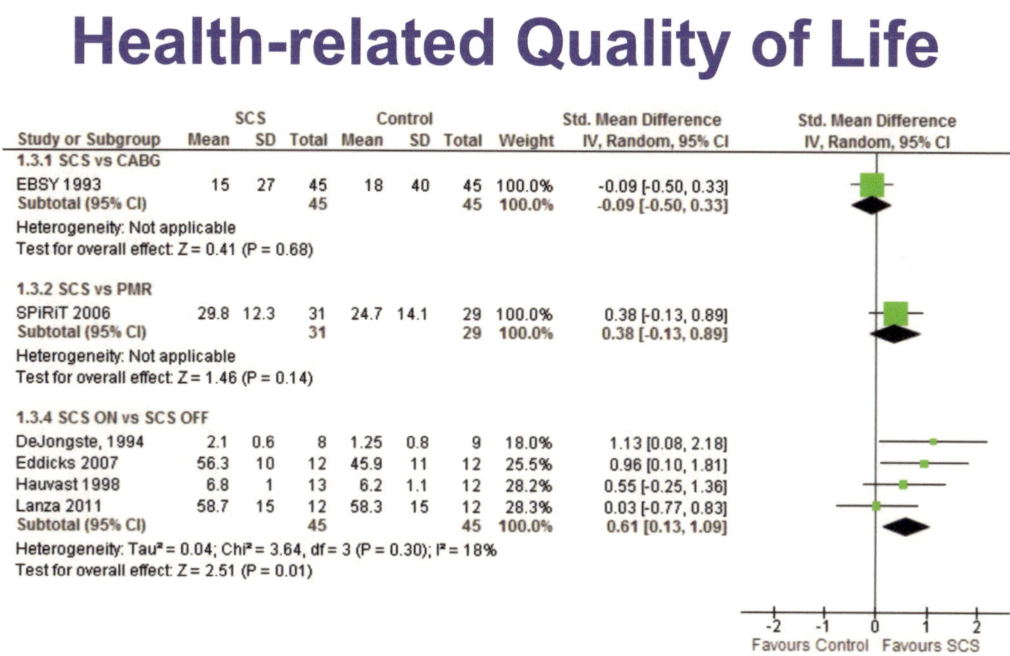

Fig. 2. Health related quality of life of 6 RCTs (adapted by R Taylor from ref. 70)

In accord with its efficacy and safety, SCS has been included in 2002 into to the ACC/AHA guidelines as an additional therapy for the treatment of this group of patients, with a class 2 indication.[71]

All modalities of electrical neuromodulation are reversible. Mainly for medico-legal reasons, combination with other devices is not advocated.[72] Divergent literature is available too, reporting on the safety in combination with artificial cardiac pacemakers[73] and implantable cardioverter defibrillators when specific measures are taken into account.[74]

With regard to the safety aspects of electrical neuromodulation, many worry as it might deprive the patients of their angina. In studies on patients with stable angina, all patients ultimately experienced angina.[59] The fear for a potentially jeopardizing situation during an acute coronary syndrome, resulting from a suppressed conduction to the brain during active neuromodulation, does not seem to be justified, since electrical neuromodulation does not seem to block nociceptive information from the heart to the brain.[33]

Accordingly electrical neuromodulation is not found to conceal complaints of angina during a myocardial infarction since the nociceptive information on ischemia from the heart to the brain is modulated but not abolished.[75,76,77] Electrical neuromodulation, rather than eliminating angina normalized the, through sensitization enhanced, angina threshold. The patients therefore experience an increase in exercise capacity and a reduction in severity of symptoms of angina, which does not adversely affect mortality nor morbidity. Regarding mortality in the population of patients treated with SCS for refractory angina pectoris, several studies report a relatively low annual mortality rate of about 5-7%.[13,78,79] We recently evaluated morbidity in this group of patients, by comparing medical history at baseline with follow-up data.[66] Our interest in morbidity was generated by the lack of improvement in quality of life indices in a substantial number of patients, after long-term implantation of

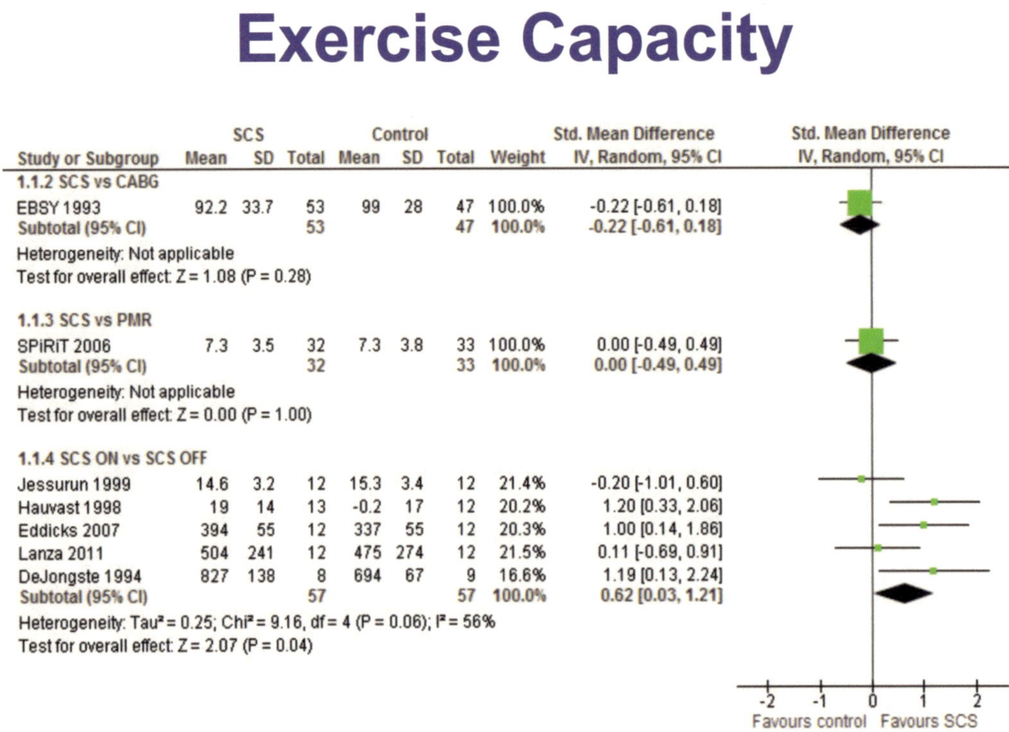

Fig. 3. Exercise tests of 7 randomized control studies (adapted by R Taylor from ref. 70)

spinal cord stimulator. We reported that in some patients the lack of improvement in quality of life was related to the presence of co-morbidities, such as respiratory diseases, musculoskeletal disorders, diabetes and obesity. As a consequence of our analysis of the effects of SCS on quality of life, we recommend that in studies on electrical neuromodulation, the effect of co-morbidities on the quality of life is taken into account.

Several cost-benefit and cost-effectiveness studies have been performed to evaluate the costs of SCS in the treatment of refractory angina. The break-even point for costs is calculated to be about three to four years.[80,81]

Given the data, electrical neuromodulation is considered as one of the best and safest adjuvant therapies to consider for patients suffocating from chronic refractory angina.[82,83]

In conclusion, studies with different designs have consistently demonstrated that electrical neuromodulation reduces complaints of angina, enabling patients to prolong their exercise, independent of the method applied. Whether or not electrical neuromodulation may improve myocardial ischemia is the subject of the next part of this chapter.

6. Electrical neuromodulation and myocardial ischemia

In the wake of many favorable outcomes on quality of life end points assessed in studies with patients suffering from chronic refractory angina pectoris, treated with electrical neuromostimulation, the debate continues whether the raise in angina threshold is associated with an improvement in ischemic tolerance.

In 1967 Braunwald *et al*, stimulating the stellate ganglion to achieve a reduction in complaints of angina, were the first to observe a concomitant reduction in myocardial ischemia during active stimulation.[39,40] The beneficial effects of electrical neuromodulation (TENS) on the resolution of ST-segment depression in patients suffering from and following an acute coronary syndrome were later confirmed by de Vries *et al*.[84,85] However, in spite of the antianginal and antiischemic effect, electrical neuromodulation was used in a rather limited number of patients. The restricted number of patients treated was attributed to the introduction of bypass surgery, at that time, making neuromodulation outdated.[40] In addition to the reduction in angina, induced through electrical neuromodulation exerted by means of stellate ganglion stimulation, its suggested antiischemic effect was later confirmed by making use of different methods, a variety of study designs, and end points. Using TENS, in the short-term limb of the study, a reduction was reported in lactated production and ST-T segment depression during pacing-induced and a long-term improvement in exercise capacity in conjunction with a persistent ST-T segment depression during maximal exercise stress tests.[43] Unfortunately, in this respect not all studies on exercise capacity are assessing ST-T segment changes,[86,87] since the recording requires either, specific filtering of the ECG signal or, temporarily withholding active stimulation during the exercise. This specific skill is related to interference of the neurostimulation induced artifacts on the ECG. Later, several observational and randomized studies, making use of this expertise to evaluate antiischemic effects of SCS, by means of bicycle or treadmill exercise stress tests as the method of choice, show consistent findings of a reduction in ST-T segment depression at maximal and at comparable work load, in conjunction with improvement in exercise duration. [57,59,61,62,63] So, in spite of a prolonged exercise duration the patients had less myocardial ischemia. However, in a meta-analysis of 5 randomized studies on exercise stress tests ST-T segment changes were not significantly altered, following SCS (Fig 4)

Some studies included in the meta-analysis used a subthreshold versus threshold stimulation, others used the design of stimulation versus no stimulation and others used stimulation versus active non-neurostimulation comparators.[70] Of note, a study only examining the duration of the work out by a 6 minute walk test was excluded from the meta-analysis.[88]

Furthermore, ambulatory ECG monitoring also showed a reduction in ischemic burden in daily life.[61,89] Studies on SCS making use of ambulatory ECG recording are more difficult to perform because of the so-called carry-over effect.[90] This observation was already reported in 1967 by Shealy *et al,* coining the phenomenon "post-stimulation prolonged analgesia after discharge".[91] The investigators reported that after subcutaneously electrical stimulation of a peripheral nerve, the central response continues for seconds up to a minute, depending among others on the duration of stimulation. Later Armour and coworkers showed this latency following electrical nerve stimulation, also to occur in the intra cardiac neurons, in the presence of myocardial ischemia.[92] Jessurun *et al* demonstrate that this post-analgesic effect may even last for weeks.[93] This prolonged stimulation effect may affect study outcomes. Moreover, specific filters are required to reduce the stimulation artifacts on the ECG.

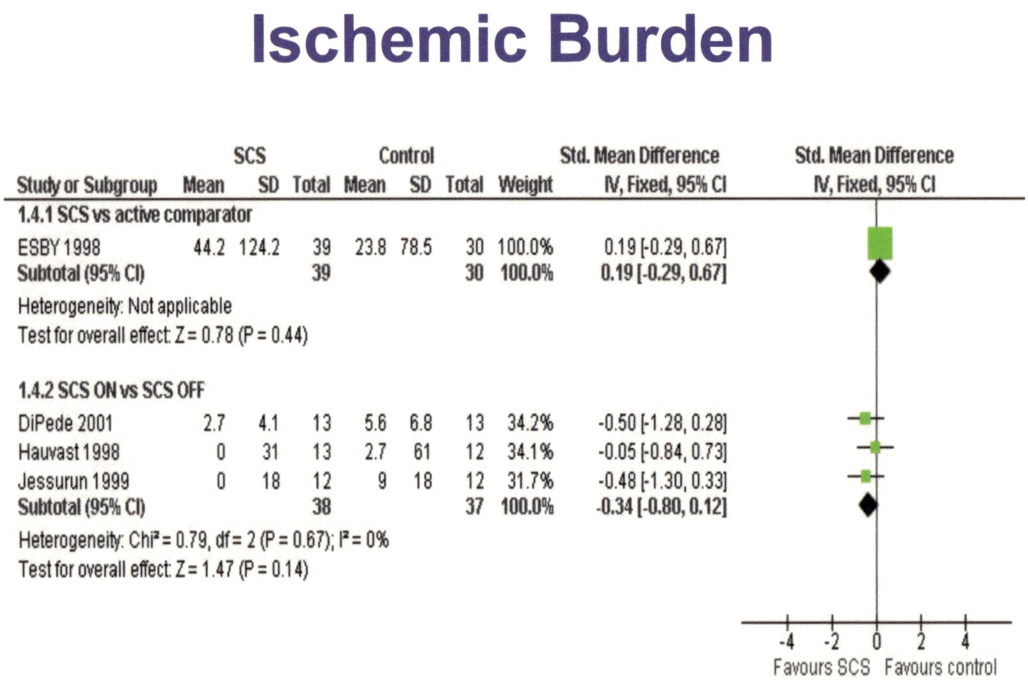

Fig. 4. Ischemic burden evaluated in 4 randomized studies (by R Taylor)

In this regard, studies on right atrial pacing showing a delayed onset of angina following active SCS also substantiates the antiischemic effect of electrical neuromodulation by reporting a reduction in ischemia at maximal exercise during active SCS and a concomitant reduction in lactate production.[94]

So, albeit that electrical neuromodulation has been found in both observational and randomized studies, using sequential ECG recordings, exercise stress tests at comparable and maximal work load, and ambulatory ECG recordings, to significantly improve ST-T segment depression, considered as a marker for myocardial ischemia, these findings raise the question which neurocardiological mechanisms are involved. Therefore, electrical neuromodulation was used to examine the neural hierarchy in cardiac control.[2,34]

Initially, the favorable effects of SCS, for other indications than angina, were attributed to a sympathicolytic effect.[75]

In 1950 Lindgren was the first to report on beneficial outcomes of bilateral upper cutting of the thoracic sympathetic nerves in patients suffering from severe angina.[95] Later modulation of nerves became more accepted than the destruction of nerves. Meglio *et al* demonstrated a reduction in heart rate in 25 patients without overt cardiac disease with a spinal cord stimulator, implanted for pain.[96] However, their early experimental finding has never been substantiated by others.

In current pharmacotherapeutical treatment of angina, ß-blocking agents have become a cornerstone for 45 years.[97] ß-Blocker agents employ their beneficial result through their effect on the sympathetic nervous system and the subsequent decrease in rate pressure product (RPP). This reduction in RPP results in a decline in myocardial oxygen demand.

Initially, the antiischemic effect of SCS was also subscribed to modulation of the autonomic nervous system, more specifically to the sympathetic limb.

Ambulatory ECG recording have not shown a change in Heart Rate Variability (HRV), a measure of autonomic function, following electrical neuromodulation.[89,98] In the setting of patients with angina, the lack of influence of SCS on HRV may be caused by the blunting effect of β-blockers on HRV in the majority of patients with angina.

Furthermore, there is scarce evidence that SCS is still active after sympathectomy (Dr Juhl G, Danmark, personal communication), no change in cardiac epinephrine spill-over was found [94,99] and SCS does not seem to affect adrenergic function as assessed by single photon emission computed tomography either (11)C-hydroxyephedrine or iodine 123- meta-iodo-benzylguanidine in patients with coronary artery disease,[100] or in patients suffering from chest pain during exercise induced ST-T segment changes but, without significant coronary artery disease (i.e. cardiac syndrome X).[101]

So, in the treatment of angina with SCS, clinical data do not support the hypothesis that electrical neuromodulation employs a β-sympaticolytic effect. The lack of sufficient evidence of a β-adrenergic effect of electrical neuromodulation does, of course, not exclude an α-sympathetic effect to be involved in changes in myocardial perfusion (vide infra).[102] There is basic evidence that SCS enhances the vagal tonus.[103] In concert with this observation, a study in patients with severe coronary artery disease demonstrates that vagal stimulation, inhibiting norepinephrine release from sympathetic nerves to the heart, may subsequently alter the sympatholytic/ vagotonic balance and so dilates cardiac microcirculatory vessels.[104]

Mannheimer and coworkers put forward the hypothesis that electrical neuromodulation reduces the myocardial oxygen demand.[94] Based on the observed reduction of ST-T segment changes at comparable work load (i.e. same RPP) the researchers hypothesized that the decrease in myocardial oxygen demand subsequently reduces symptoms associated with angina pectoris.[59] This hypothesis suggests involvement of a sympathicolytic effect. In addition, in their rapid atrial pacing study, the investigators showed an improvement in ischemic threshold during pacing induced ischemia in the presence of active SCS. In a letter to the editor of the British Medical Journal preconditioning as alternative explanation was proposed. [105] The authors based their theory on the short term between the experiment with and without SCS. In addition to ischemic preconditioning the heart is also protected during reperfusion by ischemic postconditioning, which protects the heart after the manifestation of the ischemic event through signal transduction pathways. In concert with the 'cardiac conditioning hypothesis', more plausible concepts than the reduction in myocardial oxygen demand following SCS have been postulated. These concepts are based on alterations in myocardial blood flow and subsequently in affecting myocardial perfusion.

To measure the effects in myocardial perfusion induced through electrical neuromodulation, studies have been performed with both, radionuclides and Doppler flow wires. In a study with 740 MBq 99-Technetium-MIBI an improved flow was reported in 16 out of 27 patients, only after 1 year. [106] In 10 patients no change was showed in myocardial blood flow and in one patient myocardial blood flow worsened after one year. Since, after 3 months, the investigators reported significant improvements in symptoms of angina, but not in myocardial perfusion, and after one year myocardial ischemia also improved, they concluded that "symptomatic relief precedes improvement of myocardial blood flow". In contrast to Mannheimer *et al,*[94] noticing in their rapid atrial pacing study an instantaneous reduction in myocardial ischemia, followed by a relief in angina, during SCS, in the latter study with MIBI-SPECT nuclide, a reduction in myocardial ischemia was observed only after one year. The discrepancy in latency of effects may be related to two different mechanisms.

To further evaluate the influence of SCS on myocardial ischemia, Fricke and co-workers performed a Positron Emission Tomography (PET) study with 18F-FDG as tracer to detect changes in viability and 13N-ammonia as tracer for coronary flow reserve in patients with an implanted SCS for refractory angina.[107] Irrespective of the improvement in clinical symptoms, the investigators failed to demonstrate significant alterations in coronary flow reserve. In contrast to their findings, two other observational studies, using $^{13}NH_3$ as tracer in patients with spinal cord stimulator implanted for refractory angina, reported blood flow directed from normally perfused regions to ischemic myocardial areas, in conjunction with an improvement in coronary flow reserve, resulting in a more homogenous perfused myocardium.[108, 109] This discrepancy in outcomes of the PET studies is thought to be related to differences in methodology, tracers, protocols and, tools. Furthermore, the redistribution in coronary blood flow from normally perfused to impaired perfused regions has also been observed following the administration of aminophyline, theofylline or bamiphylline and was coined "the Robin Hood phenomenon" (stealing from the "rich" non-ischemic areas and supplying the blood to the "poor" ischemic regions).[110, 111] All these three drugs are affecting adenosine handling through their interaction with Xanthine metabolisme. Further, the adenosine re-uptake inhibitor dipyridamole blunts the effect of SCS [108] and the drinking of caffeine too has been reported to reduce the effects of neuromodulation through its effect on adenosine, via xanthine metabolism.[112]

Adenosine, administered in a coronary artery provokes angina through activation of adenosine A1 receptors.[113,114] Adenosine plays a role in myocardial ischemia as well, which effect is thought to take place through activation of the A2 adenosine receptor, generating in its turn, under ischemic conditions, redistribution of local blood flow from sub-epicardial towards epicardial tissues.[115] So, the moment the critical balance between myocardial oxygen supply and demand is deferred, by either improving supply, or through a reduction in demand, a cascade of chemical reactions take place. It is conceivable that electrical neuromodulation employs its effect through interference with local adenosine handling.[116]

In addition to the increased angina threshold, which was first addressed in the rapid atrial pacing study in patients with a SCS implanted for their angina,[94] the observed antiischemic effects of SCS resluted in improvement of ischemic tolerance. Since the ischemic tolerance is considered as the result of collateral recruitment and preconditioning, the emphasis of the research was aimed at these two phenomena, in detail.

To unravel the mechanisms of action of electrical neuromodulation in cardiac performance, research was performed to the measuring of changes in coronary blood flow with Doppler flow catheters. In 1994, Chauhan *et al* showed an increase in coronary flow velocity in patients with refractory angina, during only 5 minutes' TENS.[117] In contrast to their findings, observations in an anesthetized canine preparation of SCS, in which myocardial ischemia was created through a 4 minute ligation of a coronary artery, followed by application of radiolabeled microspheres to evaluate myocardial ischemia, suggest that blood flow in the microcirculation was not affected.[118] Albeit that the occlusion was of very short duration and the canines did not show atherosclerotic coronary artery disease, this finding should not be surprising since it has been shown that the sympathetic nervous system does not seem to influence native coronary collateral vessels in canine myocardium. Other studies using Doppler flow wires confirm the initial results,[119] most likely resulting from altered coronary collateral blood flow by a so-called reversed steal, following electrical neuromodulation.[120] After the pilot phase, the recruitment of collaterals was demonstrated in a randomized control study during percutaneous coronary intervention and only 5 minutes of TENS.[121] The altered coronary blood flows does not necessarily require an increase in blood flow velocity.[122]

The other branch to improve the ischemic tolerance of the heart, (pre)conditioning, has too been subjected to mechanistic studies.[28] Initially, preconditioning was hypothesized to be induced through activation of protein kinase C cascade, which phosphorylates the mitochondrial ATP-sensitive K^+ channels. This signalling pathway leads to preconditioning through a more gradual depletion of ATP-dependent energy storage mechanism. In the present concept of preconditioning, several signaling pathways play a role. Activation of signaling pathways are suggested to take place through release of substances like neurotransmitters and vasoactive compounds, such as adenosine and endorphins. Adenosine has vasodilatory effects and is involved in nociception. Therefore, it was postulated that adenosine may be the interface between neurohumoral and cardiovascular interactions. As a result of coffee intake and dipyridamole the metabolic handling adenosine appears to be affected, in the presence of electrical neuromodulation.[108,112] Finally, electrical neuromodulation has been demonstrated both, to release beta-endorphins from the heart[123] and to affect the alpha-receptor.[124] These three prerequisites are all involved in the upregulation of G protein-coupled receptors which, in turn, activate ATP-sensitive K^+ channels, through up-regulation of protein kinase C. In an experimental set up it was demonstrated that electrical neuromodulation mitigates transient ischemia in anesthetized rabbits. The animals were all subjected to 30 minutes of coronary arterial occlusion, followed by 3 hours of reperfusion, in the presence or absence of SCS at C8-T2. Pre-emptive electrical neuromodulation was able to reduce the ischemic zone, significantly, which effect was eliminated by α-receptor blockade. A polymerase chain reaction showed an increased phosphorylation of cardiac protein kinase C. This protein is known for its role in preconditioning. Furthermore, electrical neuromodulation did not seem to affect blood pressure or heart rate. It was concluded that pre-emptive electrical neurostimulation reduces the size of infarcts induced by transient coronary artery occlusion, which cardioprotective effect involves cardiac adrenergic neurons.[124]

Both limbs involved in ischemic tolerance, collateral recruitment and preconditioning may engage similar signaling pathways at time of myocardial reperfusion, i.e. protein kinase cascades.

In conclusion, based on enhanced ischemic tolerance it is conceivable that electrical neuromodulation employs its antiischemic cardioprotective effect by improving collateral flow, enhancing preconditioning and subsequently reducing myocardial oxygen demand.

7. Final conclusions

Electrical neuromodulation is an effective adjuct treatment for patients with refractory angina. Many studies showed that it is improving the quality of life of these patients who are severely disabled by their ischemic heart disease and also enhances the ischemic threshold. The antiischemic effect is thought to take place through activation of mechanisms which induce both preconditioning and recruitment of collaterals, without either increasing mortality rate and without concealing the angina warning signal, during an acute myocardial infarction. Therefore, neuromodulation is considered as a safe therapy for patients invalidated by their refractory angina. The underlying mechanisms of action are multi-factorial and take place at different levels in heart brain axis.

8. Future developments

Electrical neuromodulation for refractory angina is lacking a feed-back option, such as is the case in a pacing device, in which you can measure the threshold through assessing the capture. The determination of objective signs of an effect shall make the therapy more widely accepted. Notwithstanding the shortcomings, the use of various applications of electrical neuromodulation for a myriad of indications will develop further. It is conceivable that for transcutaneous nerve stimulation, instead of the pads that easily come off, a shirt with built-in pads will be developed. Further, a combination of electric devices such as a spinal cord stimulator and an ICD are likely. The spinal cord stimulator may stimulate prior to the ICD to reduce the sometimes freighting discharge of the ICD for the patient. Finally, newer cardiac indications such as in the treatment for tachy-arrhythmias, heart failure, cardiac syndrome X (microvascular angina) and acute coronary syndromes will be evaluated.

9. References

[1] Natelson BH. "Neurocardiology. An interdisciplinary area for the 80s". *Arch Neurol* (1985) 42:178–84.

[2] Basic and Clinical Neurocardiology. (Eds. Armour JA; Ardell JL). Oxford University Press, NY, USA (2004)

[3] Heberden W. Some account of the breast. *Med Trans* (1772) 2:58-67
[4] Bolser DC, Chandler MJ, Garrison DW, Foreman RD. Effects of intracardiac bradykinin and capsaicin on spinal and spinoreticular neurons. *Am J Physiol* (1989) 257:H1543-50
[5] Albutaihi IA, Hautvast RW, DeJongste MJ, Ter Horst GJ, Staal MJ. Cardiac nociception in rats: neuronal pathways and the influence of dermal neurostimulation on conveyance to the central nervous system. *J Mol Neurosci* (2003) 43-52
[6] Albutaihi IA, DeJongste MJ, Ter Horst GJ. An integrated study of heart pain and behavior in freely moving rats (using fos as a marker for neuronal activation). *Neurosignals* (2004) 13:207-26
[7] Qin C, Farber JP, Miller KE, Foreman RD. Responses of thoracic spinal neurons to activation and desensitization of cardiac TRPV1-containing afferents in rats. *Am J Physiol Regul Integr Comp Physiol* (2006) 291:R1700-7
[8] Ter Horst GJ, Van den Brink A, Homminga SA, Hautvast RW, Rakhorst G, Mettenleiter TC, De Jongste MJ, Lie KI, Korf J. Transneuronal viral labelling of rat heart left ventricle controlling pathways. *Neuroreport* (1993) 4:1307-10
[9] Ter Horst GJ, Hautvast RW, De Jongste MJ, Korf J. Neuroanatomy of cardiac activity-regulating circuitry: a transneuronal retrograde viral labelling study in the rat. *Eur J Neurosci* (1996) 8:2029-41
[10] DeJongste MJ, Terhorst GJ, Foreman RD. Basic research models for the study of underlying mechanisms of electrical neuromodulation and ischemic heart-brain interactions. *Cleve Clin J Med* (2009) 76 Suppl 2:S41-6
[11] Jessurun GAJ, Meeder JG, DeJongste MJL. Defining the problem of intractable angina. *Pain Reviews*, 1997;4:89-99
[12] Mannheimer C, Camici P, Chester MR, Collins A, DeJongste M, Eliasson T, Follath F, Hellemans I, Herlitz J, Luscher T, Pasic M, Thelle D. The problem of chronic refractory angina; report from the ESC Joint Study Group on the Treatment of Refractory Angina. *Eur Heart J* (2002) 23:355-70
[13] Ten Vaarwerk IAM. Jessurun GAJ, DeJongste MJL, Andersson C, Eliasson T, Mannheimer C, Staal MJ. On behalf of the working group neurocardiology. Baseline characteristics of patients with refractory AP treated with SCS. *Heart* (1999) 82:82-9
[14] Murray S, Carson KG, Ewings PD, Collins PD, James MA. Spinal Cord Stimulation significantly decreases the need for acute hospital admission for chest pain in patients with refractory angina pectoris. *Heart* (1999) 82:89-92
[15] Vulnink NCC, Overgaauw DM, Jessurun GAJ, TenVaarwerk IAM, Kropmans TJB, Van der Schans CP, Middel B, Staal MJ, DeJongste MJL.The effects of spinal cord stimulation on quality of life in patients with therapeutically refractory angina pectoris. *Neuromodulaton* (1999) 2:1:29-36
[16] Mukherjee D, Bhatt DL, Roe MT, Patel V, Ellis SG. Direct myocardial revascularization and angiogenesis--how many patients might be eligible? *Am J Cardiol* (1999) 84:598-600
[17] DeJongste MJ, Tio RA, Foreman RD Chronic therapeutically refractory angina pectoris. *Heart* (2004) 90:225-30
[18] Schoebel FC, Frazier OH, Jessurun GA, De Jongste MJ, Kadipasaoglu KA, Jax TW, Heintzen MP, Cooley DA, Strauer BE, Leschke M. Refractory angina pectoris in end-stage coronary artery disease: evolving therapeutic concepts. *Am Heart J* (1997) 134(4):587-602

[19] Svorkdal N. Pro: anesthesiologists' role in treating refractory angina: spinal cord stimulators, thoracic epi- durals, therapeutic angiogenesis, and other emerging options. (2003) 17:536-45

[20] Gibbons RJ, Abrams J, Chatterjee K. ACC/AHA 2002 guideline update for management of patients with chronic stable angina--summary article: a report of the American College of Cardiology/American Heart Association Task Force on Practice Guidelines (Commit tee on the Management of Patients With Chronic Stable Angina). *Circulation* (2003) 107:149-58

[21] Nelson RR, Jorgenson CR, Wang Y. The rate pressure product as an index of myocardial oxygen consumption during exercise in patients with angina pectoris. *Circulation (*1987) 57:549-56

[22] Kersten JR, Pagel PS, Chilian WM, Warltier DC. Multifactorial basis for coronary collateralization: a complex adaptive response to ischemia. *Cardiovasc Res* (1999) 43:44-57

[23] A. Krogh A: The number and distribution of capillaries in muscles with calculations of the oxygen pressure head necessary for supplying tissue. *J Physiol* (1919) 52409-415
B. Krogh A: The supply of oxygen to the tissues and the regulation of the capillary circulation, *J Physiol (*1919) 52:457-474.
C. Krogh A: *Anatomy and Physiology of Capillaries.* New Haven Yale University Press. (1936)

[24] Billinger M, Fleisch M, Eberli FR, Garachemani A, Meier B, Seiler C. Is the development of myocardial tolerance to repeated ischemia in humans due to preconditioning or to collateral recruitment? *J Am Coll Cardiol* (1999) 33:1027-35

[25] Shattock MJ, Lawson CS, Hearse DJ, Downey JM. Electrophysiological characteristics of repetitive ischemic preconditioning in the pig heart. *J Mol Cell Cardiol* (1996) 28:1339-47

[26] Murry, CE; Jennings, RB, Reimer, KA. Preconditioning with ischemia: a delay of lethal cell injury in ischemic myocardium. *Circulation* (1986) 74:1124-36

[27] Garcia-Dorado D, Barba I, Inserte J. Twenty-five years of preconditioning: are we ready for ischaemia? From coronary occlusion to systems biology and back. *Cardiovasc Res* (2011) 91:378-81

[28] Hausenloy DJ, Yellon DM. The therapeutic potential of ischemic conditioning: an update. *Nat Rev Cardiol* (2011) 8:619-29

[29] Kellaway P. The William Osler Medical Essay. The part played by the electrical fish in the early history of bioelectricity and electrotherapy. *Bull Hist Med* (1946) 20:112

[30] Scheminzky, F: Recent Studies on Electronarcosis. *Wien Klin Wschr (*1936) 49:1190

[31] Melzack R, Wall PD. Pain mechanisms: a new theory. *Science* (1965) 150:971-9

[32] Rosen, S. D., Paulesu, E., Frith, C. D., Frackowiak, R. S. J., Davies, G. J. D., Jones, T. and Camici, P. G. (1994) Central nervous pathways mediating angina pectoris. *Lancet,* 344, 147–150.

[33] Hautvast RW, ter Horst GJ, DeJong B, DeJongste MJ, Blanksma PK, Paans AM, Korf J. Relative changes in regional cerebral blood flow during spinal cord stimulation in patients with refractory angina pectoris. *Eur J of Neuroscience* (1997) 9:1178-83

[34] Armour JA. Myocardial ischaemia and the cardiac nervous system. Cardiovasc Res, 1999; 41:41-54 (Review).

[35] Beecher HK. Nonspecific forces surrounding disease and the treatment of disease. *JAMA* (1962) 179:137-40
[36] Chandler MJ, Brennan TJ, Garrison DW, Kim KS, Schwartz PJ, Foreman RD. A mechanism of cardiac pain suppression by spinal cord stimulation: implications for patients with angina pectoris. *Eur Heart J (*1993) 14:96-105
[37] Foreman RD, Linderoth B, Ardell JL, Barron KW, Chandler MJ, Hull SS Jr, TerHorst GJ, DeJongste MJ, Armour JA. Modulation of intrinsic cardiac neurons by spinal cord stimulat ion: implications for its therapeutic use in angina pectoris. *Cardiovasc Res* (2000) 47:367-75
[38] Gersbach PA, Hasdemir MG, Eeckhout E, von Segesser LK. Spinal cord stimulation treatment for angina pectoris: more than a placebo? *Ann Thorac Surg* (2001) 72:S1100-4
[39] Braunwald E, Epstein SE, Glick G, Wechsler AS, Braunwald NS. Relief of angina pectoris by electrical stimulation of the carotid-sinus nerves. *New Engl J Med (*1967) 277(24):1278-83
[40] Braunwald E. Personal reflections on efforts to reduce ischemic myocardial damage. *Cardiovasc Res* (2002) 56: 332-338
[41] Moore R, Groves D, Hammond C, Leach A, Chester MR.Temporary sympathectomy in the treatment of chronic refractory angina. *J Pain Symptom Manage* (2005) 30(2):183-91
[42] Mannheimer C, Carlsson CA, Ericson K, Vedin A, Wilhelmsson C.Transcutaneous electrical nerve stimulation in severe angina pectoris. *Eur Heart J (*1982) 3:297-302
[43] Mannheimer C, Carlsson CA, Emanuelsson H, vedin A, Waagstein F, Wilhelmsson C. The effects of trans- cutaneous electrical nerve stimulation in patients with severe angina pectoris. *Circulation* (1985) 71:308-16
[44] Strobos MA, Coenraads PJ, De Jongste MJ, Ubels FL.Dermatitis caused by radio-frequency electromagnetic radiation. *Contact Dermatitis* (2001) 44:309
[45] Llamas M, Santiago D, Navarro R, Sánchez-Pérez J, García-Diez A. Unusual allergic contact dermatitis produced by a transcutaneous electrical nerve stimulator. *Contact Dermatitis* (2010) 62:189-90
[46] Shealy CN, Taslitz N, Mortimer JT, Becker DP. Electrical inhibition of pain: experimental evaluation. *Anesth Analg* (1967) 46:299-305
[47] DeJongste MJ and Staal MJ. Electrical neuromodulation for chronic refractory angina pectoris. *Res Adv in Cardiology (*2001) 1:17-12
[48] Murphy DF and Giles KE. Dorsal column stimulation for pain relief from intractable angina pectoris. *Pain* (1987) 28:365-8
[49] Eddicks S, Maier-Hauff K, Schenk M, Müller A, Baumann G, Theres H. Thoracic spinal cord stimulation improves functional status and relieves symptoms in patients with refract ory angina pectoris: the first placebo-controlled randomised study. *Heart* (2007) 93:585-90
[50] Lanza GA, Grimaldi R, Greco S, Ghio S, Sarullo F, Zuin G, De Luca A, Allegri M, Di Pede F, Castagno D, Turco A, Sapio M, Pinato G, Cioni B, Trevi G, Crea F. Spinal cord stimulation for the treatment of refractory angina pectoris: a multicenter randomized single-blind study (the SCS-ITA trial). *Pain (*2011) 152:45-52
[51] Goroszeniuk T, Kothari S Subcutaneous Target Stimulation or Peripheral Subcutaneous Field Stimulation: That Is the Question. *Neuromodulation* (2011) 14:185-185

[52] Buiten MS, DeJongste MJL, Beese U.Subcutaneous Electrical Nerve Stimulation: A Feasible and New Method for Treatment of Patients with Refractory Angina. *Neuromodulation* (2011) 14: 258-264
[53] Goroszeniuk T, Pang D, Al-Kaisy A, Sanderson K. Subcutaneous Target stimulation-peripheral subcutaneous field stimulation in the treatment of refractory angina: preliminary case reports. *Pain Practice* (2011) 11:1-9
[54] Chester MR et al. A patient-centred guide to angina. *www.agina.com*
[55] González-Darder JM, Canela P, González-Martinez V. High cervical spinal cord stimulation for unstable angina pectoris. *Stereotact Funct Neurosurg* (1991) 56:20-27
[56] Murphy DF, Giles KE. Dorsal column stimulation for pain relief from intractable angina pectoris. Pain 1987; 28,365-368
[57] Sanderson JE, Brooksby P, Waterhouse D, Palmer RBG, Neuhauser K. Epidural spinal electrical stimulation for severe angina. A study of effects on symptoms, exercise tolerance and degree of ischemia. *Eur Heart J* (1992) 13:628-33
[58] De Vries J, De Jongste MJ, Spincemaille G, Staal MJ. Spinal cord Stimulation for ischemic heart disease and peripheral vascular disease. *Adv Tech Stand Neurosurg* (2007) 32:63-89
[59] Mannheimer C, Augustinsson LE, Carlsson CA *et al.* Epidural spinal electrical stimulation in severe angina pectoris. *Br Heart J* (1988) 59:56-61.
[60] Sanderson JE, Ibrahim B, Waterhouse D *et al.* Spinal electrical stimulation for intractable angina-long-term clinical outcome and safety. *Eur Heart J (*1994) 15:810-4
[61] Hautvast RW, DeJongste MJ, Staal MJ, Gilst van WH, Lie KI. Spinal cord stimulation in chronic intractable angina pectoris: a randomized, controlled efficacy study. *Am Heart J* (1998) 136:114-20
[62] Sanderson JE, Brooksby P, Waterhouse D, Palmer RB, Neubauer K. Epidural spinal electrical stimulation for severe angina: a study of its effects on symptoms, exercise tolerance and degree of ischaemia. *Eur Heart J* (1992) 13:628-33
[63] DeJongste MJL, Hautvast RWM, Hillege H *et al.* Efficacy of spinal cord stimulation as an adjuvant therapy for intractable angina pectoris: A prospective randomized clinical study. *J Am Coll Cardiol* (1994) 23:1592-7
[64] Bagger JP, Jensen BS, Johannsen G. Long-term outcome of spinal electrical stimulation in patients with refractory chest pain. *Clin Cardiol* (1998) 21:286-8
[65] Mannheimer C, Eliasson T, Augustinsson LE, Blomstrand C, Emanuelsson H, Larsson S, Norrsell H, Hjalmarsson A. Electrical stimulation versus coronary artery bypass surgery in severe angina pectoris: the ESBY study. *Circulation* (1998) 97:1157-63
[66] Jitta DJ, DeJongste MJL, Kliphuis CM, et al. Multimorbidity, the Predominant Predictor of Quality-of-Life, Following Successful Spinal Cord Stimulation for Angina Pectoris. *Neuromodulation (*2011) 14:13-18
[67] De Vries J, DeJongste MJ, Versteegen GJ.Personality:Predictor of neurostimulation outcom es in patients with chest pain and normal coronary arteries. *Neuromodulation* (2006) 9:123-127
[68] Dobre D, van Veldhuisen DJ, deJongste MJL, et al. The contribution of observational studies to the knowledge of drug effectiveness in heart failure *Br J of Clin Pharmacol* (2007) 64: 406-14

[69] Börjesson M, Andrell P, Lundberg D, Mannheimer C. Spinal cord stimulation in severe angina pectoris--a systematic review based on the Swedish Council on Technology assessment in health care report on long-standing pain. *Pain (*2008) 140(3):501-8

[70] Taylor RS, De Vries J, Buchser E, DeJongste MJ. Spinal cord stimulation in the treatment of refractory angina: systematic review and meta-analysis of randomised controlled trials. *BMC Cardiovasc Disord* (2009) 25:9-13

[71] Gibbons RJ, Abrams J, Chatterjee K, et al. A Report of the American College of Cardiology/American Heart Association Task Force on Practice Guidelines (Committee on the Management of Patients With Chronic Stable Angina). ACC/AHA Guideline Update for the Management of Patients Stable Angina With Chronic —Summary Article. *Circulation* (2002) 107:149-58

[72] Vries J, Staal MJ, DeJongste MJL Is there a future for combinations of implantable devices in human bionics? *Neuromodulation* (2002) 5:131-132

[73] Iyer R, Gnanadurai TV, Forsey P. Management of cardiac pacemaker in a patient with spinal cord stimulator implant. *Pain (*1998) 74:333-5

[74] Enggaard TP, Andersen C, Scherer C. Spinal cord stimulation for refractory angina in pat ients implanted with cardioverter defibrillators: five case reports. *Europace* (2010) 121336-7

[75] Augustinsson LE, Eliasson T, Mannheimer C. Spinal cord stimulation in severe angina pectoris. *Stereotact Funct Neurosurg* (1995) 65:136-41

[76] Andersen C, Hole P, Oxhoj H. Does pain relief with spinal cord stimulation for angina conceal myocardial infarction ? *Br Heart J* (1994) 71:419-21

[77] Jessurun GAJ, TenVaarwerk IAM, DeJongste MJL *et al.* Sequalae of spinal cord stimulation for refractory angina pectoris. Reliabity and safety profile of long-term clinical application. *Cor Artery Dis* (1997) 8:33-7

[78] Di Pede F, Lanza GA, Zuin G, Alfieri O, Rapati M, Romanò M, Circo A, Cardano P, Bellocci F, Santini M, Maseri A; Immediate and long-term clinical outcome after spinal cord stimulation for refractory stable angina pectoris. Investigators of the Prospective Italian Registry of SCS for angina pecoris. *Am J Cardiol* (2003) 91:951-5

[79] Andréll P, Yu W, Gersbach P, Gillberg L, Pehrsson K, Hardy I, Ståhle A, Andersen C, Mannheimer C. Long-term effects of spinal cord stimulation on angina symptoms and quality of life in patients with refractory angina- results from the European Regaistry Link (EARL). *Heart* (2010);96:1132-6

[80] Simpson EL, Duenas A, Holmes MW, Papaioannou D, Chilcott J. Spinal cord stimulation for chronic pain of neuropathic or ischaemic origin: systematic review and economic evaluation. *Health Technol Assess* (2009) 13:iii, ix-x,1-154

[81] Dyer MT, Goldsmith KA, Khan SN, Sharples LD, Freeman C, Hardy I, Buxton MJ, Schofield PM. Clinical and cost-effectiveness analysis of an open label, single-centre, randomised trial of spinal cord stimulation (SCS) versus percutaneous myocardial laser revascularisation (PMR) in patients with refractory angina pectoris: The SPiRiT trial. *Trials* (2008) 9:40

[82] Mulcahy D, Knight C, Stables R, Fox K. Lasers, burns, cuts, tingles and pumps: a consideration of alternative treatments for intractable angina. *Br Heart J (*1994) 71:406-8

[83] Cameron T. Safety and efficacy of spinal cord stimulation for the treatment of chronic pain: a 20-year literature. *J Neurosurg* (2004) 100:3;Suppl:S 254-267 (review)

[84] de Vries J, Svilaas T, DeJongste MJL, et al. Impact of electrical neuro stimulation on persistent ST elevation after successful reperfusion by primary percutaneous coronary intervention. *J of Electrocardiology* (2007) 40:522-526

[85] De Vries J, DeJongste MJL, Zijlstra F, et al. Long-term effects of electrical neurostimulation in patients with unstable angina: Refractory to conventional therapies. *Neuromodulation* (2007) 10:345-48

[86] González-Darder JM, Canela P, González-Martinez V. High cervical spinal cord stimulation for unstable angina pectoris. *Stereotact Funct Neurosurg* (1991) 56:20-7.

[87] Greco S, Auriti A, Fiume D, Gazzeri G, Gentilucci G, Antonini L, Santini MSpinal cord stimulation for the treatment of refractory angina pectoris: a two-year follow-up. *Pacing Clin Electrophysiol* (1999) 22(1 Pt 1):26-32

[88] Diedrichs H, Zobel C, Theissen P, Weber M, Koulousakis A, Schicha H, Schwinger RH. Symptomatic relief precedes improvement of myocardial blood flow in patients under spinal cord stimulation. *Curr Control Trials Cardiovasc Med* (2005) 19;6:7

[89] DeJongste MJL, Haaksma J, Hautvast RW Hillege HL, Meyler PW, Staal MJ, Sanderson JE, Lie KI. Effects of spinal cord stimulation on daily life myocardial ischemia in patients with severe coronary artery disease. A prospective ambulatory ECG study. *Br Heart J (*1994) 71:413-8

[90] Murray S, Collins PD, James MA. An investigation into the 'carry over' effect of neurostimulation in the treatment of angina pectoris. *Int J Clin Pract* (2004) 58(7):669-74

[91] Shealy CN *et al*. Electrical inhibition of pain: experimental evaluation. Anesth Analg, 1967;46:299-305

[92] Armour JA, Linderoth B, Arora RC, DeJongste MJ, Ardell JL, Kingma JG Jr, Hill M, Foreman RD. Long-term modulation of the intrinsic cardiac nervous system by spinal cord neurons in normal and ischaemic hearts. A*uton Neurosci* (2002) 10;95:71-9

[93] Jessurun GA, DeJongste MJ, Hautvast RW, Tio RA, Brouwer J, van Lelieveld S, Crijns HJ.Clinical follow-up after cessation of chronic electrical neuromodulation in patients with severe coronary artery disease: a prospective randomized controlled study on putative involvement of sympathetic activity. *Pacing Clin Electrophysiol (*1999) 22:1432-9

[94] Mannheimer C, Eliasson T, Andersson B *et al*. Effects of spinal cord stimulation in angina pectoris induced by pacing and possible mechanisms of action. *Br Med J* (1993) 307:477-80

[95] Lindgrin I. Angina pectoris; a clinical study with special reference to neurosurgical treatment. *Acta Med Scand Suppl* (1950) 243:1-203.

[96] Meglio M, Cioni B, Rossi GF, Sandric S, Santarelli P. Spinal cord stimulation affects the central mechanisms of regulation of heart rate. *J Appl Neurophysiol* (1986) 49(3):139-46

[97] Balcon R, Jewitt DE, Davies JP, Oram S A controlled trial of propranolol in acute myocardial infarction. *Lanc*et (1966) 2(7470):918-20

[98] Hautvast RW, Brouwer J, DeJongste MJ, Lie KI. Effect of spinal cord stimulation on heart rate variability and myocardial ischemia in patients with chronic intractable angina pectoris--a prospective ambulatory electrocardiographic study. *Clin Cardiol* (1998) 21:33-8

[99] Norrsell H, Eliasson T, Mannheimer C, Augustinsson LE, Bergh CH, Andersson B, Waag stein F, Friberg P. Effects of pacing-induced myocardial stress and spinal cord stimulation on whole body and cardiac norepinephrine spillover. *Eur Heart J* (1997);18:1890-6

[100] Fricke E, Eckert S, Dongas A, Fricke H, Preuss R, Lindner O, Horstkotte D, Burchert W. Myocardial sympathetic innervation in patients with symptomatic coronary artery disease: follow-up after 1 year with neurostimulation. *J Nucl Med* (2008) 49(9):1458-64

[101] Spinelli A, Lanza GA, Calcagni ML, Sestito A, Sgueglia GA, Di Monaco A, Bruno I, Lamendola P, Barone L, Giordano A, Crea F. Effect of spinal cord stimulation on cardiac adr energic nerve function in patients with cardiac syndrome X. *J Nucl Cardiol* (2008)15:804-10

[102] Kudej RK, Shen YT, Peppas AP, Huang CH, Chen W, Yan L, et al Obligatory role of cardiac nerves and alpha1-adrenergic receptors for the second window of ischemic preconditioning in conscious pigs. Circ Res 2006;99:1270-1276

[103] Olgin JE, Takahashi T, Wilson E, Vereckei A, Steinberg H, Zipes DP. Effects of thoracic spinal cord stimulation on cardiac autonomic regulation of the sinus and atrioventricular nodes. *J Cardiovasc Electrophysiol* (2002) 13:475-81

[104] Zamotrinsky AV, Kondratiev B, de Jong JW. Vagal neurostimulation in patients with coronary artery disease. *Auton Neurosci* (2001) 88(1-2):109-16

[105] Marber M, Walker D, Yellon D. Spinal cord stimulation or ischemic preconditioning? *Br Med J* (1993) 307:737

[106] Diedrichs H, Zobel C, Theissen P, Weber M, Koulousakis A, Schicha H, Schwinger RH. Symptomatic relief precedes improvement of myocardial blood flow in patients under spinal cord stimulation. *Curr Control Trials Cardiovasc Med* (2005) 6:7

[107] Fricke E, Eckert S, Dongas A, Fricke H, Preuss R, Lindner O, Horstkotte D, Burchert W. Myocardial perfusion after one year of spinal cord stimulation in patients with refractory angina. *Nuklearmedizin* (2009) 48:104-9

[108] Hautvast RW, Blanksma PK, DeJongste MJ, Pruim J, van der Wall EE, Vaalburg W, Lie KI. Effect of spinal cord stimulation on myocardial blood flow assessed by positron emission tomography in patients with refractory angina pectoris. *Am J Cardiol* (1996) 1;77:462-7

[109] Mobilia G, Zuin G, Zanco P, Di Pede F, Pinato G, Neri G, Cargnel S, Raviele A, Ferlin G, Buchberger R. Effects of spinal cord stimulation on regional myocardial blood flow in patients with refractory angina. A positron emission tomography study. *G Ital Cardiol* (1998) 28:1113-9.

[110] Crea F, Pupita G, Galassi AR, el Tamimi H, Kaski JC, Davies GJ, Maseri A. Effect of theophylline on exercise-induced myocardial ischaemia. *Lancet* (1989) 1(8640):683-6

[111] Gaspardone A, Crea F, Iamele M, Tomai F, Versaci F, Pellegrino A, Chiariello L, Gioffré PA. Bamiphylline improves exercise-induced myocardial ischemia through a novel mechanism of action. *Circulation* (1993) 88:502-8

[112] Marchand S, Li J, Charest J. Effects of caffeine on algesia from transcutaneous electrical nerve stimulation. *New Eng J Med* (1995) 333:325-6

[113] Lagerqvist B, Sylvén C, Beermann B, Helmius G, Waldenström A. Intracoronary adenosine causes angina pectoris like pain--an inquiry into the nature of visceral pain. *Cardiovasc Res* (1990) 24:609-13

[114] Gaspardone A, Crea F, Tomai F, Versaci F, Iamele M, Gioffrè G, Chiariello L, Gioffrè PA. Muscular and cardiac adenosine-induced pain is mediated by A1 receptors.. *J Am Coll Cardiol* (1995) 25:251-7

[115] Berwick ZC, Payne GA, Lynch B, Dick GM, Sturek M, Tune JD. Contribution of adenosine A(2A) and A(2B) receptors to ischemic coronary dilation: role of K(V) and K(ATP) channels. *Microcirculation (*2010) 17:600-7

[116] Szentmiklósi AJ, Cseppento A, Harmati G, Nánási PP. Novel trends in the treatment of cardiovascular disorders: site- and event- selective adenosinergic drugs. *Curr Med Chem* (2011) 18:1164-87

[117] Chauhan A, Mullins PA, Thuraisingham SI, Taylor G, Petch MC, Schofield PM.. Effect of transcutaneous electrical nerve stimulation on coronary blood flow. *Circulation (*1994) 89:694-70

[118] Kingma JG Jr, Linderoth B, Ardell JL, Armour JA, DeJongste MJ, Foreman RD. Neuromodulation therapy does not influence blood flow distribution or left-ventricular dynamics during acute myocardial ischemia. *Auton Neurosci* (2001) 91:47-54

[119] Jessurun GA, Tio RT, DeJongste MJ *et al.* Coronary blood flow dynamics during transcutaneous electrical stimulation for stable angina pectoris associated with severe narrowing of one major coronary artery. *Am J Cardiol* (1998) 82:921-6

[120] De Vries J, Anthonio RL, DeJongste MJL, Jessurun GA, Tio RA, Zijlstra F. The effect of electrical neurostimulation on collateral perfusion. *Netherlands Heart J (* 2006) 14:209-14

[121] De Vries J, Anthonio RL, DeJongste MJ, Jessurun GA, Tan ES, de Smet BJ, van den Heuvel AF, Staal MJ, Zijlstra F. The effect of electrical neurostimulation on collateral perfusion during acute coronary occlusion. *BMC Cardiovasc Disord (*2007) 7:18

[122] Norrsell H, Eliasson T, Albertsson P, Augustinsson LE, Emanuelsson H, Eriksson P, Mannheimer C. Effects of spinal cord stimulation on coronary blood flow velocity. *Coron Artery Dis* (1998) 9:273-8

[123] Eliasson T, Mannheimer C, Waagstein F, Andersson B, Bergh CH, Augustinsson LE, Hedner T, Larson G. Myocardial turnover of endogenous opioids and calcitonin-gene-related peptide in the human heart and the effects of spinal cord stimulation on pacing-induced angina pectoris. *Cardiology* (1998) 89:170-7

[124] Southerland EM, Milhorn DM, Foreman RD, Linderoth B, DeJongste MJ, Armour JA, Subramanian V, Singh M, Singh K, Ardell JL. Preemptive, but not reactive, spinal cord stimulation mitigates transient ischemia-induced myocardial infarction via cardiac adrenergic neurons. *Am J Physiol Heart Circ Physiol (*2007) 292:H311-7

8

Use of Non-Invasive Brain Stimulation in Stroke

Bulent Turman[1] and Sultan Tarlaci[2]
[1]*School of Medicine, Bond University,*
[2]*Özel Ege Sağlık Hospital, Izmir*
[1]*Australia*
[2]*Turkey*

1. Introduction

Stroke is the leading cause of permanent disability in the Western world (Kolominsky-Rabas *et al.*, 2001). Clinically, stroke is defined as a neurological deficit of cerebrovascular cause that persists beyond 24 hours. The clinical outcome of a stroke depends on which part of the brain is injured and how severely it is affected. The most common symptom of a stroke is sudden weakness or numbness of the face, arm or leg, most often on one side of the body. Other symptoms include: confusion, difficulty in speech production or comprehension; visual deficits; difficulty walking, dizziness, loss of balance or coordination; severe headache with no known cause; fainting or unconsciousness. The clinical presentation is closely associated with the affected artery, which is occluded by a clot or plaque (ischemic stroke), or ruptured (hemorrhagic stroke), and the extent of tissue infarct (Amarenco *et al.*, 2009).

In recent decades, the introduction of thrombolysis and the establishment of stroke units in hospitals have led to a significant reduction of mortality rate after stroke (Howard *et al.*, 2001). However, declining mortality rate has resulted in increased proportion of patients to be left with moderate to severe disability, affecting their daily activities. It is now well-established that early rehabilitation provides more effective recovery of function than would occur in the natural course of recovery (Maulden *et al.*, 2005). However, in most cases this recovery is still incomplete. Up to 60% of patients still have impaired manual dexterity six months after the onset of stroke (Kolominsky-Rabas *et al.*, 2001; Kwakkel *et al.*, 2002).

Advances in neuroscience in the last two decades unequivocally established the brain's capacity to reorganize itself (Nudo, 2007). This has led to the development of various techniques that could potentially improve the rehabilitation of stroke patients. Most widely researched and experimented non-invasive techniques are transcranial magnetic stimulation (TMS) and transcranial direct current stimulation (tDCS).

2. Non-invasive brain stimulation methods

2.1 Transcranial Magnetic Stimulation (TMS)

In the 1980's Merton and Morton (1980) were able to stimulate the human brain non-invasively by means of transcranial electrical stimulation (TES). However, contraction of scalp muscles and activation of nociceptive fibres evoked intense unpleasant pain sensation.

Introduction of TMS by Barker, Jalinous and Freeston in 1985 instantly attracted more attention over electrical stimulation, as in this method the current in the coil could activate cortical structures without causing pain. In the following two decades there have been significant advances in this method both technologically and scientifically.

2.1.1 Basics of TMS

TMS is based on the concept of electromagnetic induction. It involves the generation of a brief but strong magnetic field capable of activating cortical elements in the brain of conscious subjects without causing pain (Wasserman *et al.,* 2008). This magnetic field is derived from a changing primary electric current circulating in a coil which then passes through the skull to induce a secondary electric current capable of altering the neurons' transmembrane potential. Rapid depolarization of the membrane leads to action potential generations (Figure 1).

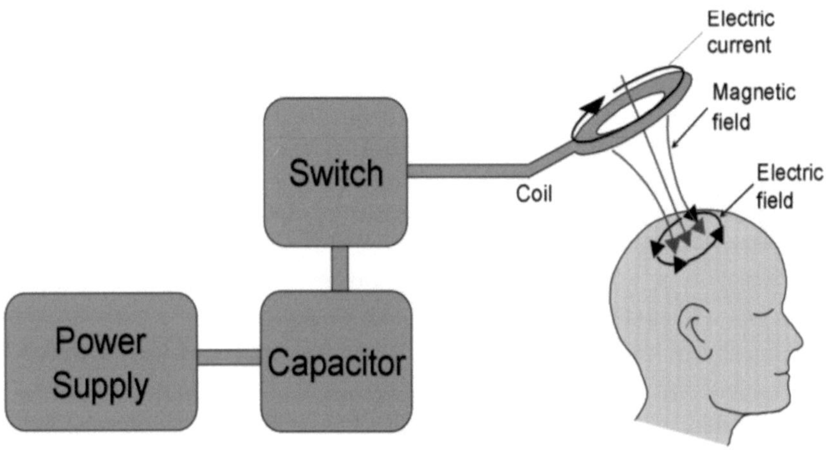

Fig. 1. TMS setup. A brief pulsed electric current passes through the coil, which results in a rapidly changing magnetic field that is perpendicular to the coil's surface. This magnetic field passes through the skull and scalp, and generates an electric field flowing in the opposite direction to the flow of current in the coil. This current leads to the activation of excitable structures in the brain tissue (from Fyre *et al.,* 2008).

The extent of activation within the cortex during magnetic stimulation is influenced by a number of variables, including the coil shape and its position over the head (Tings *et al.* 2005); number, intensity and frequency of pulses; output waveforms (monophasic vs. biphasic); induced current direction; and the anatomy of the region stimulated. For example, a circular shaped coil generates a relatively large and diffuse magnetic field over the brain, whereas a figure-of-eight (butterfly) coil produces a more focalized field (Wassermann *et al.,* 2008). More recently introduced coils, such as the double-cone coil and H-coil, were designed to stimulate deeper structures within the brain (Hayward *et al.,* 2007; Zangen *et al.,* 2005). However, in general the depth of stimulation is restricted to 2-3 cm below the scalp and the stimulated area within the cortex to around 1-3 cm^2. Increasing the stimulation intensity to activate deeper brain regions would result in wider and stronger stimulation of more superficial areas.

2.1.2 TMS techniques

A number of different stimulation techniques and paradigms have been introduced over the past two decades. Initially *single-pulse* TMS was used to primarily evaluate the excitability changes of the motor cortex and its output. It is still widely used to determine the best location (hot-spot) of recorded muscles within the motor homunculus and the active/passive motor thresholds, and to assess the effect of interventions on various intracortical influences (Wassermann *et al.,* 2008). *Paired-pulse* TMS utilizes two individual magnetic pulses, separated by a variable inter-stimulus interval (ISI). This method is used to evaluate the intracortical influences of magnetic stimulation, such as short- and long-interval intra-cortical inhibition (SICI and LICI) and intra-cortical facilitation (ICF) (for review see Reis *et al.,* 2008). The ICF of a test motor evoked potential (MEP) elicited from the target muscle can be observed at ISIs of 6-25 ms, using a subthreshold conditioning stimulus (CS) to influence the response to a subsequent suprathreshold test stimulus (TS) (Kujirai *et al.,* 1993). This effect tends to become stronger with increasing CS intensity and weaker with increasing TS intensity. A SICI on the other hand, can be observed when a subthreshold CS suppresses the MEP evoked in response to the suprathreshold TS if the interval between the stimuli is 5 ms or less (Kujirai *et al.,* 1993). In LICI a suprathreshold CS strong enough to produce an MEP in the target muscle could suppress an MEP to a later stimulus of the same intensity if the ISI was 50-200 ms.

Paired associative stimulation (PAS) technique involves applying pairs of peripheral and central stimuli repeatedly (Stefan *et al.* 2000). When around 100 peripheral electrical stimuli and central TMS pulses are paired at an ISI of 25 ms over 30 min, the cortical excitability increases. At an ISI of 10 ms a reduced cortical excitability is observed.

Technical advances in magnetic stimulator and coil designs led to more recent TMS techniques based on delivery of a series of pulses by means of multiple capacitors. This method, referred to as "repetitive transcranial magnetic stimulation" (rTMS), enabled researchers and clinicians to explore the potential benefits of TMS in clinical conditions (Pascual-Leone *et al.* 1994; Wassermann *et al.,* 2008; Hoogendam *et al.,* 2010).

2.1.3 Clinical and diagnostic applications of TMS

Since its introduction, TMS has been used to measure and evaluate the motor evoked potential (MEP) responses from target muscles and commonly applied as a non-invasive tool to clinically evaluate aspects of sensorimotor cortex and pyramidal tract function (Chen *et al.,* 2008). *Motor threshold* (MT) measurements are useful in determining the level of excitability within the motor cortex. MT is defined as the lowest stimulation required for a single pulse to produce a criterion amplitude MEP on a pre-specified fraction of consecutive trials (Wassermann *et al.,* 1998). MT measurements are also useful in establishing and following-up the hemispheric differences in clinical conditions, such as stroke. MEP *amplitude* and *onset latency* measurements are also useful parameters in the assessment and comparison of motor cortex excitability and its output. For example, in pathologies involving upper motor neurons, such as multiple sclerosis, MEP amplitudes are often reduced or absent, and central motor conduction times are prolonged (Cruz-Martínez *et al.* 2000). Somatosensory information processing at the cortical level is also influenced by TMS and can be evaluated by psychophysical measurements, such as vibration detection thresholds (Morley *et al.* 2007).

Cerebral hemispheres exert various influences on each other through interhemispheric connections. Therefore, TMS could be useful for investigating inter-hemispheric dynamics which can be investigated using paired-pulse TMS. In this paradigm, a *conditioning stimulus* is applied to one hemisphere, followed by a *test stimulus* applied to the other. Although a number of studies have reported some complex and inconsistent interhemispheric facilitatory influences dependent on background motor activity, coil position and conditioning stimulus intensity (Hanajima *et al.* 2001, Chowdhury & Matsunami, 2002), more consistent effects are observed in interhemispheric inhibition. The response to the test stimulus can be inhibited by the conditioning stimulus at inter-stimulus interval range of 6-50 ms (Ferbert *et al.*, 1992; Daskalakis *et al.* 2002). These transcallosal effects appear to be important in influencing the cortical excitability. For example, interhemispheric inhibition abnormalities have been found in patients with amyotrophic lateral sclerosis (Karandreas *et al.*, 2007).

Another method, called "*triple stimulation technique* (TST)", delivers a single magnetic pulse in association with two timed peripheral electrical pulses and is used to evaluate the integrity of neuronal pathways by means of collision (Magistris *et al.* 1999). It is reported that in amyotrophic lateral sclerosis patients TST provides a quantitative tool for assessing the upper motor neuron conduction failure and when used together with silent period measurements provides a sensitive diagnostic tool (Attarian *et al.*, 2007).

In short, TMS has been shown to be an important non-invasive diagnostic tool for evaluation of certain aspects of motor cortex function and its output. In clinical settings TMS could therefore be a useful tool to determine subclinical presentations in which clear clinical signs are not yet present or indecisive.

The most talked about adverse effect of magnetic brain stimulation is the induction of seizures. A number of cases of accidental seizures induced by rTMS have been reported over the years (total of 16 cases from 1998 to 2008). However, given the large number of subjects and patients who have undergone rTMS in over 3,000 published studies, it is suggested that the risk of rTMS to induce seizures is very low (Rossi *et al.*, 2009). Comprehensive screening of participants with regards to medication and predisposition to seizures will certainly further eliminate the possibility of this adverse effect.

2.1.4 Therapeutic applications of TMS

Since the introduction of repetitive stimulation capable stimulators, rTMS has been increasingly investigated and applied as a therapeutic tool. Using 'simple' rTMS, in which a series of regularly repeated magnetic pulses are delivered in trains and then separated by constant inter-train intervals, it is possible to induce changes to the excitability of motor cortex that outlast the stimulation period from several minutes up to 30 minutes (Touge *et al.*, 2001; Peinemann *et al.*, 2004). In this method, stimulation frequency plays a crucial role in producing selective changes in motor cortex excitability. Overall, low frequency (< 5Hz) rTMS results in suppression of corticospinal excitability, while high frequency (≥5 Hz) stimulation leads to facilitatory after-effects (for review see Siebner & Rothwell, 2003).

Another form of repetitive stimulation involves patterned stimuli. *Theta-burst stimulation* (TBS) is a burst of three to five pulses at high frequency (30-100 Hz) delivered at a repeated frequency (usually 5 Hz). This method has been shown to be safe and effective in producing changes in the excitability of motor systems (Huang & Rothwell, 2004). The typical form of TBS contains three pulse 50Hz bursts given every 200 ms (i.e. at 5 Hz) at the stimulus intensity of 80% of active motor threshold. When a 2-sec train of TBS is given every 10 sec (*intermittent TBS* - iTBS), the cortical excitability is enhanced due to a long-term potentiation (LTP) like effect. Conversely, when bursts are given every 200 ms continuously without interruption (*continuous TBS* - cTBS), the cortical excitability is suppressed due to a long-term depression (LTD) like effect (Huang *et al.*, 2005).

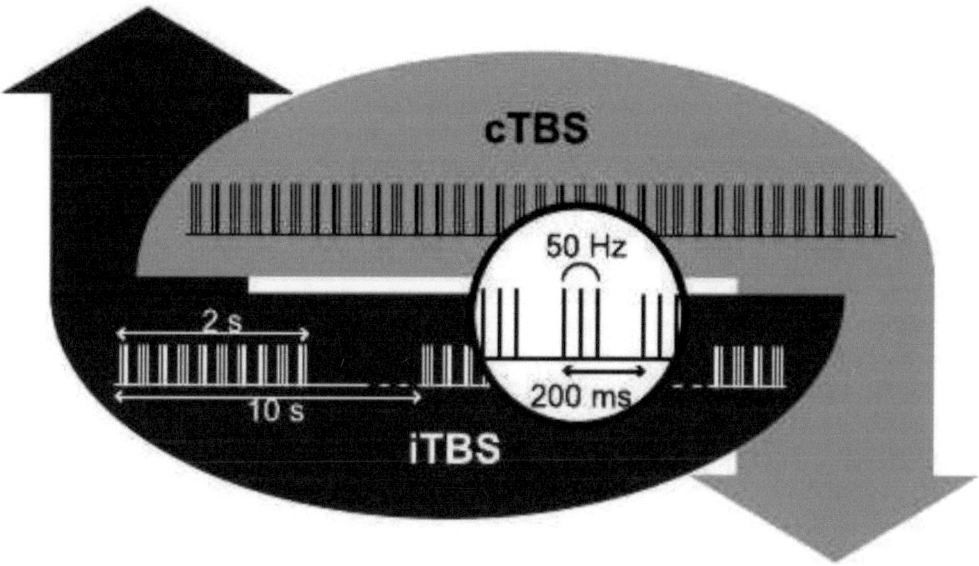

Fig. 2. Theta bust stimulation patterns. A usual TBS contains 3-pulse 50Hz bursts given every 200 ms. When a 2-sec train of TBS is given every 10 sec (iTBS), the cortical excitability is enhanced, while the excitability is suppressed when bursts are given every 200 ms continuously (cTBS) (from Huang, 2010).

More recently, *quadripulse stimulation* (QPS) has been introduced as a patterned rTMS protocol in which repeated trains of four mono-phasic pulses are separated by inter-stimulus intervals of 1.5-1250 ms to produce facilitation (at short intervals) or inhibition (at longer intervals). This protocol appears to induce long-term changes in cortical excitability, probably through a modulatory action on intracortical excitatory circuits (Hamada *et al.*, 2008).

Over the years, many studies have investigated the therapeutic use of rTMS in psychiatric disorders, particularly in depression. For this clinical condition many stimulation paradigms and durations have been trialled. At the end of 2008, the United States Food and Drug Administration (FDA) approved the NeuroStar TMS Therapy System™ for "*the treatment of Major Depressive Disorder in adult patients who have failed to achieve satisfactory improvement from one prior antidepressant medication at or above the minimal effective dose and duration in the current episode*". However, there is still no consensus on the treatment protocols and durations, and the efficacy, tolerability, cost and inconvenience of TMS over electroconvulsive therapy and medication are still debatable (Rasmussen, 2011).

Other clinical conditions in which rTMS has been investigated as a therapeutic tool include amyotrophic lateral sclerosis (ALS), dystonia, migraine and stroke. Studies on ALS patients revealed some promising preliminary data. However, recent studies have demonstrated a lack of significant long-term beneficial effects of rTMS on neurological deterioration in ALS (Dileone *et al.*, 2011).

Both inhibitory (low frequency) and excitatory (high frequency) rTMS over the primary motor cortex (M1) appear to reduce chronic pain. A number of studies have assessed the efficacy of rTMS in patients with drug-resistant chronic pain of various causes and a meta-analysis showed that rTMS was associated with a significant reduction in pain (Lima and Fregni, 2008). Analgesic effects were also shown after stimulation of other cortical areas, such as the prefrontal cortex. However, as the induced effects are relatively short duration, the therapeutic use of rTMS in chronic pain is limited, unless repeated sessions over several weeks are considered (for review see Lefaucheur *et al.*, 2008).

2.2 Transcranial Direct Current Stimulation (tDCS)

Transcranial direct current stimulation (tDCS) is a non-invasive, low-cost and easy-to-use technique that has the potential to modify cortical excitability and behavior in a range of clinical and experimental conditions. Historically, strong electrical currents have been delivered to patients for the relief of headache and epilepsy using torpedo electric fish (Kellaway, 1946). Since the rediscovery of tDCS about 10 years ago, interest in this method has grown significantly.

2.2.1 Basics of tDCS

The constant direct current delivered to the brain in tDCS is caused simply by positioning the two poles of an electric battery-based stimulator to the brain (Nitsche & Paulus, 2000). In order to stimulate the motor cortical region, the stimulating (active) electrode is placed over the motor cortex (M1) and the reference electrode over the contralateral supraorbital ridge or the neck region. More accurate stimulation of a representation within M1, such as the hand area, could be achieved after TMS assessment of the hand area's "hot spot". Two surface conductive rubber electrodes (sized 25 cm^2 - 35 cm^2) attached to the device are usually placed inside sponges soaked in NaCl solution. The sponge-electrodes are then placed and kept on their desired region by a non-conducting rubber band, which is strapped firmly around the subject's head (Figure 3). Current intensities used during sessions vary between 1 mA - 2 mA and are commonly applied for 10 to 20 minutes.

Physical modeling of currently available stimulators suggests that only around 50% of the applied current is actually delivered to the brain tissue. The remaining current is shunted across the scalp following the path of least resistance towards the other electrode (Miranda *et al.*, 2006). However, the portion of the current which does eventually reach the brain can be sufficient in altering neuronal activity (Wagner *et al.*, 2007). The current delivered by tDCS cannot directly generate action potentials in cortical neurons, as the electric field in the brain tissue is not capable of inducing a rapid depolarization (Nitsche *et al.*, 2008). Therefore, tDCS might be considered a neuromodulatory intervention. The electric field modifies the excitability of exposed cells by a tonic depolarization or repolarization of their resting membrane potential by only few millivolts. Evidence that the effects of anodal stimulation

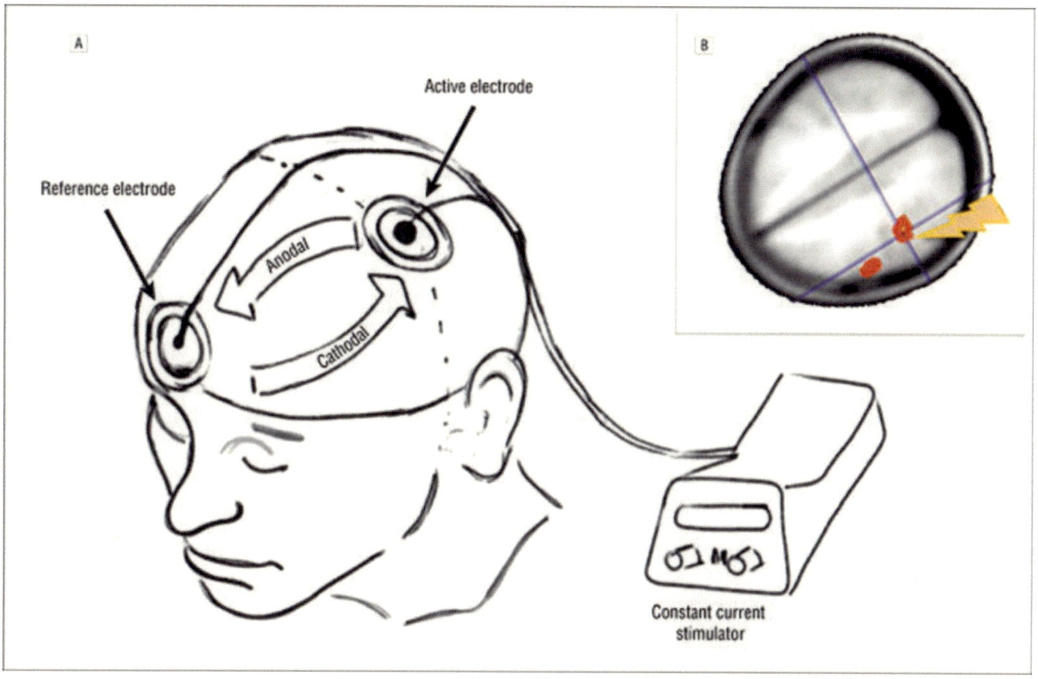

Fig. 3. tDCS setup and montage. (A) The setup using a battery-operated direct current stimulator connected with two electrodes. One electrode (active) is positioned over C3 (corresponding to the precentral gyrus), and the reference electrode is positioned over the contralateral supraorbital region. If current flows from C3 to the supraorbital region, then the tissue underlying C3 is subjected to anodal (increase in excitability) stimulation. If current is reversed, then the tissue underlying C3 is subjected to cathodal (decrease in excitability) stimulation. (B) Regional cerebral blood increases in the motor region underlying the electrode positioned over C3 after anodal stimulation. Regional cerebral blood was determined using a non-invasive arterial spin-labeling technique (from Schlaug *et al.*, 2008).

appear to be solely dependent on changes in membrane potential comes from studies using pharmacological agents. For example, while calcium channel blocker flunarizine reduces and the sodium channel blocker carbamezipine abolishes the effects of anodal stimulation, NMDA receptor antagonist dextromethorphane does not alter current-generated excitability changes (Nitsche *et al.*, 2003a). In terms of the effects of tDCS on cortical interneurons, anodal tDCS does not modify the TMS measures of either glutaminergic interneurons (intracortical facilitation - ICF) or GABAergic interneurons (short-interval cortical inhibition - SICI); suggesting that GABAergic or glutaminergic interneuronal pools are not significantly modulated (Nitsche *et al.*, 2005). During cathodal stimulation, blockade of calcium or sodium channels does not alter the effects of tDCS, suggesting a hyperpolarisation of neurons generated by tDCS itself (Nitsche *et al.*, 2003a). However, ICF and the input/output curve for TMS motor threshold were modulated during cathodal stimulation (Nitsche *et al.*, 2005), suggesting that the membrane potential of glutaminergic interneurones, rather than pyramidal neurons, is modulated by tDCS (for review see Stagg & Nitsche, 2011). Overall, the evidence so far suggests that the modulation observed with tDCS are shaped by a combination of non-synaptic mechanisms, which alter the resting membrane potential of neurons, and synaptic mechanisms, which alter the signaling strength of neurons.

2.2.2 Variables in the application of tDCS

The current density in the tissue is the quotient of current strength and electrode size. Hence, stimulation efficacy can be augmented by either increasing the current strength or reducing the electrode size (Nitsche & Paulus, 2000). Furthermore, the duration of stimulation sessions also affects the strength of the tDCS induced response; longer session durations result in prolonged after-effects (Nitsche & Paulus, 2001; Nitsche *et al.*, 2003b).

The direction of current flow is another parameter that influences the electrical stimulation effects. The population of neurons exposed to the electrical field and the shifts in their membrane potential depend mainly on the positions of the electrodes and their polarity. In tDCS, both positive electrode (anode) and negative electrode (cathode) are used for stimulation. In this circuit the current flows from the cathode to the anode. The positioning of these electrodes on the scalp is important in determining the overall effects elicited in the underlying cortex. For example, during anodal tDCS of the primary motor cortex, the anode is generally placed over the primary motor cortex (M1) and the cathode over the contralateral supraorbital region. In this montage most studies report an increase in the cortico-motor excitability (Nitsche & Paulus, 2001; Jeffery *et al.*, 2007). Conversely, reversing the current flow (cathodal stimulation) generally diminishes the cortical excitability (Ardolino *et al.*, 2005).

In the literature, so far over 100 studies with tDCS in healthy and patient populations have been published; with no serious side effects. At the start of stimulation, most subjects report a slight itching sensation, which then normally fades. It is possible to reduce or avoid this sensation by ramping the current up and down at the beginning and end of session. Poreisz *et al.*, (2007) in a group of 567 subjects, reported most commonly a mild tingling sensation (~70%), moderate fatigue (~35%) and slight itching under the electrode (~30%), and in ≤10% of cases, headache, nausea and insomnia. Other studies, for example evidence of neuronal damage as assessed by serum neuron-specific enolase, MRI measures of edema using contrast-enhanced and diffusion-weighted MRI measures, EEG waveform analyses and neuropsychological measures, reported no evidence of neural damage or brain pathology (for review see Stagg & Nitsche, 2011).

The large size of stimulating electrodes could result in the stimulation of a larger cortical region then intended. Furthermore, as the reference electrode is not physiologically inert because of current flow between electrodes, there might be modulatory effects in remote brain areas. Therefore, other brain regions and structures between electrodes should be taken into consideration during the application of tDCS. Moreover, modulations of cortical excitability can be focused by reducing the size of the stimulating electrode and by increasing the size of the reference electrode (Nitsche *et al.*, 2007). An extracephalic (e.g. neck region) reference could be used to avoid the undesirable effects of two electrodes with opposite polarities over the brain (Nitsche & Paulus, 2000).

As subjects only occasionally experience any sensation related to the stimulation, controlled placebo sessions could be conducted without the need for additional equipment or attachments. During sham stimulation the stimulator can be initially ramped up (around 10 sec), and after a 30 sec period of stimulation it can be slowly turned down (within 10 sec). With this method placebo and real stimulation sessions are indistinguishable (Gandiga *et al.*, 2006). It should be noted that with motor cortex stimulation, strong cognitive effort by the subject unrelated to the stimulated area, as well as strong activation of the stimulated motor cortex by voluntary prolonged muscle contraction abolishes the effects of tDCS (Antal *et al.*, 2007)

2.2.3 Time course and after-effects of tDCS

With short duration (seconds) tDCS, changes in cortical excitability are observed during the stimulation period, but these effects do not outlast the stimulation itself (Nitsche & Paulus, 2000). However, when applied for several minutes longs lasting excitability shifts are produced. For example, around 10 minutes of tDCS can produce stable effects for up to an hour (Nitsche & Paulus, 2001).

The changes in cortical output measures that outlast a tDCS session are dependent on membrane depolarization. The after-effects induced by anodal stimulation could be abolished by calcium or sodium channel blockers or prolonged by NMDA receptor agonists (Nitsche *et al.*, 2003a, 2004). Results from other studies using TMS mediated measures and neuropharmacological applications suggest that the after-effects of anodal tDCS are dependent on modulation of both GABAergic and glutaminergic synapses, and these effects are modulated by acetylcholine, serotonin and catecholamines (for review see Stagg & Nitsche, 2011).

In order to achieve relatively stable changes in cortical function, repeated sessions of tDCS is necessary. For example, recently it was reported that tDCS enhances motor skill acquisition over multiple days through an effect on consolidation (Reis *et al.*, 2009). However, the optimal number and duration of sessions, as well as intersession intervals will depend on the objective of the study or therapeutic application, and requires more research.

2.2.4 Therapeutic applications of tDCS

tDCS has been shown to have beneficial effects in a wide range of clinical pathologies; such as refractory epilepsy (Fregni *et al.*, 2006), stroke (Fregni *et al.*, 2005; Hummel *et al.*, 2005) and various pain conditions (for review see O'Connell *et al.*, 2011), as well as psychiatric conditions, like depression and addiction (Arul-Anandam & Loo 2009; Utz *et al.*, 2010). However, the measurable effects induced in a single session are usually short lived. With repeated session tDCS, growing number of clinical trials is reporting long-term benefits, in particular for depression. For example, in a recent double-blind clinical trial with 40 patients with major depression, significantly large reductions in depression scores were reported after dorsolateral prefrontal cortex (DLPFC) anodal tDCS applied for 10 sessions during a 2-week period (Boggio *et al.*, 2008). These results suggest promising potential for tDCS as an antidepressant treatment.

3. Use of non-invasive brain stimulation in stroke

Following stroke, the neuroplastic changes within the brain lead to reorganization that is attributable to spontaneous recovery of function. Possible mechanisms of such reorganization include; axonal and/or dendritic regeneration or sprouting, reorganization within the lesioned cortical region by means of synaptic modulation, and remapping of functional representations from the lesioned region onto neighboring unaffected areas surrounding the lesion or homologous areas within the unaffected hemisphere.

During local ischemia various cytotoxic and metabolic reactions result in the loss of structural and functional integrity of neural tissue (Schallert *et al.*, 2000). However, early repair mechanisms, such as expression of developmental proteins and other substrates of molecular plasticity, as well as structural changes, such as regeneration and sprouting, modulation of synaptic plasticity, changes in cortical excitability due to neurotransmitter alterations take place locally and in remote areas of the brain (Witte & Stoll 1997). There is increasing evidence that suggests functional reorganization in both hemispheres. Functional magnetic resonance imaging (fMRI) studies reveal bilateral activation in recovered stroke patients (Gerloff *et al.*, 2006; Nair *et al.*, 2007).

A network of cortical and subcortical areas constitutes the motor system. The final motor output is determined by complex interactions between multiple excitatory and inhibitory circuits within and between these areas. After stroke, the balance in this system could be vitally disturbed as a result of damage to neurons or their fibers within the white matter which connects these areas. For example, in recovered stroke cases, magnetic stimulation over the dorsal premotor cortex, the superior parietal lobe, as well as the primary motor cortex results in significant interference with recovered finger movement performance (Lotze *et al.*, 2006). Furthermore, experimental results using TMS in stroke patients suggest that the motor output from the lesioned hemisphere could be further reduced by pathologically enhanced inhibitory influences from the intact hemisphere (Murase *et al.*, 2004; Duque *et al.*, 2005; Hummel & Cohen, 2006). Although the exact mechanism of this interhemispheric interaction is still unclear, the possibility that suppressing the inhibitory influences exerted by the intact hemisphere could improve recovery has gained interest in recent years.

As stated earlier, depending on the stimulation parameters, cortical excitability can be reduced (inhibition) or enhanced (facilitation). Therefore, non-invasive brain stimulation could accelerate, facilitate or potentiate the functional recovery process and provide better rehabilitation outcomes. TMS and tDCS are the most extensively researched methods in stroke recovery and rehabilitation (for review see Nowak *et al.*, 2010). These techniques not only cause a local change in cortical excitability, but can also evoke changes within remote parts of the cortical motor system, hence improve recovery after stroke (Nowak *et al.*, 2008; Ameli *et al.*, 2009; Grefkes *et al.*, 2010).

3.1 Application of TMS in stroke

In the last decade a number of studies using rTMS in stroke patients have been conducted. These include, single session interventions, in which patients are assessed before and after rTMS and longer term treatment strategies in which patients are given daily sessions of rTMS for up to two weeks. In multiple session interventions rTMS is usually combined with conventional physical therapy to assess and compare the benefits of rTMS in rehabilitation (for review see Khedr & Abo-El Fetoh, 2010; Nowak *et al.*, 2010). Majority of these studies have been conducted in chronic stroke patients whose baseline performance is likely to be stable, compared to acute and subacute stroke cases.

So far, there have been over twenty clinical studies conducted using low or high frequency simple rTMS, or theta-burst stimulation (TBS) of the lesioned or intact hemisphere in acute or chronic patients (for review see Khedr & Abo-El Fetoh, 2010). For example, Koganemaru *et al.*, (2010) used 5 Hz rTMS of the upper-limb area of the primary motor cortex, combined with extensor motor training, and suggested that combining motor training with rTMS can facilitate use-dependent plasticity and achieve functional recovery of motor impairments that cannot be accomplished by either intervention alone. Overall, rTMS gives a 10-30% improvement over sham in a range of performance measures, from simple reaction times to timed behavioral tests. In addition, the effects of multiple session intervention tend to be similar in size but longer lasting than those seen in single session trials.

Even more complex intervention protocols, by stimulating multiple target areas have been trialed. For example, in a group of thirty chronic stroke patients, comparison of unilateral and bilateral rTMS (1 Hz over intact hemisphere and 10 Hz over affected hemisphere) revealed improved motor training effect on the paretic hand after bilateral rTMS (Takeuchi *et al.*, 2008).

Although still relatively few, there are studies conducted to investigate the possible benefits of rTMS in other disabilities associated with stroke; such as, dysphagia, aphasia and hemispatial neglect. The underlying concept of rTMS treatment is based on "upregulating" the lesioned hemisphere or "downregulating" the intact hemisphere (for review see Platz & Rothwell, 2010). Altered connectivity within the cortex as a result of stroke influences the modulatory effects of afferent inputs (Tarlaci *et al.*, 2010). Therefore, combining TMS intervention with afferent inputs, such as vibrotactile stimuli could also be effective.

Overall, the application of rTMS as a therapeutic tool is still in its infancy. According to available evidence, cortical magnetic stimulation could be an effective method for improving functional recovery of acute and chronic stroke. Table 1 summarizes the studies undertaken using rTMS. Although the majority of results report improvements in various behavioral functions, the overall methodology remains to be optimized, in particular regarding the number and duration of rTMS sessions, the site, frequency and intensity of stimulation and the exact timing of rTMS application after stroke

3.2 Application of tDCS in stroke

Human studies using electrical brain stimulation can be divided into invasive and non-invasive. The invasive method principally involves implantation of epidural electrodes through a small craniotomy around a "hot spot" within the perilesional area determined by fMRI. Cortical stimulation is then applied together with physical therapy. Initial cortical stimulation feasibility studies in combination with a motor rehabilitation training targeting the affected arm and hand reported significant improvements compared to control patients receiving only rehabilitation (Brown *et al.*, 2006; Levy *et al.*, 2008). However, in a subsequent larger, multi-center study (Everest Clinical Trial) involving 174 chronic stroke patients (implant and control groups) who underwent six weeks of upper limb rehabilitation, the outcome measures did not meet its primary efficiency end-point at 4-week follow-up, with improvement of 30% in both implant and control groups (Harvey & Winstein, 2009). It is clear that more basic and clinical research into the efficacy of invasive cortical electrical stimulation is needed.

Study	Stimulation Side	Lesion location	Time of stroke	Stimulus	Behavioral results on affected hand
Khedr et al., 2005	IL	26 cortical, 26 subcortical	acute	3 Hz, 10 daily stimulation sessions	Improved hand function (Scandinavian Stroke Scale, National Institute of Health Stroke Scale Scale, Barthel index)
Mansur et al., 2005	CL	10 subcortical	subacute, chronic	1 Hz	Shortened simple and choice reaction times, improvement of hand function (Purdue Pegboard Test)
Takeuchi et al., 2005	CL	20 subcortical	chronic	1 Hz	Improved peak pinch acceleration
Boggio et al., 2006	CL	one subcortical	chronic	1 Hz	Improved hand function (clinical testing), no change in spasticity (modified Ashworth scale for spasticity)
Fregni et al., 2006	CL	2 cortical, 13 subcortical	chronic	1Hz , 5 daily stimulation sessions	Shortening of simple and choice reaction times, improvement of hand function (Jebsen-Taylor Hand Function Test, Purdue Pegboard Test)
Kim et al., 2006	IL	5 cortical, 10 subcortical	chronic	10 Hz	Improved movement accuracy and movement time (sequential finger movement task)

Study	Stimulation Side	Lesion location	Time of stroke	Stimulus	Behavioral results on affected hand
Malcom et al., 2007	IL	11 cortical, 8 subcortical	chronic	20 Hz, followed by constraint induced movement therapy, 10 daily stimulation sessions	Improved hand function (Wolf Motor Function Test, Motor Activity Log) after constraint induced movement therapy, no additive effect of rTMS
Talelli et al., 2007	CL	3 cortical, 3 subcortical	chronic	continuous theta burst stimulation	No change in acceleration and amount of peak grip force
Talelli et al., 2007	IL	3 cortical, 3 subcortical	chronic	intermittent theta burst stimulation	Improved movement speed, no effect on peak grip force
Nowak et al., 2008	CL	15 subcortical	subacute	1 Hz	Improved grasping movements (kinematic motion analysis)
Takeuchi et al., 2008	CL	20 subcortical	chronic	1 Hz, stimulation session with metronome-paced pinching between index finger and thumb	Improved of pinch acceleration and peak pinch force
Dafotakis et al., 2008	CL	12 subcortical	subacute, chronic	1 Hz	Improved timing and efficiency of grasping (kinctic motion analysis)
Liepert et al., 2007	CL	12 subcortical	acute	1 Hz	No change in peak grip force, improved hand function (Nine Hole Peg Test)

Study	Stimulation Side	Lesion location	Time of stroke	Stimulus	Behavioral results on affected hand
Kirton et al., 2008	CL	10 children with subcortical stroke	chronic	1 Hz, 8 daily stimulation sessions	Improved hand function (Melbourne assessment of upper extremity function)
Carey et al., 2009	CL	1 subcortical, 1 cortical	chronic	1 Hz primed by 6Hz	Improved hand function (clinical testing)
Carey et al., 2009	CL	10 cortical	chronic	1 Hz primed by 6Hz	No change in hand function (clinical testing); transiently deteriorated verbal learning (Hopkins Verbal Learning Test-Revised)
Khedr et al., 2009	IL	48 subcortical and cortical	acute	3 Hz or 10 Hz, 5 daily stimulation sessions	Improved hand function 1,2,3 and 12 months after rTMS
Yozbatiran et al., 2009	IL	No detailed information	subacute, chronic	20 Hz	Improved grip strength, improved hand function (Nine hole peg test)
Koganemaru et al., 2010	IL	9 subcortical	chronic	5 Hz	Better improvement of extensor movement when rTMS is combined with extensor motor training
Grefkes et al., 2010	CL	11 subcortical	subacute	1 Hz	Improved hand function supported by fMRI

Table 1. A summary of studies and their outcomes conducted with rTMS in stroke patients IL: ipsilesional, CL: contralesional. Time of stroke after symptom onset; acute: < 1month, subacute 1-6 months, chronic > 6 months (modified from Nowak *et al.*, 2010).

Introduction of tDCS as a research tool a decade ago also attracted attention for its clinical application in stroke. tDCS would have advantages over direct cortical stimulation by stimulating a wider region of brain involving not only the primary motor cortex but also premotor, supplementary motor and somatosensory areas, all of which have been

Study	Stimulation side	Lesion location	Time of stroke	Stimulus	Behavioral results on affected hand
Fregni et al., 2005	IL	2 cortical, 4 subcortical	chronic	anodal	Improved hand function (Jebsen-Taylor Hand Function Test)
Fregni et al., 2005	CL	3 cortical, 3 subcortical	chronic	cathodal	Improved hand function (Jebsen-Taylor Hand Function Test)
Hummel and Cohen., 2005	IL	1 subcortical	chronic	anodal	Improved hand function (Jebsen-Taylor Hand Function Test, peak pinch force), shortened simple reaction times
Hummel et al., 2005	IL	1 cortical, 5 subcortical	chronic	anodal	Improved hand function (Jebsen-Taylor Hand Function Test)
Hummel et al., 2006	IL	No detailed information	chronic	anodal	Shortened simple reaction time, increased peak pinch force
Boggio et al., 2007	IL	1 subcortical	chronic	anodal	Improved hand function (Jebsen-Taylor Hand Function Test)
Boggio et al., 2007	CL	9 subcortical	chronic	cathodal, 5 daily stimulation sessions	Improved hand function (Jebsen-Taylor Hand Function Test)
Hesse et al., 2007	IL	8 cortical, 2 subcortical	acute, subacute	anodal, followed by robotassisted arm training, 6 daily stimulation sessions	Improved hand function (Jebsen-Taylor Hand Function Test, Medical Research Council score)
Celnik et al., 2009	IL	9 cortical and subcortical	chronic	anodal, followed by peripheral nerve stimulation to the affected hand and a key pressing task	Improved key pressing task performance
Lindenberg et al., 2010	IL	20 cortical and subcortical	chronic	bihemispheric (anodal on IL, cathodal on CL)	Improved key pressing task performance

Table 2. A summary of studies and their outcomes conducted with tDCS in stroke patients IL: ipsilesional, CL: contralesional. Time of stroke after symptom onset; acute: < 1month, subacute 1-6 months, chronic > 6 months (modified from Nowak *et al.*, 2010).

implicated in the recovery process (Nair *et al.*, 2007). Furthermore, as a non-invasive technique, tDCS is less risky, portable and flexible in its montage parameters. Studies investigating the effects of anodal tDCS of the lesioned hemisphere on rehabilitation measures suggest limited benefits of this intervention. For example, Hummel *et al.* (2005, 2006) reported beneficial effects of anodal tDCS on reaction times and a set of hand functions that mimic activities of daily living in the paretic hand of patients with chronic stroke. However, in a study involving robot-assisted arm training during anodal tDCS of ten stroke patients, the arm function of only three patients improved significantly (Hesse *et al.*, 2007). Based on the concept of modulation of corticomotor excitability by peripheral sensory inputs (Kaelin-Lang *et al.*, 2002), Celnik *et al.*, (2009) investigated the effects of tDCS and peripheral nerve stimulation (PNS) on motor training in chronic stroke patients and reported a significant facilitatory effect of combing tDCS with PNS compared with each intervention alone.

In recent years, most clinical studies have been designed with the concept of interhemispheric competition. Hence, abnormal interhemispheric inhibition is the hypothetical model for these experimental therapies. It is possible to modulate cortical excitability within motor areas of the lesioned and intact hemispheres by means of tDCS, as well as rTMS. These modulatory influences may induce synaptic plasticity and/or interfere with maladaptive processes that could develop after stroke. Although still limited, studies so far with cathodal stimulation of the intact hemisphere and/or anodal stimulation of the lesioned hemisphere suggest improvements in hand function (Fregni *et al.*, 2005; Boggio *et al.*, 2007; Lindenberg *et al.*, 2010).

In summary, research on the efficacy of tDCS as a therapeutic intervention is well underway. Table 2 summarizes the cases, stimulation protocols and outcomes of tDCS studies in stroke patients. It is clear that more clinical data are required to establish efficient protocols, including the optimal stimulation locations, dose, duration and frequency of treatment.

4. Controversies

In a recent review, the key opinion leaders in the area of brain stimulation identified and addressed the controversial aspects of "therapeutic" cortical stimulation in stroke (Hummel *et al.*, 2008). These controversies include the following:

1. *Mechanism of effect*: Increased cortical excitability with brain stimulation suggests plastic changes in glutaminergic and GABAergic intracortical networks, resembling the mechanism of LTP-like changes at the cellular level. However, these assumptions are indirect and have not been proven directly. With regards to inhibitory stimulation of the intact hemisphere to suppress transcallosal inhibition, clinical reports are encouraging, but still there are relatively few studies and the exact neuronal mechanism of this interhemispheric interaction is not clear.
2. *Site of stimulation*: There is evidence of beneficial clinical outcomes from stimulation of the lesioned, as well as the intact hemisphere. Although theoretically susceptibility to seizures with lesioned hemisphere stimulation is possible, so far no such incident has been reported. Other possible adverse effects include the excitotoxicity and metabolic changes in the vicinity of the lesion due to induced hyperexcitability and the current

shunting effects of the scar tissue within brain. In this regard, targeting the intact rather than the lesioned hemisphere as the site of stimulation could have advantages. However, if post-stroke reorganizational changes leading to functional recovery are, at least in part, due to inputs originating from the intact hemisphere, reducing the activity of this region with excitability-decreasing stimulation could have unintended consequences and lead to impaired performance of the paretic hand (Lotze *et al.*, 2006). Interaction between multiple cortical areas, such as premotor and supplementary areas, and the posterior parietal cortex during motor performance makes these regions a possible target for up-regulation or down-regulation during stroke recovery. However, our understanding of the role and interaction of these areas is still limited, and more basic research is necessary.

3. *Type of stimulation and its parameters*: Although epidural electrical stimulation has advantages over non-invasive methods due to its proximity to the cortical tissue, still more patient data is needed to establish its benefits. In terms of practical use, tDCS is advantageous over TMS because it is safer, easier to apply, portable and well-tolerated by patients. It is also a cheaper option as a device. However, technological advances and expending markets will certainly lead to cheaper and more portable magnetic stimulators in the near future.

   Currently, most stimulation parameters for stroke patients are based on the effectiveness of polarity, electrode/coil size, stimulus amplitude, frequency, duration, and session repetition and interval reported in previous studies, in particular in healthy subjects. As more data become available on the efficacy of clinical studies using different parameters, eventually consensus on this controversy will be reached.
4. *Combining stimulation techniques*: Studies so far indicate that stimulation alone might not produce significant improvement in motor function. If combined with other interventional techniques, such as peripheral nerve stimulation (Celnik *et al.*, 2009), better outcomes could be achieved. However, studies that combined brain stimulation with constrained-induced movement therapy (Malcolm *et al.*, 2007) or robot-aided training (Hesse *et al.*, 2007) failed to show clear additive effects. Clearly, more clinical studies are needed in order to determine which combinations could produce better clinical outcomes of motor function.
5. *Commencement of stimulation*: As mentioned earlier, most clinical studies are conducted on chronic stroke patients (>6 months). Although in the chronic stage the deficits are stable and it is easier to assess motor function, within the brain the scar tissue has already formed and natural reorganizational changes have occurred. On the other hand, interference during the acute stage when there is NMDA-induced calcium influx, which might be involved in neuronal toxicity, could result in unintended changes in the brain. Several studies report dynamic changes in neural activation patterns within both lesioned and intact hemispheres during the functional recovery process (for review see Hummel *et al.*, 2008). Therefore, as we better understand the exact mechanisms of post-stroke reorganization, it will be easier to determine the optimal commencement times for intervention by non-invasive brain stimulation. There are a number of variable factors that can influence the magnitude and direction of plastic changes induced during and after non-invasive brain stimulation. These include; age, sex, genetic profile, regular daily activity level, attention, use of neuropharmacological drugs and time of

day (for review see Ridding & Ziemann, 2010). Future therapeutic application of brain stimulation will most likely be part of personalized medicine which takes into account all these variable factors.

6. *Effect size*: Reports so far on the effectiveness of brain stimulation on various motor tasks indicate an improvement of only 10-30% over placebo (for review see Khedr & Abo-El Fetoh, 2010). The transient nature of these improvements is also a shortcoming and raises the question that if these outcomes are obvious improvements to daily activities of patients. As the controversies outlined above are resolved in time, the effect size of clinical measures will also improve and produce accepted meaningful functional improvements after stroke.

5. Conclusion

In the last two decades, non-invasive brain stimulation techniques have been increasingly employed as a therapeutic tool in the rehabilitation of stroke patients. However, these methods are still experimental and there are many questions and unknowns to be addressed before agreed intervention prescriptions are determined for optimal and desired outcomes. In conclusion, non-invasive brain stimulation techniques are novel and promising but still in their infancy as universally accepted clinical tools.

6. References

Amarenco, P., Bogousslavsky, J., Caplan, L.R., Donnan, G.A. & Hennerici, M.G. (2009). Classification of stroke subtypes. *Cerebrovasc Dis.* 27, 493-501.

Ameli, M., Grefkes, C., Kemper, F., Riegg, F.P., Rehme, A.K., Karbe, H., Fink, G.R. & Nowak, D.A. (2009). Differential effects f high-frequency repetitive transcranial magnetic stimulation over ipsilesional primary motor cortex in cortical and subcortical middle cerebral artery stroke. *Ann Neurol.* 66, 298-309.

Antal, A., Terney, D., Poreisz, C. & Paulus, W. (2007). Towards unravelling task- related modulations of neuroplastic changes induced in the human motor cortex. *Eur J Neurosci.* 26, 2687-2691.

Ardolino, G., Bossi, B., Barbieri, S. & Priori, A. (2005). Non-synaptic mechanisms underlie the after-effects of cathodal transcutaneous direct current stimulation of the human brain. *J Physiol.* 568, 653-663.

Arul-Anandam, A. & Loo, C. (2009). Transcranial direct current stimulation: A new tool for the treatment of depression? *J Affective Disorders.* 117, 137-145.

Attarian, S., Verschueren, A. & Pouget, J. (2007). Magnetic stimulation including the triple-stimulation technique in amyotrophic lateral sclerosis. *Muscle Nerve.* 36, 55-61.

Barker, A., Jalinous, R. & Freeston, I. (1985). Non-invasive magnetic stimulation of human motor cortex, *Lancet,* 1(8437), 1106-1107.

Boggio, P.S., Nunes, A., Rigonatti, S.P., Nitsche, M.A., Pascual-Leone, A., & Fregni, F. (2007). Repeated sessions of noninvasive brain DC stimulation is associated with motor function improvement in stroke patients. *Restor Neurol Neurosci.* 25, 123-129.

Boggio, P.S., Rigonatti, S.P., Ribeiro, R.B., Myczkowski, M.L., Nitsche, M.A., Pascual-Leone, A., & Fregni, F. (2008). A randomized, double-blind clinical trial on the efficacy of cortical direct current stimulation for the treatment of major depression. *Int J Neuropsychopharmacol.* 11, 249–254.

Brown, J.A., Lutsep, H.L., Weinand, M. & Cramer, S.C. (2006). Motor cortex stimulation for the enhancement of recovery from stroke: a prospective, multicenter safety study. *Neurosurgery*. 58, 464-473.

Celnik, P., Paik, N.J., Vandermeeren, Y., Dimyan, M. &Cohen, LG. (2009). Effects of combined peripheral nerve stimulation and brain polarization on performance of a motor sequence task after chronic stroke. *Stroke*. 40, 1764-1771.

Chen, R., Cros, D., Curra, A., Di Lazzaro, V., Lefaucheur, J., Magistris, M.R., Mills, K., Rösler, K.M., Triggs, W.J., Ugawa, Y. & Ziemann, U. (2008). The clinical diagnostic utility of transcranial magnetic stimulation: Report of an IFCN committee. *Clin Neurophysiol*. 119, 504-532.

Chowdhury, S.A. & Matsunami, K.I. (2002). GABA-B-related activity in processing of transcallosal response in cat motor cortex. *J Neurosci Res*. 68, 489-495.

Cruz–Martínez, A., González-Orodea, J.I., López Pajares, R. & Arpa, J. (2000). Disability in multiple sclerosis. The role of transcranial magnetic stimulation. *Electromyogr Clin Neurophysiol*. 40, 441-447.

Daskalakis, Z.J., Christensen, B.K., Fitzgerald, P.B., Roshan, L. & Chen, R. (2002). The mechanisms of interhemispheric inhibition in the human motor cortex. *J Physiol* 543, 317–326.

Dileone, M., Profice, P., Pilato, F., Ranieri, F., Capone, F., Musumeci, G., Florio, L., Di Iorio, R. & Di Lazzaro, V. (2011). Repetitive transcranial magnetic stimulation for ALS. *CNS & Neurological Disorders Drug Targets*. 9, 331-334.

Duque, J., Hummel, F., Celnik, P., Murase, N., Mazzocchio, R. & Cohen L.G. (2005). Transcallosal inhibition in chronic subcortical stroke. Neuroimage. 28, 940 –946.

Ferbert, A., Priori, A., Rothwell, J.C., Day, B.L., Colebatch, J.G. & Marsden, C.D. (1992). Interhemispheric inhibition of the human motor cortex. *J Physiol* 453, 525–546.

Fregni, F., Boggio, P., Mansur, C., Wagner, T., Ferreira, M., Lima, M., Rigonatti, S.P., Marcolin, M.A., Freedman, S.D., Nitshe, M.A. & Pascual-Leone, A. (2005). Transcranial direct current stimulation of the unaffected hemisphere in stroke patients. *Neuroreport*. 16, 1551–1555.

Fregni, F., Thome-Souza, S., Nitsche, M.A., Freedman, S.D., Valente, K.D., Pascual-Leone, A. (2006). A controlled clinical trial of cathodal DC polarization in patients with refractory epilepsy. *Epilepsia*. 47, 335–42.

Fyre, R., Rotenberg, A., Ousley, M. & Pascual-Leone, A. (2008). Transcranial magnetic stimulation in child neurology. *J Child Neurol*. 23, 79-96.

Gandiga, P.C., Hummel, F.C. & Cohen, L.G. (2006). Transcranial DC stimulation (tDCS): a tool for double-blind sham-controlled clinical studies in brain stimulation. *Clin Neurophysiol*. 117, 845-850.

Gerloff, C., Bushara, K., Sailer, A., Wassermann, E.M., Chen, R., Matsuoka, T., Waldvogel, D., Wittenberg, G.F., Ishii, K., Cohen, L.G. & Hallett, M. (2006). Multimodal imaging of brain reorganization in motor areas of the contralesional hemisphere of well recovered patients after capsular stroke. *Brain*. 129, 791-808.

Grefkes, C., Nowak, D.A., Wang, L.E., Dafotakis, M., Eickhoff, S.B. & Fink, G.R. (2010). Modulating cortical connectivity in stroke patients by rTMS assessed with fMRI and dynamic causal modeling. *Neuroimage*. 50, 233-242.

Hamada, M., Terao, Y. Hanajima, R., Shirota, Y., Nakatani-Enomoto, S., Furubayashi, T., Matsumoto, H. & Ugawa, Y. (2008). Bidirectional long-term motor cortical plasticity and metaplasticity induced by quadripulse transcranial magnetic stimulation. *J Physiol.* 586, 3927-3947.

Hanajima, R., Ugawa, Y., Machii, K., Mochizuki, H., Terao, Y., Enomoto, H., Furubayashi, T., Shiio, Y., Uesugi, H. & Kanazawa, I. (2001). Interhemispheric facilitation of the hand motor area in humans. *J Physiol.* 531, 849–859.

Harvey, R.L. & Winstein, C.J. (2009) Everest Trial Group. Design for the Everest randomized trial of cortical stimulation and rehabilitation for arm function following stroke. *Neurorehabil Neural Repair.* 23, 32-44.

Hayward, G., Mehta, M.A., Harmer, C., Spinks, T.J., Grasby, P.M. & Goodwin, G.M. (2007). Exploring the physiological effects of double-cone coil TMS over the medial frontal cortex on the anterior cingulate cortex: an H2(15)O PET study. *Eur J Neurosci.* 25, 2224-2233.

Hesse, S., Werner, C., Schonhardt, E.M., Bardeleben, A., Jenrich, W. & Kirker, S.G. (2007). Combined transcranial direct current stimulation and robot-assisted arm training in subacute stroke patients: a pilot study. *Restor Neurol Neurosci.* 25, 9-15.

Hoogendam, J.M., Ramakers, G.M. & Di Lazzaro V. (2010). Physiology of repetitive transcranial magnetic stimulation of the human brain. *Brain Stimul.* 3, 95-118.

Howard, G., Howard, V.J., Katholi, C., Oli, M.K. & Huston, S. (2001). Decline in USstroke mortality: an analysis of temporal patterns by sex, race, and geographic region. *Stroke.* 32, 2213- 2220

Huang, Y. & Rothwell, J. (2004). The effect of short duration bursts of high frequency, low intensity transcranial magnetic stimulation on the human motor cortex. *Clin Neurophysiol.* 115, 1069-1075.

Huang, Y. (2010). The modulation of cortical motor circuits and spinal reflexes using theta burst stimulation in healthy and dystonic subjects. *Restor Neurol Neurosci.* 28, 449-457.

Huang, Y., Edwards, M., Rounis, E., Bhatia, K. & Rothwell, J. (2005). Theta burst stimulation of the human motor cortex. *Neuron.* 45, 201-206.

Hummel, F.C. & Cohen, L.G. (2006). Non-invasive brain stimulation: a new strategy to improve neurorehabilitation after stroke? *Lancet Neurol.* 5, 708 –712.

Hummel, F., Celnik, P., Giraux, P., Floel, A., Wu, W., Gerloff, C., & Cohen, L.G. (2005). Effects of non-invasive cortical stimulation on skilled motor function in chronic stroke. *Brain.* 128, 490–499.

Hummel, F.C., Celnik, P., Pascual-Leone, A., Fregni, F., Byblow, W.D., Buetefisch, C.M., Rothwell, J., Cohen, L.G. & Gerloff, C. (2008). Controversy: Noninvasive and invasive cortical stimulation show efficacy in treating stroke patients. *Brain Stimul.* 1, 370–382.

Hummel, F.C., Voller, B., Celnik, P., Floel, A., Giraux, P., Gerloff, C. & Cohen, L.G. (2006). Effects of brain polarization on reaction times and pinch force in chronic stroke. *BMC Neuroscience.* 7, 73.

Jeffery, D.T., Norton, J.A., Roy, F.D. & Gorassini, M.A. (2007). Effects of transcranial direct current stimulation on the excitability of the leg motor cortex. *Exp Brain Res.* 182, 281–287.

Kaelin-Lang, A., Luft, A.R., Sawaki, L., Burstein, A.H., Sohn, Y.H. & Cohen, L.G. (2002). Modulation of human corticomotor excitability by somatosensory input. *J Physiol.* 540, 623–633.

Karandreas, N., Papadopoulou, M., Kokotis, P., Papapostolou, A., Tsivgoulis & G., Zambelis, T. (2007). Impaired interhemispheric inhibition in amyotrophic lateral sclerosis. *Amyotroph Lateral Scler*. 8, 112-118.

Kellaway, P. (1946). The part played by electric fish in the early history of bioelectricity and electrotherapy. *Bull Hist Med*. 20, 112–37.

Khedr, E.M. & Abo-El Fetoh, N. (2010). Short- and long-term effect of rTMS on motor function recovery after ischemic stroke. *Restor Neurol Neurosci*. 28, 545-559.

Koganemaru, S., Mima, T., Thabit, M.N., Ikkaku, T., Shimada, K., Kanematsu, M., Takahashi, K., Fawi, G., Takahashi, R., Fukuyama, H. & Domen, K. (2010). Recovery of upper-limb function due to enhanced use-dependent plasticity in chronic stroke patients. *Brain*. 133, 3373-3384.

Kolominsky-Rabas, P.L.,Weber, M., Gefeller, O., Neundörfer, B.& Heuschmann, P.U. (2001). Epidemiology of ischemic stroke subtypes according to the TOAST criteria: incidence, recurrence, and long-term survival in ischemic stroke subtypes: a population-based study. *Stroke*. 32, 2735-2740.

Kujirai, T., Caramia, M.D., Rothwell, J.C., Day, B.L., Thompson, P.D., Ferbert, A., Wroe, S., Asselman, P. & Marsden, C.D. (1993). Corticocortical inhibition in human motor cortex. *J Physiol*. 471, 501-519.

Kwakkel, G., Kollen, B.J. & Wagenaar RC. (2002). Long-term effects of intensity of upper and lower limb training following stroke: a randomised trial. *J Neurol Neurosurg Psychiatry*. 72, 473-479.

Lefaucheur, J.P., Antal, A., Ahdab, R., de Andrade, D.C., Fregni, F., Khedr, E.M., Nitsche, M. and Paulus, W. (2008). The use of repetitive transcranial magnetic stimulation (rTMS) and transcranial direct current stimulation (tDCS) to relieve pain. *Brain Stimul*. 1, 337–344.

Levy, R., Ruland, S., Weinand, M., Lowry, D., Dafer, R. & Bakay, R. (2008). Cortical stimulation for the rehabilitation of patients with hemiparetic stroke: a multicenter feasibility study of safety and efficacy. *J Neurosurg*. 108, 707-714.

Lima, M.C. & Fregni, F. (2008). Motor cortex stimulation for chronic pain: systemic review and meta-analysis of the literatura. *Neurology*. 70, 2329-2337.

Lindenberg, R. Renga, V. Zhu, L.L. Nair, D. & Schlaug, G. (2010). Bihemispheric brain stimulation facilitates motor recovery in chronic stroke patients. *Neurology*. 75, 2176-2184.

Lotze, M., Markert, J., Sauseng, P., Hoppe, J., Plewnia, C. & Gerloff, C. (2006). The role of multiple contralesional motor areas for complex hand movements after internal capsular lesion. *J Neurosci*. 26, 6096-6102.

Malcolm, M.P., Triggs, W.J., Light, K.E., Gonzalez Rothi, L.J., Wu, S., Reid, K. & Nadeau, S.E. (2007). Repetitive transcranial magnetic stimulation as an adjunct to constraint-induced therapy: an exploratory randomized controlled trial. *Am J Phys Med Rehabil*. 86, 707–715.

Magistris, M.R., Rösler, K.M., Truffert, A., Landis, T. & Hess, C.W. (1999). A clinical study of motor evoked potentials using a triple stimulation technique. *Brain*. 122, 265-279.

Maulden, S.A., Gassaway, J., Horn, S.D., Smout, R.J. & DeJong, G. (2005). Timing of initiation of rehabilitation after stroke. *Arch Phys Med Rehabil*. 86. S34-S40.

Merton, P. & Morton, H. (1980). Stimulation of the cerebral cortex in the intact human subject. *Nature*, 285, 227.

Miranda, P.C., Lomarev, M. & Hallett, M. (2006). Modeling the current distribution during transcranial direct current stimulation. *Clin Neurophysiol.* 117, 1623–1639.

Morley, J. W., Vickery, R.M., Stuart, M. & Turman A.B. (2007). Suppression of vibrotactile discrimination by transcranial magnetic stimulation of primary somatosensory cortex. *Eur J Neurosci.* 26, 1007-1010.

Murase, N., Duque, J., Mazzocchio, R. & Cohen L.G. (2004). Influence of interhemispheric interactions on motor function in chronic stroke. *Ann Neurol.* 55, 400–409.

Nair, D.G., Hutchinson, S., Fregni, F., Alexander, M., Pascual-Leone, A. & Schlaug, G. (2007). Imaging correlates of motor recovery from cerebral infarction and their physiological significance in well-recovered patients. *Neuroimage.*34, 253-263.

Nitsche, M. & Paulus, W. (2000). Excitability changes induced in the human motor cortex by weak transcranial direct current stimulation. *J Physiol.* 527, 633–639.

Nitsche, M. & Paulus, W. (2001). Sustained excitability elevations induced by transcranial DC motor cortex stimulation in humans. *Neurology.* 57, 1899–1901.

Nitsche, M., Cohen, L.G., Wassermann, E., Priori, A., Lang, N., Antal, A., Paulus, W., Hummel, F., Boggio, P.S., Fregni, F. & Pascual-Leone, A. (2008). Transcranial direct current stimulation: state of the art 2008. *Brain Stimul.* 1, 206–223.

Nitsche, M.A., Doemkes, S., Karaköse, T., Antal, A., Liebetanz, D., Lang, N., Tergau, F. & Paulus, W. (2007). Shaping the effects of transcranial direct current stimulation of the human motor cortex. *J Neurophysiol.* 97, 3109-3117.

Nitsche, M.A., Fricke, K., Henschke, U., Schlitterlau, A., Liebetanz, D., Lang, N., Henning, S., Tergau, F. & Paulus, W. (2003a). Pharmacological modulation of cortical excitability shifts induced by transcranial direct current stimulation in humans. *J Physiol.* 553, 293–301.

Nitsche, M.A., Jaussi, W., Liebetanz, D., Lang, N., Tergau, F. &, Paulus, W. (2004). Consolidation of human motor cortical neuroplasticity by D-cycloserine. *Neuropsychopharmacology.* 29, 1573–1578.

Nitsche, M.A., Schauenburg, A., Lang, N., Liebetanz, D., Exner, C., Paulus, W. & Tergau, F. (2003b). Facilitation of implicit motor learning by weak transcranial direct current stimulation of the primary motor cortex in the human. *J Cogn Neurosci.* 15, 619–626.

Nitsche, M.A., Seeber, A., Frommann, K., Klein, C.C., Nitsche, M.S., Rochford, C., Liebetanz, D., Lang, N., Antal, A., Paulus, W. & Tergau F. (2005). Modulating parameters of excitability during and after transcranial direct current stimulation of the human motor cortex. *J Physiol.* 568, 291–303.

Nowak, D.A., Bösl, K., Podubeckà, J. & Carey, J.R. (2010). Noninvasive brain stimulation and motor recovery after stroke. *Restor Neurol Neurosci.* 28, 531-544.

Nowak, D.A., Grefkes, C., Dafotakis, M., Eickhoff, S., Küst, J., Karbe, H. & Fink, G.R. (2008). Effects of low-frequency repetitive transcranial magnetic stimulation of the contralesional primary motor cortex on movement kinematics and neural activity in subcortical stroke. *Arch Neurol.* 65, 741-747.

Nudo, R.J. (2007). Postinfarct cortical plasticity and behavior recovery. *Stroke.* 38, 840-845.

O'Connell, N.E., Wand, B.M., Marston, L., Spencer, S. & DeSouza, L.H. (2011). Non-invasive brain stimulation techniques for chronic pain. *Cochrane Database Syst Rev.* Vol.6, 2011.

Pascual-Leone, A., Valls-Solé, J., Wassermann, E.M. & Hallett , M. (1994). Responses to rapid-rate transcranial magnetic stimulation of the human motor cortex. *Brain*.117, 847–858.

Platz, T. & Rothwell, J.C. (2010). Brain stimulation and brain repair - rTMS: from animal experiment to clinical trials - what do we know? *Restor Neurol Neurosci*. 28, 387-398

Peinemann, A., Reimer, B., Loer, C., Quartarone, A., Munchau, A., Conrad, B. & Siebner, H.R. (2004). Long-lasting increase in corticospinal excitability after 1800 pulses of subthreshold 5 Hz repetitive TMS to the primary motor cortex. *Clin Neurophysiol*. 115, 1519-1526.

Poreisz, C., Boros, K., Antal, A. & Paulus, W. (2007). Safety aspects of transcranial direct current stimulation concerning healthy subjects and patients. *Brain Res Bull*. 72, 208–214.

Rasmussen, K. (2011). Some considerations in choosing electroconvulsive therapy versus transcranial magnetic stimulation for depression. *The Journal of ECT*. 27, 51-54.

Reis, J., Schambra, H.M., Cohen, L.G., Buch, E.R., Fritsch, B., Zarahn, E., Celnik, P.A. & Krakauer, J.W. (2009). Noninvasive cortical stimulation enhances motor skill acquisition over multiple days through an effect on consolidation. *Proc Natl Acad Sci U S A*. 106, 1590–1595.

Reis, J., Swayne, O.B., Vandermeeren, Y., Camus, M., Dimyan, M.A., Harris-Love, M., Perez, M.A., Ragert, P., Rothwell, J.C. & Cohen, L.G. (2008). Contribution of transcranial magnetic stimulation to the understanding of cortical mechanisms involved in motor control, *J Physiology*. 586, 325-3351.

Ridding, M.C. & Ziemann, U. (2010). Determinants of the induction of cortical plasticity by non-invasive brain stimulation in healthy subjects. *J Physiol*. 588, 2291–2304.

Rossi, S., Hallett, M., Rossini, P.M., Pascual-Leone, A. & The Safety of TMS Consensus Group. (2009). Safety, ethical considerations, and application guidelines for the use of transcranial magnetic stimulation in clinical practice and research. *Clin Neurophysiol*. 120, 2008-2039.

Schallert, T., Leasure, J.L. & Kolb, B. (2000). Experience-associated structural events, subependymal cellular proliferative activity, and functional recovery after injury to the central nervous system. *J Cereb Blood Flow Metab*. 20, 1513-1528.

Schlaug, G., Renga, V. & Nair, D. (2008). Transcranial direct current stimulation in stroke recovery. *Arch Neurol*. 65, 1571-1576.

Siebner, H.R. & Rothwell, J. (2003). Transcranial magnetic stimulation: new insights into representational cortical plasticity. *Exp Brain Res*. 148, 1-16.

Stagg, C.J. & Nitsche, M.A. (2011). Physiological basis of transcranial direct current stimulation. *The Neuroscientist*. 17, 37-53.

Stefan, K., Kunesch, E., Cohen, L,G., Benecke, R. & Classen, J. (2000). Induction of plasticity in the human brain by paired associative stimulation. *Brain* 123, 572-584.

Takeuchi, N., Tada, T., Toshima, M., Takayo, C., Matsuo, Y. & Ikoma, K. (2008). Inhibition of the unaffected motor cortex by 1 Hz repetitive transcranial magnetic stimulation enhances motor performance and training effect of the paretic hand in patients with chronic stroke. *J Rehabil Med*. 40, 298-303.

Tarlaci, S., Turman, B., Uludag, B. & Ertekin, C. (2010). Differential effects of peripheral vibration on motor-evoked potentials in acute stages of stroke. *Neuromodulation: Technology at the Neural Interface*. 13, 232-237.

Tings, T., Lang, N., Tergau, F., Paulus, W. & Sommer, M. (2005). Orientation-specific fast rTMS maximizes corticospinal inhibition and facilitation. *Exp Brain Res.* 163, 3233-333.

Touge, T., Gerschlager, W., Brown, P. & Rothwell, J.C. (2001). Are the after-effects of low-frequency rTMS on motor cortex excitability due to changes in the efficacy of cortical synapses? *Clin Neurophysiol.* 112, 2138–2145.

Utz, K.S., Dimova, V., Oppenländer, K. & Kerkhoff, G. (2010). Electrified minds: Transcranial direct current stimulation (tDCS) and Galvanic Vestibular Stimulation (GVS) as methods of non-invasive brain stimulation in neuropsychology - A review of current data and future implications. *Neuropsychologia.* 48, 2789-2810.

Valls-Sole, J., Pascual-Leone, A., Wassermann, E.M. & Hallett, M. (1992). Human motor evoked responses to paired transcranial magnetic stimuli. *Electroencep Clin Neurophysiol.* 85, 355-364.

Wagner, T., Fregni, F., Fecteau, S., Grodzinsky, A., Zahn, M. & Pascual-Leone, A. (2007). Transcranial direct current stimulation: a computer-based human model study. *Neuroimage.* 35, 1113–1124.

Wassermann, E.M. (1998). Risk and safety of repetitive transcranial magnetic stimulation: report and suggested guidelines from the International Workshop on the Safety of Repetitive Magnetic Stimulation. *Electroencep Clin Neurophysiol.* 108, 1-16.

Wassermann, E.M., Epstein, C., Ziemann, U., Walsh, V., Paus, T. & Lisanby, S. (eds) (2008). *The Oxford Handbook of Transcranial Stimulation*, Oxford University Press, Oxford.

Witte, O.W. & Stoll, G. (1997). Delayed and remote effects of focal cortical infarctions: secondary damage and reactive plasticity. In: Freund HJ, Sabel BA, Witte OW, eds. *Brain Plasticity, Volume 73: Advances in Neurology.* Philadelphia, PA: Lippincott-Raven, 207–227.

Zangen, A., Roth, Y., Voller, B. & Hallett, M. (2005). Transcranial magnetic stimulation of deep brain regions: evidence for efficacy of the H-coil. *Clin Neurophysiol.* 116, 775-779.